Clinical Examination of the Hand

An Evidence-Based Approach

Edited by
J. Terrence Jose Jerome

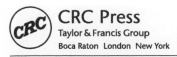

CRC Press
Taylor & Francis Group
Boca Raton London New York

CRC Press is an imprint of the
Taylor & Francis Group, an **informa** business

First edition published 2022
by CRC Press
6000 Broken Sound Parkway NW, Suite 300, Boca Raton, FL 33487-2742

and by CRC Press
2 Park Square, Milton Park, Abingdon, Oxon, OX14 4RN

© 2022 Taylor & Francis Group, LLC
CRC Press is an imprint of Taylor & Francis Group, LLC

Library of Congress Cataloging-in-Publication Data

Names: Jerome, J. Terrence Jose, editor.
Title: Clinical examination of the hand : an evidence-based guide / edited by J. Terrence Jose Jerome.
Description: First edition. | Boca Raton, FL : CRC Press, 2022. | Includes bibliographical references and index. | Summary: "This handbook brings together the basic elements of hand and upper limb case, from examination to clinical diagnosis of various hand and upper limb related diseases. It improvises the examination skills of the reader with proficiency to arrive for a provisional diagnosis for the given hand surgery and related diseases"-- Provided by publisher.
Identifiers: LCCN 2021049770 (print) | LCCN 2021049771 (ebook) | ISBN 9780367647186 (hardback) | ISBN 9780367647162 (paperback) | ISBN 9781003125938 (ebook)
Subjects: MESH: Hand Injuries--diagnosis | Hand--physiology | Physical Examination--methods | Evidence-Based Medicine
Classification: LCC RD559 (print) | LCC RD559 (ebook) | NLM WE 830 | DDC 617.5/75044--dc23/eng/20211101
LC record available at https://lccn.loc.gov/2021049770
LC ebook record available at https://lccn.loc.gov/2021049771

ISBN: 9780367647186 (hbk)
ISBN: 9780367647162 (pbk)
ISBN: 9781003125938 (ebk)

DOI: 10.1201/9781003125938

Typeset in Palatino
by Deanta Global Publishing Services, Chennai, India

Access the Support Material: www.routledge.com/9780367647162

Dedicated to my wife, Dr Thirumagal; my daughters Shruthika and Dharshana; dad; mom; father and mothers-in-law and Josewa Florence, who have been a source of great pride.

Table of Contents

Foreword

Several years ago, in an editorial in the *Journal of Hand and Upper Extremity*, I posed the question, "Has the contemporary electronic medical record made the comprehensive hand examination obsolete?" How timely and appropriate, therefore, is this comprehensive text, *Evidence-Based Clinical Examination of the Hand*, edited by Dr J Terrence Jose Jerome? Assembling a group of internationally recognized contributors, this text comprehensively expands from the basics of history taking, inspection and general palpation to move to in-depth descriptions and illustrations of motor, sensory, vascular and peripheral nerve palsy, including the claw hand associated with Hansen's disease, as well as the important methods of the wrist. The final chapters include key features of evaluating radiographs, the requirements and indications for special diagnostic tests.

Having started my orthopaedic residency at a time when the importance of the physical examination was continuously emphasized, it soon became apparent to me that many clinical diagnoses of conditions of the hand and upper limb will be realized just from careful patient history and systematic hand examination. While technology continues to improve the reliability of diagnosis, do we always require a 3D CT scan of the wrist to tell us the fracture pattern, an EMG to confirm the diagnosis of carpal tunnel syndrome when the history and physical examination presents a very clear picture of the patient's condition or an MRI angiogram to show an occlusion of the ulnar artery at the wrist which could be predicted by routinely including Allen's test with our standard hand examination?

Finally, the efforts to spend the time needed to perform a thorough history and physical examination provides an additional benefit which is to be able to spend more time with our patient, the careful laying on of hands and to establish the remarkable patient–doctor relationship which is a unique part of our chosen profession.

Jupiter J. "Has the Contemporary Electronic Medical Record Made the Comprehensive Hand Examination Obsolete?" *J Techniques of Hand and Upper Extremity Surgery.* 2017; 21: 75–6

Dr Jesse B Jupiter
Past President, American Shoulder and Elbow Surgeons; Past President, American Association of Hand Surgeons, Hansjoerg Wyss/AO Professor, Harvard Medical School; Visiting Orthopedic Surgeon, Massachusetts General Hospital, Boston, MA, US

Preface

The journey of a thousand miles begins with a single step. It is a baby step towards imparting knowledge to the next generation. I believe experience is power and to be shared. This sharing of wisdom came from an immense struggle in understanding the concept by various means. This includes eminent teachers, various conference meetings, continuing medical education (CME), instructional courses and international experts. Gaining knowledge is the first step to wisdom. Sharing is the first step to humanity. A candle loses nothing by lighting another candle. This book on **evidence-based clinical examination of the hand** is the first step to society. It has a well-defined object for orthopaedic surgeons, plastic surgeons, hand surgeons, general surgeons, trauma surgeons, emergency specialists, aspiring surgeons and hand therapists. It is not to serve as a textbook of hand surgery. Instead, it will impart the basics on hands and upper limbs to readers to understand the applied anatomy and biomechanics concerning its use and absence. The book also improvizes the examination skills of the reader with the proficiency to arrive at a provisional diagnosis for the given hand surgery and related diseases. It is by the sole hard work and passion from all contributors worldwide to bring this state-of-the-art book that would be a "must carry" for all clinics and practices. The chapters are presented with simple language and down-to-earth understanding of clinical pictures and videos, which are embedded for readers to obtain the most benefit.

We have also tried to bring together all of the essential elements resulting in the clinical diagnosis of various hand- and upper limb-related diseases and discussed in brief the differential diagnosis and possible intervention. It would always be an asset for trainees, graduates, postgraduates and fellows who intend to brush up their basics and excel in hand surgery.

"Think of this book as bait – If I can catch them, then you can train them" – quoted Paul W Brand.

Adding to it, this book would be a victorious accomplishment and an educational bait!

Dr J Terrence Jose Jerome

Acknowledgements

Learning is not attained by choice; it must be sought with ardour and attended to with diligence. All that is new in this book has been worked out for succinct learners to have it as a handbook for clinics as well as the substantial hand surgery textbooks available on the market. Clinical examination is an art, and this book serves to meet the necessary and relevant facts in making the art more interesting and efficacious.

Dr Mathew Varghese, Director of Orthopaedics, St Stephen's Hospital, New Delhi, India, has been my teacher and the soul behind this book. His ideas and innovative clinical acumen are beyond compare. All these are converted into print in this book. A special thanks to all my teachers, who have imparted me with fundamentals and technical nuances in the clinical diagnosis of hand injuries.

We also appreciate the advice and help of Dr K Thirumagal, Dr Vijay Malshikare and Dr Anil K Bhat, who have read parts or all of the manuscript.

My patients, who have been the fundamental pillar of this book, have a special place in my heart and thoughts.

Editor

J Terrence Jose Jerome, MBBS, FRCS, DNB, MNAMS, FICS, European Diploma in Hand Surgery, FNB (Hand and Microsurgery), PGDMLE (National Law School), MCh(Ortho)

Dr J Terrence Jose Jerome has been the Editor in Chief of the *Journal of Hand and Microsurgery* for 13 straight years since its inception. He did his undergraduate studies at the Government Medical College, Thanjavur, India; postgraduate studies in Orthopaedic Surgery at St Stephen's Hospital, New Delhi, India; and his Fellowship in Hand and Microsurgery at Ganga Hospital, Coimbatore, India. Since then, he has been very active in his private practice in hand and reconstructive microsurgery. He worked as a full-time consultant in Apollo Speciality Hospitals and visits premier institutions in India. He owns a hospital with 30 beds, state-of-the-art operating microscopes, operating theatres and intensive care units. His primary interest is brachial plexus injuries, free flaps, reconstructive microsurgery in the hand and upper limb, distal radius, elbow, carpal and hand fractures. He received his FRCS (Glasgow) in 2020. He is the first Indian to qualify for a European Diploma in Hand Surgery, in 2010. He is the first Indian to be awarded the prestigious ASSH International Travelling Fellow, in 2019. He has more than 80 peer-reviewed publications and delivered 200 paper presentations, 60 guest lectures at various national and international platforms. He is the master brain behind the Tamil Nadu Orthopaedic Association mobile app, website administration and is currently serving as the IT wing secretary. He worked efficiently as an executive committee member in the Tamil Nadu Orthopaedic Association. He received many gold medals at various conferences held in India. He is a teaching expert in the scientific and PG teaching committee of state and national orthopaedic associations. He was the Convener of the Indo-Japan Hand Meet held in 2019. He is the secretary of the Society for Indian Hand Surgery and Microsurgeons. Recently he started a monthly journal club for the *Journal of Hand and Microsurgery*, inviting eminent speakers like Jesse Jupiter, Asif Ilyas, Charles Goldfarb, Amy Moore, Patrick Houvet, Christophe Mathoulin and renowned speakers from across the globe to deliver talks on exciting topics.

Contributors

Ashwath M Acharya, MS(Ortho), FNB(Hand & Microsurgery)
Department of Orthopaedics
Kasturba Medical College
Manipal, India

Nikhil Agrawal, MD
Department of Orthopaedic Surgery
Harvard Medical School
Boston, MA
and
Massachusetts General Hospital
Boston, MA

Mohammed Tahir Ansari, MS(Ortho), DNB, MRCS, European Diploma in Hand Surgery
Department of Orthopaedics
All India Institute of Medical Sciences
New Delhi, India

Anil K Bhat, MS(Ortho)
Department of Orthopaedics
Kasturba Medical College
Manipal, India

Jorge G Boretto, MD
Orthopaedic and Traumatology Department
Hospital Italiano de Buenos Aires
Buenos Aires, Argentina

Samuel Cohen-Tanugi, MD
Department of Hand Surgery
Ortho Carolina Hand Center
Charlotte, NC

Neal Chen, MD
Orthopaedic Hand and Arm Center
Massachusetts General Hospital
Boston, MA

Franco De Cicco, MD
Orthopaedic and Traumatology Department
Hospital Italiano de Buenos Aires
Buenos Aires, Argentina

Bassem Elhassan, MD
Department of Orthopaedic Surgery
Massachusetts General Hospital
Boston, MA

Mithun Pai G, MS(Ortho), FNB(Hand & Microsurgery)
Department of Orthopaedics
Kasturba Medical College
Manipal, India

Rohit Garg, MD
Department of Orthopaedic Surgery
Massachusetts General Hospital
Boston, MA

R Glenn Gaston, MD
Department of Hand Surgery
Ortho Carolina Hand Center
Charlotte, NC

Devansh Goyal, MS(Ortho)
Department of Orthopaedics
All India Institute of Medical Sciences
New Delhi, India

Theodore Guild, MD
Harvard Combined Orthopaedic Residency Program
Boston, MA

Janice Hc, MD
Department of Orthopaedic Surgery
Massachusetts General Hospital
Boston, MA

Patrick Houvet, MD
Department of Orthopaedic Surgery
Institut Français de Chirurgie de la Main
Paris, France

Santanu Kar, MS(Ortho)
Department of Orthopaedics
All India Institute of Medical Sciences
New Delhi, India

G Karthikeyan, MS, MCh(Plastic Surgery)
Institute for Research and Rehabilitation of Hand and Department of Plastic Surgery
Stanley Medical College and Government Hospital
Chennai, India

Rajesh Malhotra, MBBS, MS, FRCS, FACS, FICS, FIMSA, FAMS, FNASc
Department of Orthopaedics
All India Institute of Medical Sciences
New Delhi, India

Vijay A Malshikare, FRCS(G), DO, FCPS
18.52 North Hospital
Pune, India

Chaitanya S Mudgal, MD, MS(Orth.), M. Ch(Orth.)
Harvard Medical School
Massachusetts General Hospital
Boston, MA

Raj Murali, FRCS(Edin), FRCS(Lond)
Wrightington, Wigan and Leigh NHS
    Foundation Trust
Wigan, UK
and
Edge Hill University
Ormskirk, UK

Usama Farghaly Omar, MD
Department of Orthopaedic Surgery
Khoo Teck Puat Hospital
Singapore

Vaikunthan Rajaratnam, FRCS
Department of Orthopaedic Surgery
Khoo Teck Puat Hospital
Singapore

Dyuti Deepta Rano, MS(Ortho)
Department of Orthopaedics
All India Institute of Medical Sciences
New Delhi, India

Ignacio Rellán, MD
Orthopaedic and Traumatology Department
Hospital Italiano de Buenos Aires
Buenos Aires, Argentina

Shav Ru pasinghe, MD
Wrightington Hospital
Wigan, UK

Takehiko Takagi, M.D., Ph.D.
Department of Surgical Specialties
National Center for Child Health and
    Development
Tokyo, Japan

Timothy Teo Wei Wen, MD
Department of Orthopaedic Surgery
Khoo Teck Puat Hospital
Singapore

Dafang Zhang, MD
Department of Orthopaedic Surgery
Brigham and Women's Hospital
Boston, MA
and
Harvard Medical School
Boston, MA

Abbreviations

AVN	avascular necrosis
TFCC	triangular fibro cartilage
CMC	carpometacarpal
USG	ultrasound
MRI	magnetic resonance imaging
EDC	extensor digitorum communis
EPL	extensor pollicis longus
ECRL	extensor carpi radialis longus
ECRB	extensor carpi radialis brevis

1 Introduction

J Terrence Jose Jerome

CONTENTS

HAND

The hand is unique and versatile on its own. Its uniqueness in adaptability to the given circumstances makes it one of the fascinating organs of the body. It is a highly specialized structure possessing sensation and is capable of grasping and manipulating objects with power and position. It recognizes form, assesses size and appreciates texture through the property of tactile gnosis [1]. The mysteries of its functions reflect the principle that the whole is greater than the sum of its parts, and its functions are controlled by the brain, which makes decisions and initiates actions [2].

HAND ARCHITECTONIC

The primitive five-digit hand was modified gradually to adapt to its changing functions from an arboreal to a terrestrial habitat. The assumption of the upright position was the primary stimulus for the development of the forelimbs to perform free and complicated activities. The skeletal structure of the hand was also modified to permit specialized

DOI: 10.1201/9781003125938-1

1

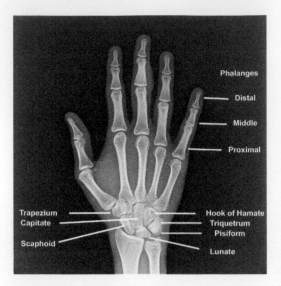

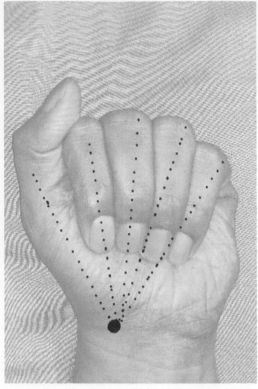

Figure 1.1 Shows the anatomy and normal X-ray. The five rays of the hand. Each ray has multiple joints. The thumb has two joints. The metacarpophalangeal and interphalangeal joints are formed by the first metacarpal and two phalanges. The rest of the fingers have three joints formed with the metacarpal and proximal phalanx as MCP joint, proximal and middle phalanx as PIP joint, middle and distal phalanx as DIP joint. There are altogether 19 bones and muscles with 17 joints in the hand, almost making it the most crucial part of the body.

movement with the help of extrinsic and intrinsic muscles. The critical anatomical attributes of the human hand are shown in Figure 1.1.

1. The thumb possesses an independent and wide range of movements made possible by the saddle-shaped metacarpal trapezial joint (first carpometacarpal joint).

2. The index finger possesses independent movement in several planes because of increased mobility of the second metacarpophalangeal joint.

3. A less fixed unit is composed of the middle, ring and little fingers, fourth and fifth metacarpal bones. The contour and angles of the fourth and fifth metacarpophalangeal joint allow approximately 25° of internal rotation of the little finger and about 15° of internal rotation of the ring finger which enables each finger to point towards the scaphoid tubercle when it is flexed (Figures 1.2 and 1.3).

4. A fixed unit composed of a distal carpal row and second and third metacarpal bones provides the base that supports these mobile units.

Figure 1.2 The picture shows the oblique flexion of the middle, ring and little fingers. The most important feature is when the index, middle and ring fingers are flexed at the MCP and PIP joints, their axis converges towards scaphoid tuberosity. The index finger alone flexes in a sagittal plane whereas the middle, ring and little fingers have oblique flexion towards the scaphoid tubercle. The more you go far away (little finger) the finger flexes more obliquely towards the median axis.

5. Mobile proximal carpal row provides the base for wrist movements.

HAND SURFACES

The dorsum of the hand is convex with dorsal skin and nails, which are aesthetically important. It has less subcutaneous fat with more venous plexus up to the upper limb. Dorsal venous arches are seen in thin-built individuals. They are quite variable in arrangement and patterns. The basilic vein originates from the ulnar side of the hand and ascends to the upper limb.

In contrast, the dorsal arch on the radial side forms the cephalic vein routinely used for intravenous cannulation. The dorsal skin is thin and allows free flexion and extension of the fingers and wrist. The

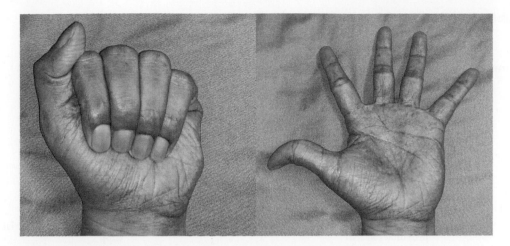

Figure 1.3 The fingers extend and abduct while opening the hand with thumb short in length and separated from the index finger and others. They flex and adduct while forming a closed fist or closing the hand following the oblique axis of flexion.

knuckles are the metacarpophalangeal (MCP) joint and the metacarpal heads are prominent over the dorsum of the hand when making a fist.

The dorsal skin over the knuckles allows unfettered mobility of extensor tendons during flexion and extension of the metacarpophalangeal (MCP) joint. The palmar surface or the volar aspect of the hand is concave in structure and functionally important with well-connected palmar fascia. The palmar fascia is the shock absorber allowing free movement and safeguarding underlying vital structures. The pulp

and the palm provide the best grip during all hand movements. There are various creases in the fingers and the palm with little value as references (look for extensor tendon and flexor tendon anatomy and zone description) (Figure 1.4) (Table 1.1).

Radial borders along the thumb and little finger form the ulnar border (Figures 1.5 and 1.7). The radial side refers to the area close to the thumb and the ulnar side close to the little finger. We prefer to name them as radial or ulnar for the lateral or medial sides, respectively, as far as the hand is concerned. Over the palm, the radial aspect is the thenar eminence

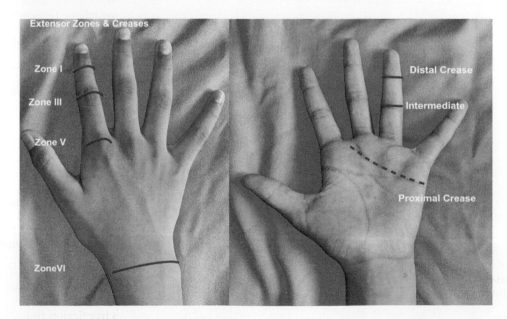

Figure 1.4 Picture showing the dorsum of hand and the volar aspect of the hand.

Table 1.1: Zones of Tendon Injury [33]

Extensor Tendon Zones

Zones	Location	Injury/Remarks
I	Area from the DIP joint to the fingertip	Mallet finger
II	Encompasses the middle phalanx	
III	Refers to the PIP joint	Boutonniere deformity
IV	Area over the proximal phalanx	
V	Refers to the MP joint	Human bite injuries, sagittal band rupture
VI	Encompasses the metacarpal	Fist injuries
VII	Area over the wrist	
VIII	Forearm	Wrist drop
IX	Muscular area of the extensor mechanism at the middle and proximal forearm	Neurological injury, wrist drop

Flexor Tendon Zones

Zones	Location	Injury/Remarks
I	Area distal to the insertion of the FDS tendon	Jersey finger
II	Area where both flexor tendons (FDP, FDS) run together in a fibrous tunnel commencing at proximal aspect of the A1 pulley to Zone I	
III	The palmar section of the sheath where fibrous tunnel is absent and has the origin of the lumbricals from the FDP tendon	
IV	The flexor tendons within the carpal tunnel. Distal to the transverse carpal ligament at approximately the level of the superficial palmar vascular arch, the lumbrical tendons take their origin from the FDP tendons	Spaghetti wrist
V	Extends from the muscle-tendon junction to the proximal aspect of the carpal tunnel	

Note: The palmar creases, which are often used as landmarks, do not in fact overlie the joints whose flexion induces them to fold (Figure 1.4). Only the middle digit creases coincide with the proximal interphalangeal joints; the distal crease lies just distal to the distal interphalangeal joint and the proximal crease lies almost halfway down the proximal phalanx.

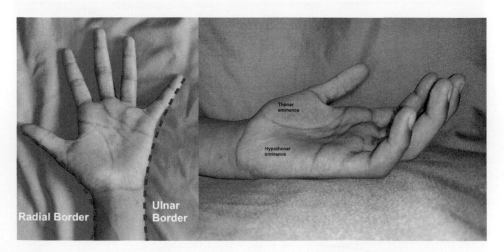

Figure 1.5 Picture showing the radial, ulnar border of the hand, thenar and hypothenar eminence.

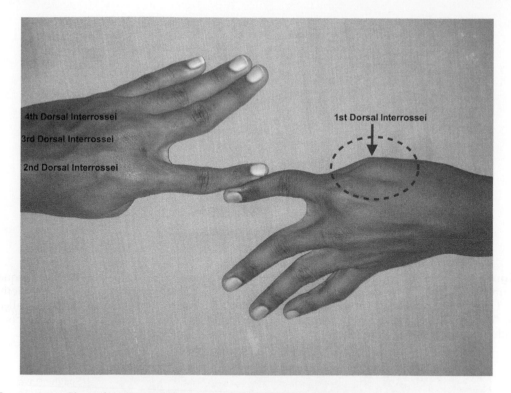

Figure 1.6 Clinical pictures showing the dorsal interossei in the hand.

which is formed by the muscles that act on the thumb (abductor pollicis brevis, opponens pollicis and flexor pollicis brevis). The ulnar aspect is the hypothenar eminence and consists of muscles acting on the little finger (abductor digiti minimi, flexor digiti minimi and opponens digiti minimi).

On the dorsal side, forced spreading out of the index finger against resistance shows the prominence of first dorsal interossei muscle. The second and third dorsal interossei can be seen and felt on either side of the middle finger. The fourth interossei can be seen and felt between the ring and little fingers (Figure 1.6).

On the volar side lies the palmar interossei, which are smaller than dorsal interossei and cannot be felt or seen. The middle finger has no palmar interossei. The thumb and index finger interossei originate from the ulnar aspect of the entire metacarpal and are inserted into the dorsal expansion. The ring and little finger interossei originate from the radial aspect of the entre metacarpal and insert into the third and fourth lumbrical respectively and also the base of the proximal phalanx [3].

SKELETON OF THE WRIST AND HAND

The hand skeleton comprises of carpal bones, metacarpal and phalanges. There are eight carpal bones. Four in the proximal and four in the distal row. The scaphoid, lunate, triquetral and pisiform form the proximal row. The scaphoid, lunate and triquetrum form a convex arch and articulate with distal radius and inferior radioulnar joint. The pisiform articulates with triquetrum alone. The trapezium, trapezoid, capitate and hamate form the concave distal carpal row. The distal row and fourth and fifth metacarpal are a less mobile unit (Figure 1.7).

OSSIFICATION OF BONES

The hand and wrist have 27 bones. The thumb has the shortest metacarpal articulating with the proximal phalanx to perform various vital functions (Figure 1.8). It has two phalanges and one metacarpal articulating with the trapezium. The trapezium is angled out in front of the carpal plane. The angle made by the first metacarpal to the second is about 45°, and this is the reason for more delicate movements of thumb in the given circumstances (Figure 1.9). The index, middle, ring and little fingers have an unequal length with one metacarpal and three phalanges each (Table 1.2).

MOVEMENTS OF WRIST AND HAND JOINTS

Movements are quintessential for the complex functions of hand. Overall functions have been classified based on the joints, which are mobile

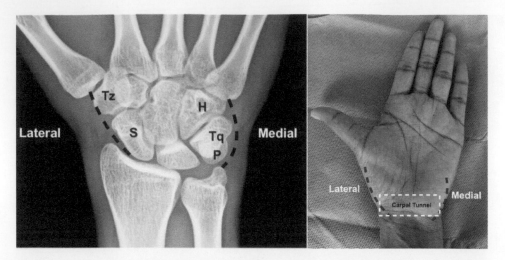

Figure 1.7 (a) The X-rays of the wrist. The medial projections are formed by the pisiform triquetrum and the hook of the hamate. The scaphoid tuberosity and trapezium form lateral projections. (b) These two projections form the carpal groove which is converted into an osseous tunnel called the "carpal tunnel." The carpal tunnel has nine flexor tendons and the median nerve as contents under the flexor retinaculum.

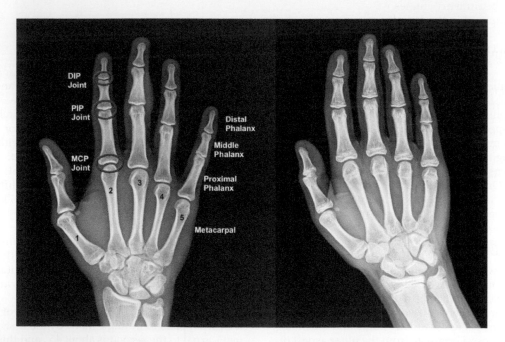

Figure 1.8 X-rays of the hand. (a) The thumb has one metacarpal and two phalanges forming MCP and IP joints. The rest of the fingers have metacarpal, proximal, middle- and ring-finger phalanges starting MCP, PIP and DIP joints, respectively. (b) The growing ends (epiphyseal plates) are located in the proximal ends of thumb metacarpal and proximal ends of proximal, middle and distal phalanges in the index, middle, ring and little fingers. The metacarpals in the index, middle, ring and little fingers have epiphyseal plates at their base (end).

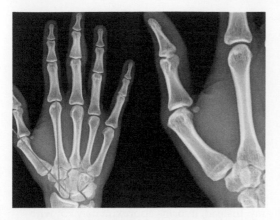

Figure 1.9 Radial aspect of the hand. The index metacarpal is the longest with the thumb being the shortest of all metacarpals. These two metacarpals form 45° because of the orientation of the trapezium. The carpometacarpal joint is saddle-shaped and opposite to the articular surface of the trapezium and base of the first metacarpal. The trapezium articulates with the proximal row scaphoid in the radial aspect of the wrist.

and fixed. The thumb and little finger joints are mobile but less rigid, compromising the stability. The index, middle and ring fingers are rigid, stable and less mobile. The architectures of the hand are so delicate and complicated that every movement is dependent on the neighbouring joints to some extent to get better hand function [4].

HAND GEOMETRY

The metacarpal base articulates with the distal carpal row (trapezium on the lateral to hamate on the ulnar side). The distal carpal row articulates with the proximal carpal row bones. This proximal carpal row gives wrist flexion, extension, radial deviation and ulnar deviation movements (Figure 1.10). The proximal carpal row articulates with the radius and ulna to form an inferior (distal) radioulnar joint. It is a uniaxial pivot joint providing pronation and supination (Figure 1.11). Interestingly, the wrist has three axes of movement, allowing the hand to be positioned in any spatial configuration and enabling it to be placed as needed for grip, prehensile and grasping [5].

CLOSING THE HAND

The fingers are not of the same length. This is because of the difference in the metacarpal and phalanges. When you attempt to close the fingers, all of them flex and move in a direction towards the thenar eminence. Similarly, when they try and catch objects, all the fingers flex towards the pulp of the thumb to make different pinches and grasps.

The radial aspect is the thumb, and the medial aspect is the little finger. In closing action, the fingers move away from the median axis towards scaphoid tubercle. This is because the ring and little fingers are short in length and have adaptive flexion movement of 10 and 15° at their Carpometacarpal (CMC) joint, making it mobile towards the thenar eminence. So ulnar digits move obliquely far away from the median axis as they approach the palm. Try looking at your hand and experience the closing and opening hand actions! (Figure 1.12).

OPENING THE HAND

Opening the hand or fist is an ingenious mechanism involving a coordinated fashioned

Table 1.2: Ossification of Bones

Bones at Birth	1.5–2.5 years	Ossification Appearance 3 years	4 years	5 years	9–10 years	Fusion Years (Union of the Ossification Centres with the Shaft)
Capitate, hamate		Triquetrum	Lunate	Scaphoid, trapezium, trapezoid	Pisiform	9–12 years
Five metacarpals and phalanges in thumb and fingers	Second to fifth metacarpal heads					15–19 years
	Thumb metacarpal base All phalanges base					15–17 years

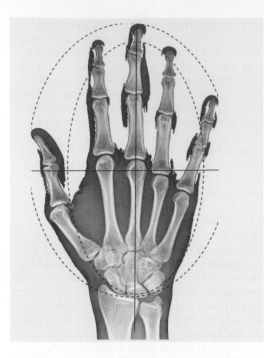

Figure 1.10 Hand geometry. The shape and size about its property of space were studied by multiple circles drawn keeping the fingers wide, abducted and extended. The fingertips lie on the circumference of a circle whose centre is in the third metacarpal head, and the circle also runs along the articular surface of the distal radius. The carpus lies within a smaller circle with the capitate head as the centre. The longitudinal axis of the hand passes through the middle finger, the third metacarpal and the capitate head.

movement at Distal interphalangeal (DIP), proximal interphalangeal (PIP), MCP and wrist joints. Extensor expansion is the key factor responsible for opening and occurs where it allows different muscles to act by linking different levels of mechanism.

The transverse axis of the palm is formed by a line joining the MCP joints in the palm. Interestingly, the line is not straight but oblique, which starts more distal to the MCP joint of the index finger and ends more proximal to MCP joint of the little finger. This is contrary to one's expectation of a straight line joining all MCP joints and a perpendicular axis to the median ray. Instead, it forms approximately 75° with the longitudinal axis. This has to be borne in mind when applying splints or cast immobilization so due care is given that MCP joint is flexed in an oblique line (Figure 1.13).

THE ARCHES OF THE HAND

1. Transverse arches:
   a. Transverse carpal arch (Figure 1.14)
   b. Transverse metacarpal arch (Figure 1.15)

2. Longitudinal arch (Figure 1.16)
3. Oblique arch (between thumb and each of the fingers) (Figures 1.17–1.21)

There is longitudinal and transverse concavity in the hand created by these arches. It resembles a cup with a palmar concavity when the thumb is placed next to the index finger. The cup shape becomes a gutter when the thumb opens out to grasp an object. Here the major oblique axis follows the thumb crease. For the

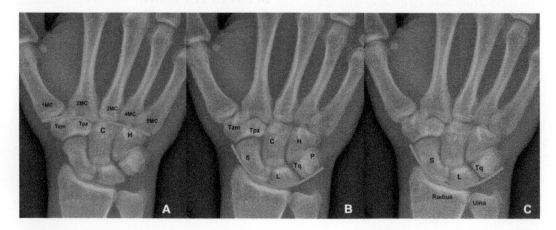

Figure 1.11 (a), (b) and (c) These show the articulation at the metacarpal base, distal carpal, proximal carpal row and radioulnar joint.

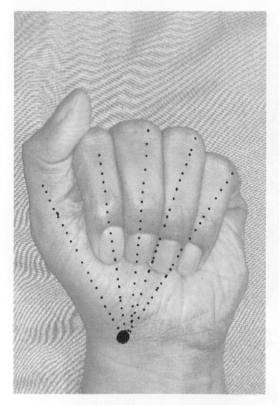

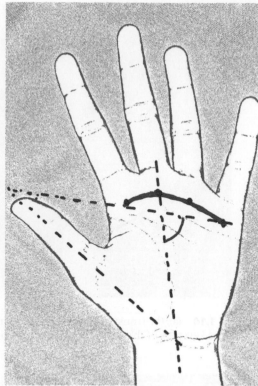

Figure 1.12 The oblique flexion of the ulnar three digits. Only the index ray flexes in a sagittal plane. The more ulnar the digit, the more obliquely it flexes toward the median axis. The last four digits flex at the metacarpophalangeal and proximal interphalangeal joints; their axes converge toward the scaphoid tubercle.

Figure 1.13 A pictorial diagram showing the obliquity of the transverse palmar axis. The axis (transverse) passes along the line from the second to the fifth metacarpal head forming 75° with the longitudinal axis (middle finger ray). The transverse axis in the palm is oblique and follows the thumb crease.

better function of prehension, these curvatures have to be kept in as very essential in their longitudinal and transverse axis.

BASIC HAND POSTURES
Figures 1.22–1.25 show the basic hand postures.

SYNERGY
Extension and flexion of wrist produce synergy movements (Figure 1.26) (Video 1.1).

The most exciting aspect of the wrist and hand is synergism. Let us do an exercise to feel this in our normal hand. The wrist should be held in a relaxed and mid-pronated position with the elbow flexed at 90°. Now rotate the forearm to complete pronation. The wrist will fall into flexion, and fingers automatically extend. Again, turn the wrist to full supination and note the wrist goes to dorsiflexion and fingers into flexion. A simple and easy way is to ask the patient to flex and extend the wrist and notice this synergy.

1. Extension of the wrist permits full flexion of the digits:

The transverse carpal arch keeps the flexor tendons close to the axis of flexion-extension of the wrist. This arch is responsible for the synergistic action of the extensors and flexors of the wrist. The transverse carpal arch is disturbed in cases of synovitis wrist where the flexor tendons displace volar causing reduced wrist extension and negligible synergy.

2. Wrist flexion places the long extensors under tension and automatically extends the digits.

HAND MOVEMENTS AND FUNCTIONS
Movements may be simple or complex, which are accomplished by the continuous change of posture as the hand performs different

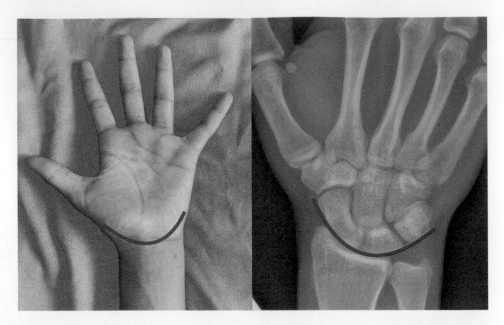

Figure 1.14 (a), (b) Transverse carpal arch (the transverse arch of the distal carpal row is much more rigid. The keystone of this arch is formed by the capitate, which moves with the fixed metacarpals).

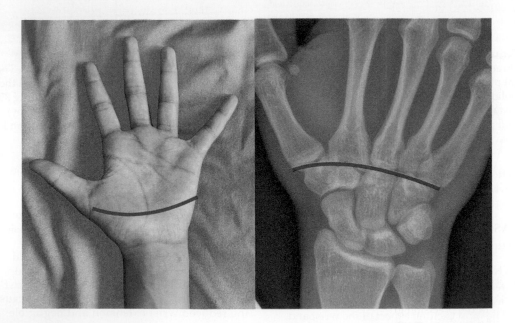

Figure 1.15 (a) and (b) The transverse metacarpal arch forms the sides of the cup or the palmar gutter. It can deepen the concavity when they move over the fixed third metacarpal. The second and third metacarpal bones are fixed and rigid. There is 10° of mobility at the fourth metacarpal and 20° at the fifth metacarpal.

actions. Changes occur for accommodating objects of varying size, shape and consistency with variable strength exerted to maintain their required degree of force for holding an item. Purposeful movements are not executed by the action of a single muscle but are produced by the combined efforts of a group comprising agonist, antagonist fixators and stabilizers. Stability, balance, synergism, coordination and synchronism are essential for smooth execution of movements [6, 7]. The functions of the hand are broadly divided

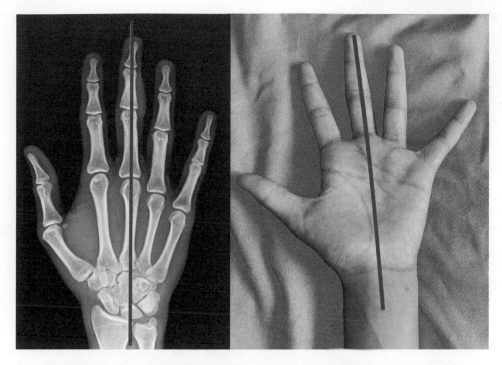

Figure 1.16 (a), (b) The longitudinal arches are composed of a fixed portion, the carpometacar-pal, and a mobile portion, the digits. For every ray, there is a longitudinal arch. It extends from the concavity on the volar surface of the metacarpal shaft to the tip of the fingers.

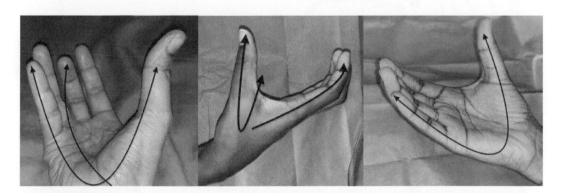

Figure 1.17 (a), (b), (c) The thumb forms four different oblique arches of opposition. The most important and functionally competent is the oblique arch between the thumb and index finger used in the precision grip (arrows). The arch between the thumb and little finger establishes a locking mechanism on the ulnar side of the hand in power grips.

into two categories: Prehensile and non-prehensile. Prehensile activities are further classified into precision handling and power grip [1].

Precision handling consists of subtle moments performed mainly by the thumb and index finger and occasionally assisted by the middle finger. The position will be specific to humans and higher primates and is controlled by the recently evolved cortico-motoneuronal spinal tract. Animals like squirrel monkeys have a less developed cortico-spinal tract and no thumb opposition – "ape thumb" deformity.

The force required for precision action is approximately one quarter that needed for the power group. It is accomplished by a variety of pinch mechanisms (Figure 1.27) namely:

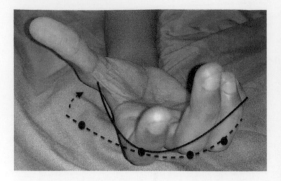

Figure 1.18 The hollowness or concavity of the palm depends on the changes in the position of the transverse metacarpal arch. Flexing and adducting the first and fifth metacarpal heads increases the concavity of the arch. At the same time, the heads of the second and third metacarpal are fixed and produce no change in the arch.

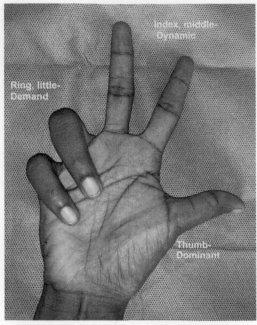

Figure 1.20 3 Ds classifying the functional zones of the hand. 1) D – Dominant thumb. 2) D – Dynamic index- and middle-finger [precision grip]. 3) D – Demand ring and little finger (power grip against the palm).

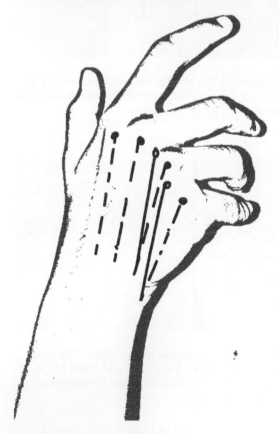

Figure 1.19 The rigidity and mobility seen in metacarpals. The second and third metacarpals are rigid and stable. No movements are possible. The fourth metacarpal has 10° of flexion at its carpal articulation. The fifth metacarpal has 20° of flexion. It is also accompanied by a slight lateral rotational movement in the longitudinal axis of the hand.

- The execution of integrated movements to achieve pinch and grasp (Figures 1.28 and 1.29)

- Actions of a fixed nature performed with either an open or closed hand like pushing, pulling hooking and resting the hands on the knuckles or palm

- Moments utilizing the fingertips or the entire hand to produce percussive actions such as those employed to play the piano, type or box

PROPERTIES OF THE HAND IN REACHING AND GRASPING

The motion of the hand without references to force causing reaching and grasping an object develops in parallel as a function of the object's position, size and orientation with smooth velocity profile. The hand has the unique capacity to pre-shape itself before grasping any objects. It configures itself by nature of activities. Overall, the hand can reach or grasp an object by this inbuilt nature which again depends on the size, shape and location of the object [8–12]. Example: It pre-shapes itself to take a pen or write with a bigger pen.

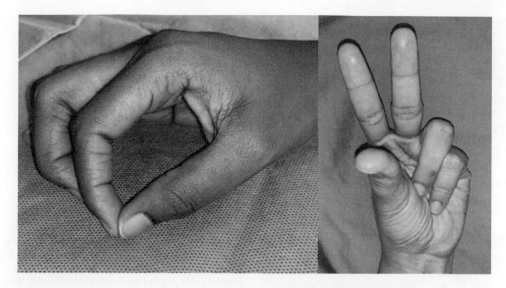

Figure 1.21   (a), (b) The three-finger configuration. Thumb, index and middle fingers always work in close association for all grips. They do not require force but work synergically for more refined movements. It is called the "dynamic tripod."

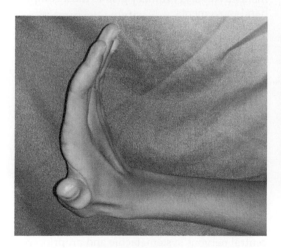

Figure 1.22   Extension of the metacarpophalangeal (MCP) joint: Pushing objects.

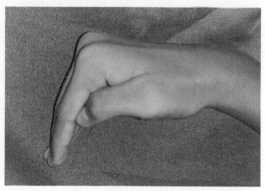

Figure 1.23   Flexion of the metacarpophalangeal joint and extension of the interphalangeal joint (lumbrical muscle action).

MOVEMENTS OF THE THUMB

Figures 1.30 and 1.31 show the basic thumb movements.

Significance of the Index Finger

- The index finger never does any particular work.

- The index finger acts as a stabilizer for any external stimulus. Example: Catching a ball where index fingers exert the stabilizing mechanism to minimize ball roll.

- The index finger is a "navigator" and assists the thumb and most importantly in opposition axis. The thumb is the "pilot" for computation of a hand trajectory towards a target [13, 14].

- In addition to the stabilizing role, the thumb and index finger together have a stronger force production capability compared to the other digits [15, 16].

THE HAND IS THE MASTERSTROKE OF PERFORMANCE

The hand is a highly specialized organ of execution. One size fits all. It is more prudent to say the hand fits all daily activities. Either it is an expression or variety of instruments for use, it has no light of its own. It is "a device

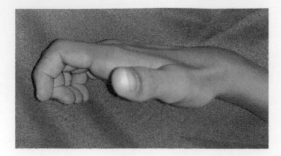

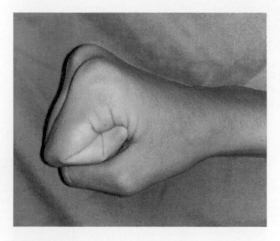

Figure 1.24 Extension of the metacarpophalangeal joint and flexion of the interphalangeal joints (hook).

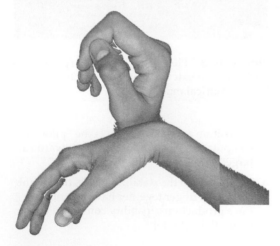

Figure 1.25 Flexion of the metacarpophalangeal joint and the interphalangeal joints (IP) – fist.

 Video 1.1 Video of the hand synergism.

www.routledge.com/9780367647162.

HAND FUNCTIONS

The functions of the hand can be described based on their utilization. They are passive, percussive and functions that require a greater deal of mobility. The passive functions are opening the fingers for carrying, lifting or making a cup in the palm or flattening the palm. The percussive functions include tabla percussions, drums, tapping fingers, clapping hands or pounding fists. Immobile PIP and DIP joints achieve this because the motions start from the MCP joint and more proximally. The functions require a great deal of mobility such as Namaste, Vanakkam, symbolic, expressive gestures, prehensible gestures, grasps, intricate manoeuvres and ordinary grip to most complex hand movements.

GRIP AND PREHENSION

Prehension is a combination of various complex activities used by the hand in grasping and reaching for an object. The functions can be communication, writing, feeding, cleaning, working, hunting, making tools, participating in cultural and social activities where the hand is innate as an irreplaceable organ for its multifaceted functions. The movement of the thumb and other fingers to grasp an object is an integral part of prehension. Prehension is not purely a motor act like holding items with these fingers. It involves an intention to do, sensory control and, finally, implementation of a motor act such as grip. The central nervous system, tactile and proprioceptive sensibility, controls the prehension.

TYPES OF GRIP

The two types of grip are static grip and dynamic grip.

PHASES OF PREHENSION

The simple task of lifting a phone narrates the components of prehension (Figure 1.32).

1. Regard (intention/approach)
2. Reach
3. Grasp/grip
4. Manipulation (maximize the efficiency)
5. Release of grip (regulation of grip)

Figure 1.26 Synergy pictorial presentation.

that can, in turn, strike, receive and give, feed, take an oath, beat a musical rhythm, read for the blind, speak for the mute, reach to a friend, stop a foe, and become a hammer, pincer, alphabet ..." [17].

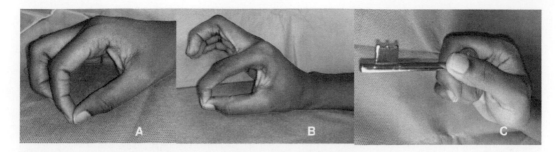

Figure 1.27 The power group, on the other hand, utilizes all the digits to exert a strong force with which to grasp an object. The primary motor functions are the hand. (a) The pulp to full contact between the end of the thumb and index finger. (b) The nail to the nail pinch. (c) The lateral pinched between the pulp of the thumb on the side of the index finger.

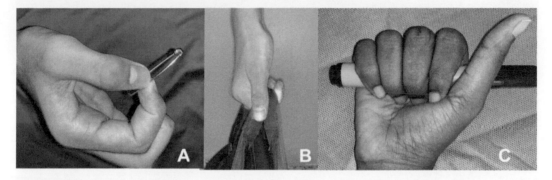

Figure 1.28 (a) Palmar grasp (pluri-digital). (b) Hook or snap grasp. (c) Palmar grasp (multi-pulpar).

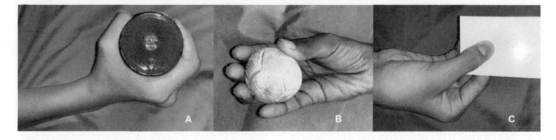

Figure 1.29 Various grips of the hand. (a) Cylindrical grasp. (b) Spherical grasp. (c) Lateral grasp.

THE GRIP CONSISTS OF THREE STAGES

We know well that grip is the motor component of prehension. This can be divided into a power grip and a precision grip. They are self-explanatory (Figure 1.33).

1. Power grip: Let us see the example of an orthopaedic surgeon holding the chisel and hammering it as an innate of his operative skills.
2. Precision grip: Let us see the precision work again in the picture. This time the surgeon is focused extensively to achieve accuracy.

TYPES OF GRIP

1. Thumb–finger grip

The thumb–finger pinch is one of the more delicate movements of the thumb which needs a strong opposition, good webspace and intact neuromuscular function. Thumb tries to oppose to grip on the object by movements occurring at various levels. The first metacarpal adducts in the longitudinal plane of the palm and then pronate towards the item. The

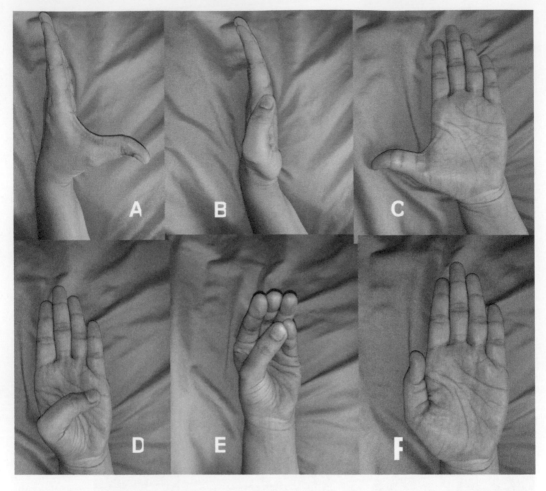

Figure 1.30 Movements of the thumb. (a) Thumb abduction. (b) Adduction. (c) Thumb extension. (d) Flexion. (e) Thumb opposition. (f) Retropulsion.

proximal phalanx flexes, pronates and radially deviates, and the distal phalanx flexes to a variable degree with pronation required to grip the object. An excellent first webspace, intact ligaments and musculotendinous coordination are essential to make this grip efficient. The termino–terminal pinch is used for small items, where the tip of the thumb opposes the touch of the pulp of the index finger (Figure 1.34(a)). This pinch is precisely the contact between the tips of two fingers whereas the other fingers flex to form a regular "O."

The pulp of thumb pronates and pinches the supinated opposed index finger's pulp with distal phalanges of both fingers with incomplete extension to form a subterminal pulpar pinch (Figure 1.34(b)).

The lateral pinch is between the distal phalanx of the thumb and the lateral aspect of the index finger. It is quite a strong pinch compared

to the above. It is of three types: Thumb-distal phalanx of index, thumb-middle phalanx and thumb-proximal phalanx depending upon the need (Figure 1.35).

Kapandji has proposed 11 stages for evaluating thumb opposition. It is based on the movement of thumb–finger pinch at various levels of opposition (Figure 1.36). The test is valid when the thumb passes every stage of the wide course it has been passed through.

2. Interdigital grip

When there is spastic thumb or thumb weakness, the rest of the fingers adapt to use the interdigit as a form of gripping object. The less powerful finger abductors and adductors augmented by the long flexors provide interdigital grip in holding small and light items (Figure 1.37(a)).

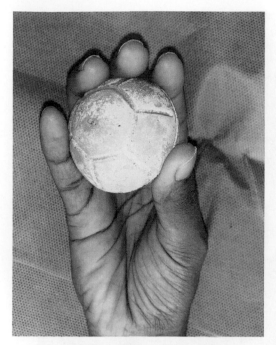

Figure 1.31 The thumb is stable at full pronation, full opposition because of the maximum ligament tension, muscle contraction and joint congruence. Holding a ball makes the thumb in a plane perpendicular to the other fingers. It is short and more mobile with various vital functions across the palm to the ulnar border of the hand.

3. Composite grip

In addition to the tripod grip, an additional fourth point is required for some actions to have stability. Usually, the palm provides stability and remains the fourth point (Figure 1.37(b)).

4. Hook grip

Hook grips occur when all fingers are flexed at the PIP joints with the thumb adducted. Carrying a bag or lifting heavy objects or post-surgical PIP joint arthrodesed fingers have this hook grip (Figure 1.37(c)).

5. Digito-palmar grip

There are certain circumstances where the thumb may not be needed for the grip (Figure 1.37(c)). The index, middle, ring and little fingers flex first at the PIP joint, then at the MCP joint and finally at the DIP joint to lift objects against the palm which is very firm and consistent in performing this task.

6. Tripod grip/fixation

The work formed by the thumb, index and middle fingers is called a tripod grip or tridactyl. Examples are writing, holding a cup handle or fork, buttoning shirts, etc. They do not require much force, but precision is mandated in performing this accurate work (Figure 1.38).

HOW ONE SELECTS A GRIP

It is the pattern of work which determines the selection of grip. They can be precision or powerful. Precision work needs less power which is supplemented by the thumb, index and middle fingers. These do not need the palm. Most professionals like doctors and engineers need this precision for their daily activities. The power is given by ulnar fingers (ring and little fingers) and palm. Manual labourers need power to do their jobs and less precision in their work (Figure 1.39).

The positioning of the hand to grasp and adapt to its form is complex. More important is the regulation of the force of the grip. The force of grip must be varied depending upon the weight of the object, fragility (glass), surface characteristics (slippery, rough) and its utilization (Figure 1.40). Also, Pacinian corpuscles play a semi-automatic role in measuring and regulating the grasping force. Interestingly, there is always an overshoot of forces in the initial/first grasp of an unknown object, then the second/subsequent grasp automatically regulates the level of force required for prehension. In leprosy, the hand has lost its sensory safety signals, forcing the hand to non-healing wounds/ulcers by excessive pressure.

ESSENTIALS IN THE MECHANISM OF GRIP

Figures 1.39–1.43 are the mechanism of a grip.

QUINTESSENTIAL FOR GRIP (GOOD SENSATION IN THE PREHENSILE ZONE AND FREE MOBILITY OF FINGERS)

The sensory functions of the hand are essential for prehension, various specific grips (digito-palmar, lateral pinch), correct positioning, spatial orientation, holding objects and protecting it from injury. The most important part of the hand (thumb, index finger and middle finger) is supplied with the median nerve (Figure 1.44). The most important part of the hand for power grips (ring and little finger) is supplied with the ulnar

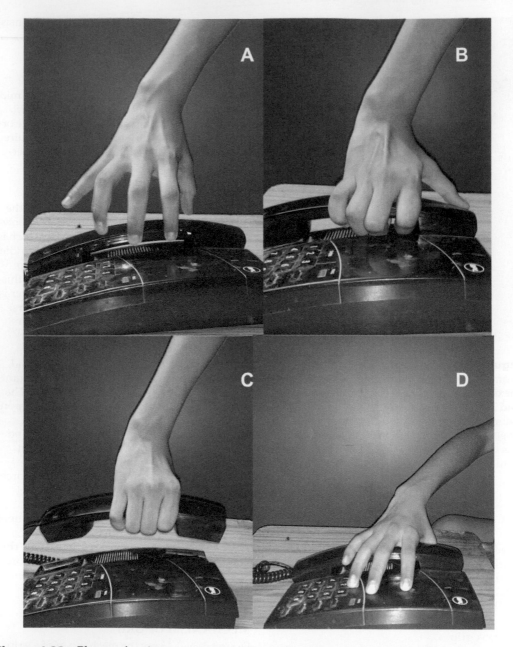

Figure 1.32 Phases of prehension. It has the "regard" as the visual attention of the phone receiver, perceiving the location and size of the receiver. (a) Reach: Preparing the upper limb position to reach the receiver with elbow extension and forearm pronated and reshaping the hand to pick up the phone. (b) Grasp/grip: The act of closing the hand to lift the phone receiver and stabilizing it to prevent it from falling out of the hand. (c) Manipulation: The hand always maximizes its efficiency to hold the object, adjusts the hand within the hand and manipulates to its convenience until the end of the task. (d) Release of grip: It is how the phone receiver leaves the hand.

nerve. Median and ulnar nerve paralysis results in sensory loss and motor loss to varying degrees.

APPLIED ANATOMY

The extrinsic and intrinsic muscles of the hand and the wrist play an important role in hand function. Let us understand the applied anatomy of these two groups of muscles.

1. The extrinsic muscles (muscles which originate in the forearm and have their insertion in the fingers, controlling their

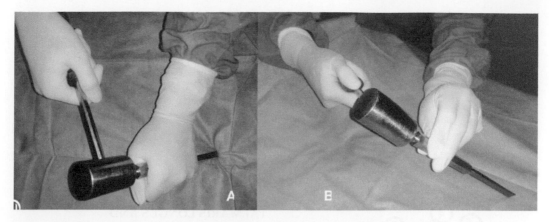

Figure 1.33 The surgeon has to hold the hammer tight so that it does not slip or fall away from his precision. He keeps the right wrist in ulnar deviation. The FCU is the prime force and stabilizer for his wrist action and power grip. The thumb adducts to hold the hammer within the fingers and reinforces the grip. (a) The surgeon then hammers the chisel through sequential movements at his shoulder, elbow and wrist. Also note the left hand, where the chisel is held within the first webspace by thumb adduction and wrist dorsiflexion to perform the task efficiently. The role of the palm is to hold the hammer and the chisel within its reach. Here the palm's participation is negligible. (b) The right hand holds the hammer. The thumb and the index finger have lateral grip; the ulnar fingers holding the hammer give power by the palmar grip. Similarly, the left hand holds the chisel with precision by multiple pulp grips (index, middle, ring and little fingers) holding between the thumb and other fingers, through numerous pulp grips between the fingers and the thumb.

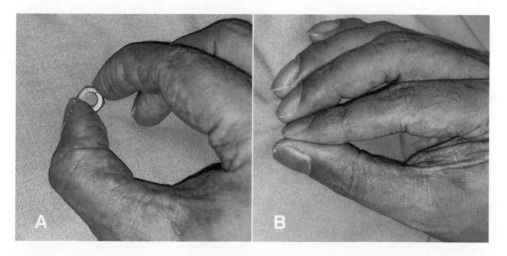

Figure 1.34 The thumb-finger pinch (a) termino-terminal pinch. (b) subterminal pulpar pinch.

movement, e.g., wrist flexors and extensors, finger extensor and flexor tendons, palmaris longus).

2. The intrinsic muscles (muscles which originate within the hand and insert into the fingertips and control their movement, e.g., lumbricals).

EXTRINSIC MUSCLES
Long Digital Flexor Tendons

The flexor digitorum superficialis (FDS) and flexor digitorum profundus (FDP) are the long digital flexor tendons. The FDS originates from the forearm and divides into two slips to each finger with independent flexion movement

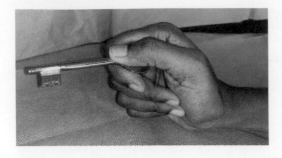

Figure 1.35   Lateral pinch.

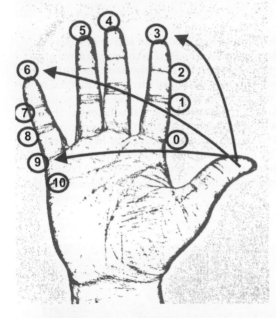

Figure 1.36   Kapandji's stage of opposition.

at the proximal interphalangeal joint. It is a potential donor for tendon transfers because of its independence [18]. The FDP originates as a single muscle mass in the forearm and divides into four tendons to activate flexion at the distal interphalangeal joint of the fingers simultaneously. Its action has been compared to a charioteer who drives a quadriga (Roman chariot) without independent control and movement [19] (Figure 1.45). The FDP is most efficient when the excursion of all its tendons is equal and in unison and remains poor for tendon transfers.

PALMARIS LONGUS AND LITTLE FINGER FDS

The palmaris longus is a muscle of the superficial flexor compartment of the forearm. It inserts into the distal half of the flexor retinaculum and palmar aponeurosis. It is supplied by the median nerve. It acts as a tensor of the palmar aponeurosis and a weak wrist flexor. This muscle is phylogenetically degenerated and has been reported quite extensively for its anatomical variability and variation in the prevalence of absence in different ethnic groups. It is an expendable tendon used as a tendon graft in various reconstructive surgeries of the upper limb. Its absence has been reported in literature as 16% unilateral and 9% bilateral [20]. Considering its potential use and demand for tendon reconstruction, its presence has to be checked routinely in any clinical practice. There have been various methods described in literature to check the presence of palmaris longus (Figures 1.46–1.49).

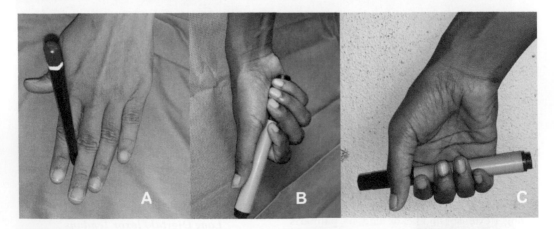

Figure 1.37   (a) Interdigital grip. (b) This is a picture of the hand holding large objects. The hand accommodates the large items in its palmar groove, which is oblique in axis and longer in area of contact. So, the object assigns itself in the oblique way along the transverse palmar axis to get control more than the grip. (c) This is the picture of the hook grip where the digits and the palm hold the object without the thumb. This digito-palmar grip needs MCP and IP joint flexion complementing each other.

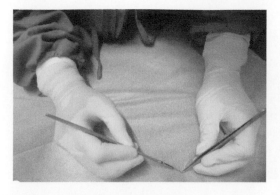

Figure 1.38 Pictures of precision handling involving thumb and index finger, tripod precision handling (surgeon holding the knife and finer instruments).

The routine clinical checking of an FDS in the little finger in practice makes an impact about its significance. The absence of FDS function in the little finger is a congenital anomaly with an incidence of 6.8% in unilateral and 6.0% bilateral [21]. In such absence, the FDP takes care of flexion at the DIP and indirectly at the PIP and MCP joint by its long course of passage and action. Hence, a patient with a flexor tendon injury to the little finger has to be dealt meticulously considering the absence factor and due attention and care has to be given to repair both tendons if available and in the absence of the FDP alone. There is no significance in the relationship between absent palmaris longus and absent FDS of the little finger. Standard methods can test the presence or absence (Video 1.2). Look for the flexion at the proximal interphalangeal joint (PIP) (Figures 1.50 and 1.51).

INTRINSIC MUSCLES

The intrinsic muscles of the hand are divided into palmar, thenar and hypothenar groups. The palmar group is comprised of the lumbrical and the interossei muscles which have a greater concentration of muscle spindle than any other muscles in the body to carry out fine and precision activities [22].

PRIME FUNCTION AND ROLE OF LUMBRICALS

- With the aid of its FDP tendon, each lumbrical adds materially to the force of flexion of the metacarpophalangeal joint.

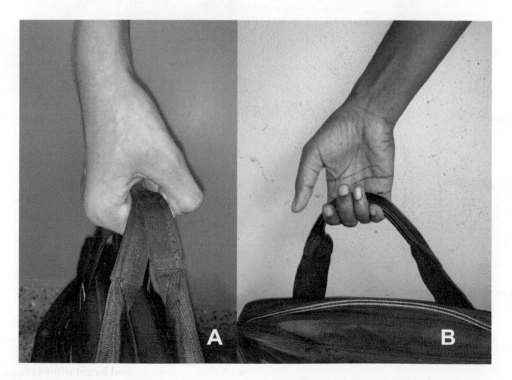

Figure 1.39 The picture of powerful grip and a fatigue hook. (a) There is a full closure of the hand around an object, involving the thumb with flexion at the MCP and IP joints. (b) The grip becomes a hook of the IP joints because of fatigue losing the precision.

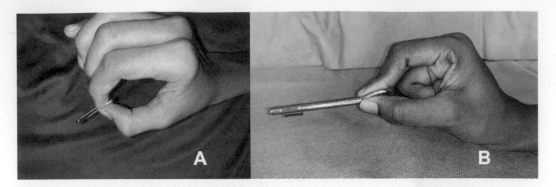

Figure 1.40 (a) Terminal pinch (holding pin). (b) Subterminal or pulpar pinch (holding key).

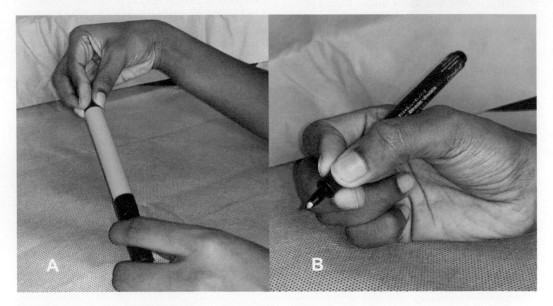

Figure 1.41 (a), (b) The precision becomes more perfect when the third digit is added (writing and opening up).

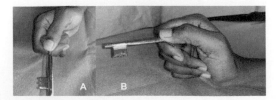

Figure 1.42 Thumb-index finger grip. This is called a lateral pinch. It's between the thumb and lateral border of the index finger used in daily activities like key pinch and visiting card holding position.

- As the tips of the fingers close in normal grasp, the tension on the lumbricals progressively increases. When grasp is almost completed, the lumbricals are physiologically in position to contribute most to the flexion of the MCP joint and grasp.

- The lumbricals certainly join forces with the interossei in performing the timely coordinated movements of the fingers in such action as needle-threading.

- They stabilize the MCP joint and contribute to the force of the final phase of the grasp.

- As the lumbricals contract, the FDP tendon is pulled distally to prevent flexion of the IP joints. Conversely, the lumbricals become inactive as the FDP begins to contract. These

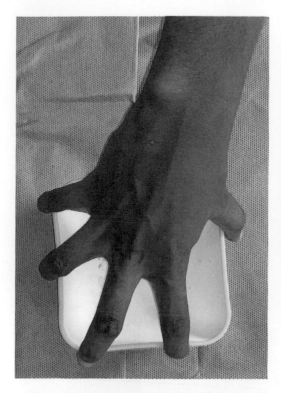

Figure 1.43 The maximum opening of the hand to reach large objects depends on the webspace (between thumb and little finger) and length of the other digits.

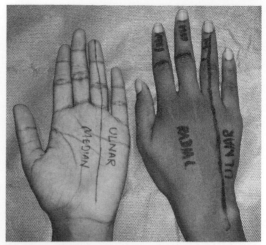

Figure 1.44 (a) Dorsal surface. (b) Volar surfaces of the hand with outlines depicting the borders of sensory innervation via the median, radial and ulnar nerves.

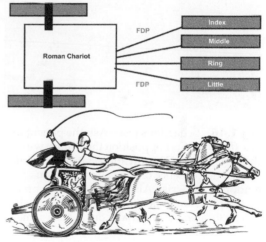

Figure 1.45 Quadriga.

actions indicate that FDP and lumbricals do not contract simultaneously. Interestingly, activity of both muscles may be seen during prehensile functions [23].

SIGNIFICANCE OF INTEROSSEI

The role of the first dorsal interossei during the mechanism of pinch and various other prehensile activities is crucial and indispensable. It is challenging to replace it with surgical interventions (tendon transfers) when the muscle is paralyzed (Figure 1.52).

There exists a synergistic antagonism between the intrinsic musculature and the extensor digitorum communis at the metacarpophalangeal (MCP) joint. Distal to the proximal interphalangeal joint, the anatomical configuration and the functional potentiality of both the extensor digitorum communis and the intrinsic musculature inserting into the aponeurosis are the same (both cause IP extension alone). With the MCP joint stabilized by either the extensor digitorum communis or the intrinsics, the other is capable of completing the extension of the digit (normal function of interossei is MCP flexion and IP extension. Either EDC or intrinsics

have to stabilize the MCP joint first to get this done).

THE EXTENSOR EXPANSION

It is formed from the expansion of the tendon of the extensor digitorum (EDC) at the proximal interphalangeal joint (PIPJ) (Figure 1.53) [24].

The tendon is split into three parts:

- One central: Inserted into the base of middle phalanx

- Two laterals: Inserted into the base of the distal phalanx

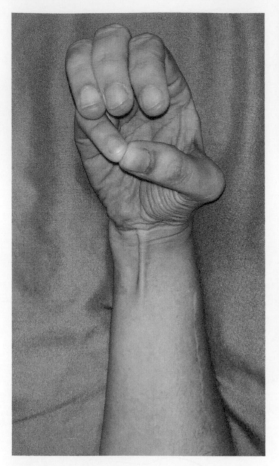

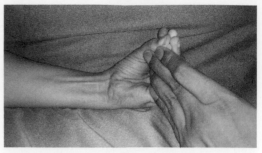

Figure 1.48 Test II: The patient is asked to abduct the thumb against resistance with the wrist in slight palmar flexion. Look and feel for the palmaris longus.

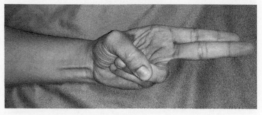

Figure 1.49 "Two-finger sign" method: The patient is asked to extend the index and middle finger fully. The wrist, ring and little fingers are flexed. Finally, the thumb is entirely opposed and flexed. Look and feel for the palmaris longus tendon.

Fig 1.46 Schaeffer's test – Ask the patient to flex the wrist and opposition the thumb with the little finger. One can appreciate the prominence and presence of the palmaris longus tendon at the wrist. Also, do not misinterpret by the presence of flexor carpi radialis, which can be located more radially during the same manoeuvre.

The expansion receives the insertions of:

1. Corresponding interosseous muscle (on each side)
2. Lumbrical muscle (on the radial side)

Three pairs of ligamentous components join the assembly from either side. The proximal wing, the phalangeal component, is made up of the dorsal interossei muscle which possesses a bifid insertion. One slip inserts into the phalangeal tubercle of the proximal phalanx. The other slips insert into the central tendon to form the hood (dossier) over the proximal phalanx. The intermediate wing is placed on the radial side of the fingers whilst the palmar interossei are attached to the ulnar side of the index finger and the radial side of the ring and little fingers [25]. The most distal component is the retinacular Landsmeer ligament which arises from the flexor sheath in the region of the proximal phalanx and courses volar to the PIP joint to join

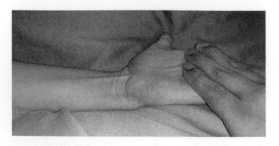

Figure 1.47 Test I: The examiner passively hyperextends the metacarpophalangeal joints of all fingers. The patient is asked to flex the wrist. Look for the prominence of palmaris longus on the ulnar aspect of the wrist.

Video 1.2   Video demonstrating the absence of PIP joint flexion in little finger caused by the FDS tendon. Also, note that movements of ring and little finger show that the little finger flexes the DIP joint (FDP tendon) and not the PIP joint (FDS tendon). The FDP tendon flexes the DIP joint first and subsequently the entire finger passing the flexion momentum to the PIP joint thereby indirectly flexing it.

www.routledge.com/9780367647162.

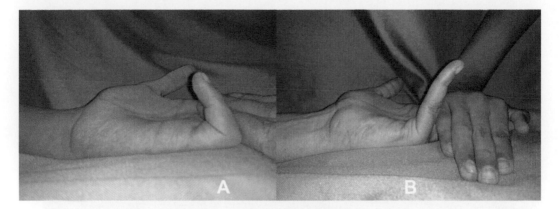

Figure 1.50   (a) The demonstration of little finger FDS function. The examiner prevents the flexion of other fingers and actively allows the patient to flex the little finger. (b) Picture demonstrating the absence of the little finger FDS on modified testing.

the common terminal extensor that inserts into the base of the distal phalanx. The Landsmeer ligament prevents hyperextension of the PIP joints. Three characteristic deformities of the fingers are due to an imbalance caused by interference with the extensor expansion mechanism. They are the boutonniere, swan-neck and mallet deformities [26].

HAND IN SPACE

The hand in space gives the real-time picture of the hand put to use in human being. The entire upper limb functions as a vector with the hand at its distal-most part remaining distinctive and unique. The hand functions in a well-organized and systematic way provided the proximal joints are stable and mobile without deformities and shortening. During the entire movement, the hand remains under vision control.

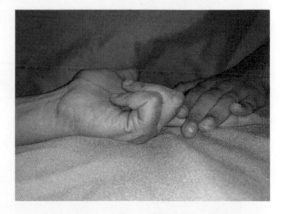

Figure 1.51   Modified test of showing the function of the FDS. By masking the index and middle fingers, the patient can flex the ring and little fingers at the PIP joint.

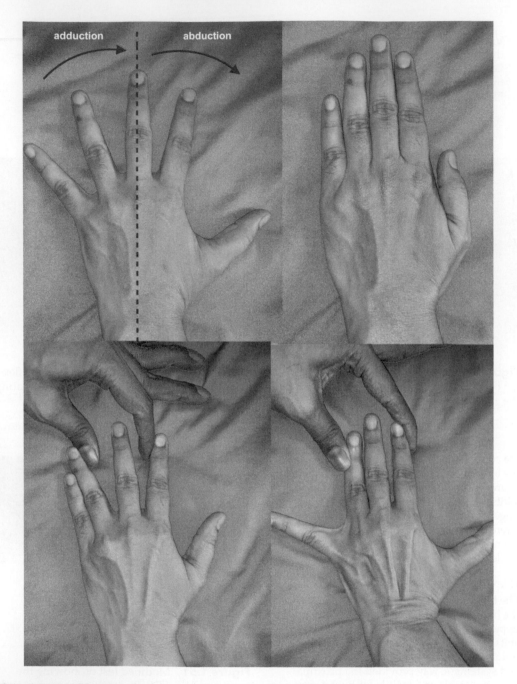

Figure 1.52 Function of interossei. Finger abduction and adduction.

The hand is so integrated with other parts of the body; it must be studied exclusively and thoroughly [27–30] (Figure 1.54).

THE HAND AND THE CENTRAL NERVOUS SYSTEM

The brain is the master control of hand movement, and the hand is the brain for all movements. The primary motor cortex, subcortical

cerebellar and pontomedullary circuits control the functions of the hand. A complex system admixed with a lot of desirable sensory information; muscular coordination created a larger area of representation in the motor cortex. The hand occupies a third of the primary motor cortex (junction of upper and lower thirds). A unique and vast area of representation is seen for the thumb and fingers exclusively in this

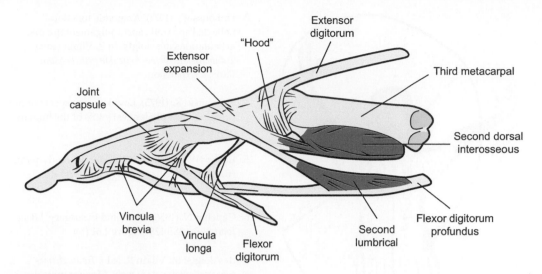

Figure 1.53 Extensor expansion lateral view.

motor cortex. For a long time there have been numerous theories and philosophical interpretations analyzing the relationship between the brain and the hand. Many criticize that the hand is just an evolution of the modern human's comprehensive actions to the demand and some portray the hand as a multi-talented organ distinctively characteristic of man and an agent of conscious activity. Technically, "The mind makes the hand; the hand makes the mind" [31, 32].

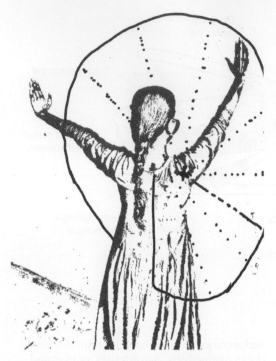

Figure 1.54 This is a picture of a girl with a wide-open hand and upper limb placed in the space to appreciate its spatial orientation. The entire movement is spherical-centred at the shoulder. Hand circumduction: To reach the mouth (feeding, eating, drinking, etc.). With movements, the hand is in a position close to the ipsilateral thigh, which is the end of the sphere and its functional limit in the space. The upper limit of the space if when the shoulder is in maximum abduction and extension. Hand moving to the posterior aspect (dorsal zone): the arm is carried backwards and inwards, elbow flexed and the forearm pronated or supinated for the lower half of the body and supinated for the upper half of the body and perineal region (personal hygiene care). Hand moving to the same side head: Shoulder externally rotated and elbow flexed to reach the back of the head. Hand moving to the opposite shoulder: Hand crosses the opposite side of the body to reach shoulder and head (left side).

FUNDING: NIL

REFERENCES

1. Napier J. (1980). *Function of the Hand*. In Hands Ch. 3, pp. 67–83, Pantheon, New York.

2. Wheeler RH. (1929). *The Science of Psychology*. Thomas Crowell Publishers, New York.

3. Dubousset J. (1971). Anatomie fonctionnelle de l'appareil capsulo-ligamentaire des articulations des doigts. In R. Vilain (eds.), *Traumatismes Ostéo-Articulaires de la Main*. Paris: L'Expansion.

4. Kuczynski K. (1975). Less-known aspects of the proximal interphalangeal joints of the human hand. *Hand*, 7:31–3.

5. Littler JW. (1960). The physiology and dynamic function of the hand. *Surg Clin North Am.*, 40:259.

6. Capener N. (1956). The hand in surgery. *J Bone Joint Surg.*, 38B:128 (Figure 1.61 (b)).

7. des doigts. In: Vilain R. (ed.), *Traumatismes osteo-articulaires de la main*. Monographic du GEM. Expansion Scientifique Française, Paris.

8. White RL. (1960). Restoration of function and balance of the wrist and hand by tendon transfers. *Surg Clinics North Am.*, 40:427–59.

9. Jeannerod M. (1988). *The Neural and Behavioural Organization of Goal-Directed Movements*. Clarendon Press, Oxford.

10. Paulignan Y, Jeannerod M, MacKenzie C and Marteniuk R. (1991). Selective perturbation of visual input during prehension movements. 2. The effects of changing object size. *Exp Brain Res.*, 87(2):407–20.

11. Santello M, Flanders M and Soechting JF. (1998). Postural hand synergies for tool use. *J Neurosci.*, 18(23):10105–15.

12. Mason DR, Gomez JE, and Ebner TJ. (2001). Hand synergies during reach-to-grasp. *J Neurophysiol.*, 86:2896–910.

13. Santello M, Bianchi M, Gabiccini M, Ricciardi E, Salvietti G, Bicchi A et al. (2016). Hand synergies: Integration of robotics and neuroscience for understanding the control of biological and artificial hands. *Phys Life Rev.*, 17:1–23. doi:10.1016/j.plrev.2016.02.001

14. Wing AM and Fraser C. (1983). The contribution of the thumb to reaching movements. *Q J Exp Psychol A.*, 35:297–309.

15. Galea MP, Castiello U and Dalwood N. (2001). Thumb invariance during prehension movement: Effects of object orientation. *Neuroreport*, 12:2185–7.

16. Kinoshita H, Kawai S and Ikuta K. (1995). Contributions and coordination of individual fingers in multiple finger prehension. *Ergonomics*, 38:1212–30.

17. Valery P. (1938). Discours d'ouverture au Congres de Chirurgie. Nouvelle Revue Française, Paris.

18. Shrewbury MM and Kuczynski K. (1974). Flexor digitorum superficialis tendons in the fingers of the human hand. *The Hand*, 6:121–33.

19. Verdan C. (1960). Syndrome of the quadriga. *Surg Clinic North Am.*, 40:425–26.

20. Thompson NW, Mockford BJ, Rasheed T and Herbert KJ. (2002). Functional absence of flexor digitorum superficialis to the little finger and absence of palmaris longus--is there a link? *J Hand Surg Br.*, 27(5):433–4.

21. Townley W, Swan MC and Dunn RL. (2010). Congenital absence of flexor digitorum superficialis: Implications for assessment of little finger lacerations. *J Hand Surg Eur.*, 35(5):417–8.

22. Eyler DL and Markee JE. (1954). The anatomy and function of the intrinsic musculature of the fingers. *J Bone Joint Surg Am.*, 36-A (1):1–9.

23. Close J. Robert and Kidd Caroline C. (1969). The functions of the muscles of the thumb, the index, and long fingers: Synchronous recording of motions and action potentials of muscles. *JBJS*, 51(8):1601–20.

24. Fowler SB. (1949). Extensor apparatus of the digits. *Bone Joint Surg.*, 31-B: 477.

25. Landsmeer JMF. (1955). Anatomical and functional investigation of the articulations of the human fingers. *Acta Anat.* Supp24.

26. Elliot RA. (1970). Injuries of the extensor mechanism of the hand. *Orthop clinics North Am.*, 1:335–54.

27. Kapandji A1. (1963). *Physiologie articulaire*, volume 1. Librarie Maloine, Paris.

28. Santello M, and Soechting JF. (2000). Force synergies for multifingered grasping. *Exp Brain Res.*, 133:457–67.

29. Forster O. (1934). The motor cortex in man in the light of Hughlings Jackson's doctrines. *Brain*, 59:135–59.

30. Penfield WG and Boldney EV. (1937). Somatic motor and sensory representation in the cerebral cortex of man as studied by electrical stimulation. *Brain*, 60:389–443.

31. Penfield WG and Rasmussen T. (1950). *The Cerebral Cortex of Man*. Macmillan, New York.

32. Focillon H. (1947). Eloge de la main. In: *Vie des formes*. Presses Universitaires de France, Paris.

33. Kleinert HE and Verdan C. Report of the Committee on Tendon Injuries. *J Hand Surg (Am).* 1983;8:794–798.

2 Clinical Evaluation

History Taking and Arriving at a Clinical Diagnosis

J Terrence Jose Jerome

CONTENTS

DOI: 10.1201/9781003125938-2

HISTORY TAKING

Hand examination is an art, and it is not impossible to make it better by proper clinical examination. All you need is to gain the confidence of the patient who is sitting in front of you. He is the guidance for all his complaints, and you need patience to listen and a simple understanding of it. There may be instances where you may feel lost, but to gain his confidence you need to travel a bit in his direction and turn him later towards your goal.

CHIEF COMPLAINTS (ASCENDING CHRONOLOGY DURATION)

1. Pain

2. Weakness

3. Numbness, tingling sensation

4. Deformity

5. Loss of movement

6. Stiffness

7. Trigger symptoms

HISTORY OF PRESENTING COMPLAINTS

1. Pain

Pain is the most common presenting complaint in patients with hand and upper limb problems; it is an unpleasant sensory and emotional experience associated with actual or potential tissue damage. Pain is a complex personal experience that is difficult to measure objectively. The clinical assessment of pain can assist with our understanding of its basis and can assist with evaluating the effectiveness

of treatment. Let us see the objective behind this symptom and how we can progress to a diagnosis.

WHAT IS THE DURATION OF PAIN?

Constant – infection, arthritis
Intermittent – morning stiffness (rheumatoid arthritis), at the end of the day (osteoarthritis)

HOW IS IT EXPERIENCED?

Localized – abscess, cellulitis
Radiating – radiculopathy (C5–C6 disc is the most common symptom in younger patients)

WHETHER ASSOCIATED WITH PARAESTHESIA, NUMBNESS?

Yes – cervical disc prolapse is associated with numbness and paraesthesia.

Pattern of cervical spine nerve roots distribution and affections in radiculopathy [1, 2] (Table 2.1).

HOW TO DIFFERENTIATE BETWEEN CARPAL TUNNEL SYNDROME AND C6 RADICULOPATHY?

Provocative Tests

1. Spurling's test

It is designed to reproduce symptoms and is performed by laterally flexing, rotating and compressing the patient's head toward the side of the symptoms (weight approx. 7kg). This effectively causes the pathologic foramen to close and should reproduce the symptoms. This test is very reproducible and extremely specific but is not sensitive. If this induces radiating pain and paraesthesia into the symptomatic extremity, it strongly suggests nerve

Table 2.1: Pattern of Cervical Radiculopathy

Level	Root	Pain Distribution	Sensory Involvement (Numbness, Paraesthesia, Burning, Tingling or Both)	Motor Involvement (Weakness)	Reflexes Lost
C4–5	C5	Medial scapular border, lateral upper arm to elbow	Shoulder, lateral upper arm	Deltoid, supraspinatus, infraspinatus	Biceps
C5–6	C6	Lateral forearm, thumb and index finger	Lateral forearm, thumb, index	Biceps, brachioradialis, wrist extensors	Biceps/ Brachioradialis absent
C6–7	C7	Medial scapula, posterior arm dorsum of forearm, middle finger	Posterior forearm, middle finger	Triceps, wrist flexors, finger extensors	Triceps absent
C7–T1	C8	Shoulder, ulnar side of the forearm, little finger	Ulnar aspect of forearm, little finger	Thumb flexors, adductor pollicis, finger flexors Abduction, finger intrinsics, grip	-

Table 2.2: Difference between C6 Radiculopathy and Carpal Tunnel Syndrome

	C6 Radiculopathy	Carpal Tunnel Syndrome
Symptoms	Present throughout and affected by activities	Worse in the early morning. Night handshakes amidst sleep disturbances. **The patient often flaps or flicks the hands to get relief.**
Motor deficits	Biceps weakness. Biceps jerk absent. Minimal wrist extensor weakness	Abductor pollicis brevis which is innervated by the recurrent branch of the median nerve atrophy. Thenar atrophy.
Additional tests	Spurling's manoeuvre will exacerbate C6 radicular pain.	Tinel's at the wrist, Durken's median nerve test, and wrist flexion will exacerbate.

root compression, usually secondary to disk herniation. It should be noted that lateral head movement away from the symptomatic extremity sometimes can accentuate pain and paraesthesia in the symptomatic upper extremity secondary to stretching of a compressed nerve root (Table 2.2) (Figure 2.1).

Scratch collapse test

The scratch collapse test is another clinical test that may be used to identify a site of nerve compression and has been shown to have good psychometric properties. This test is unique in that it uses a response independent of the sites of compression in the upper extremity. The examiner is positioned in front of the patient with their arms in a neutral shoulder rotation, 90° of elbow flexion, wrists in a neutral position and fingers extended. The examiner assesses isometric shoulder external rotation strength by applying a force to both forearms, and the patient applies an equal resisted force of external shoulder rotation to maintain the arms in a static

position. The skin over the site of nerve compression to be assessed is lightly scratched and a similar force is applied to the forearms to resist isometric shoulder external rotation. A loss of shoulder external rotation strength will result in "collapse" of the arm toward the abdomen.

Significance of scratch collapse test:

a) A positive response relies on the loss of muscle strength (shoulder external rotation) and therefore provides an outcome unrelated to the site of nerve compression.

b) This test has been shown to have good positive and negative predictive values in the assessment of patients with carpal and cubital tunnel syndrome with abnormal nerve conduction studies.

c) This test is particularly useful in patients with diffuse symptoms, multiple levels of nerve compression, and normal nerve conduction studies.

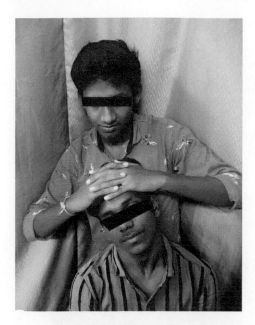

Figure 2.1 Spurling sign. Axial compression of the spine and rotation to the ipsilateral side of symptoms reproduces or worsens cervical radiculopathy. Pain on the side of rotation is usually indicative of foraminal stenosis and nerve root irritation.

2. Durken's median nerve test

The examiner exerted an even pressure on the flexor retinaculum (directly to the median nerve) in the carpal tunnel with both thumbs (Figure 2.2). The interval from the application of compression to the onset of numbness, pain or paraesthesia in the distribution of the median nerve distal to the level of the carpal tunnel should be recorded [3].

AN ADDITIONAL TEST FOR CARPAL TUNNEL SYNDROME AND ITS SIGNIFICANCE

The readers can see additional tests for carpal tunnel (Table 2.3).

How to Differentiate between C8 and Ulnar Neuropathy?

The readers can see the difference shown in Table 2.4.

3. Neck "distraction" test

The patient is made to lie in supine and the examiner holds the chin and occiput and applies gradual pulling force. A positive test reduces the cervical spinal nerve compression and thereby reduces upper extremity pain and paraesthesia.

4. Valsalva test

Like low back pain/sciatica, the Valsalva maneuver with resultant increased intrathecal pressure can sometimes accentuate the neck and upper extremity symptoms due to underlying cervical radiculopathy.

As with low back pain/sciatica, the Valsalva manoeuvre with resultant increased intrathecal pressure can sometimes accentuate the neck and upper extremity symptoms when due to underlying cervical radiculopathy.

5. Lhermitte's test

In patients with myelopathy affecting the posterior columns, neck flexion can produce paresthesia, usually in the back, but sometimes into the extremities (Figure 2.3 arrow). Lhermitte's test is most commonly associated with an inflammatory process such as multiple sclerosis, but it is sometimes noted with spinal cord compression.

6. Adson's and hyperabduction tests

Long used in the evaluation of suspected thoracic outlet syndrome, these tests are nonspecific and unreliable. With the patient sitting erect, the upper extremities at the side (Adson) or symptomatic upper extremity abducted and extended (hyperabduction), the radial pulse is palpated. Each test is positive if the pulse disappears, and paraesthesia develops in the hand of the symptomatic extremity. Also, an upper limb tension test is sensitive for diagnosing thoracic outlet syndrome (Figure 2.4).

7. Tinel's sign

Compression or percussion over the site of entrapment often will trigger or reproduce the sensory symptoms distal to the entrapment site, a phenomenon called Tinel's sign (dysesthesias produced by tapping over the nerve) (Figure 2.5).

CERVICAL MYELOPATHY

Clinicians should also inquire about symptoms of myelopathy. These may occasionally be subtle (e.g., diffuse hand numbness and clumsiness, which are often attributed to peripheral neuropathy or carpal tunnel syndrome, difficulty with balance and sphincter disturbances presenting initially as urinary urgency or frequency rather than as retention or incontinence) (Table 2.5).

MRC – Medical Research Council scale

PAIN AND ASSOCIATED SYMPTOMS

The characteristic presence of fever, chills, unexplained weight loss, unremitting night pain, previous cancer, immunosuppression or intravenous drug use should alert clinicians to a more serious disease like tumour or infection [4] (Table 2.6).

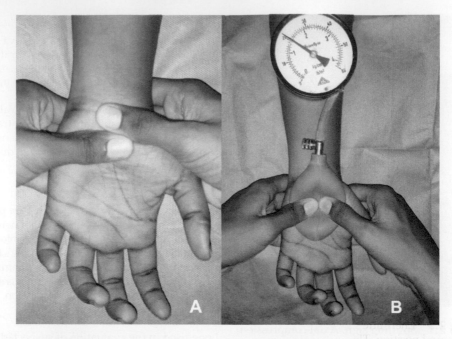

Figure 2.2 (A) The carpal compression test is performed by the examiner exerting even pressure, with both thumbs, to the median nerve in the carpal tunnel. A positive sign means the reproduction of symptoms. (B) The test consists of direct compression of the median nerve running deep to the flexor retinaculum, is being performed with a device that consists of a rubber atomizer-bulb connected to a pressure manometer from a sphygmomanometer. A pressure of 150 mm of mercury (20 kPa) is applied to the area of the carpal tunnel for as long as thirty seconds. A positive sign means the reproduction of symptoms.

Table 2.3: Carpal Tunnel Syndrome Tests Significance

Test	Sensitivity (%)	Specificity (%)
Durken's median nerve test (carpal compression test)	87	90
Phalen's test	70	84
Tinel's sign	56	80

Table 2.4: Differences between C8 Radiculopathy and Ulnar Neuropathy

	C8 Radiculopathy	Ulnar Neuropathy (Most Common at Cubital and Less Common at Guyon's Canal/Entrapment Syndrome)
Sensory deficits (burning, tingling or both). Tinel's sign: pain that radiates down into your little finger when you bang your ulnar nerve at the elbow, called "hitting your funny bone."	Inferior medial aspect of the arm into the entire ring and little fingers.	Ulnar half of ring and little finger. Absent sensation over the dorso-ulnar aspect of the wrist (dorsal branch of ulnar nerve involvement seen in cubital tunnel syndrome). This feature differentiates between cubital tunnel syndrome and Guyon's canal compression of the ulnar nerve.
Motor deficits.	Same.	Weakness, atrophy, hand clumsiness.
Additional tests (Spurling's test)	1. Absent response with local anaesthesia at wrist level.	1. Local anaesthetic block at the entrapment site abolishes the sensory disturbance and Tinel's sign in the entrapment neuropathies. 2. Positive Tinel's at the elbow. 3. Elbow flexion test (flexion of the arm may trigger tingling sensation into the little finger).

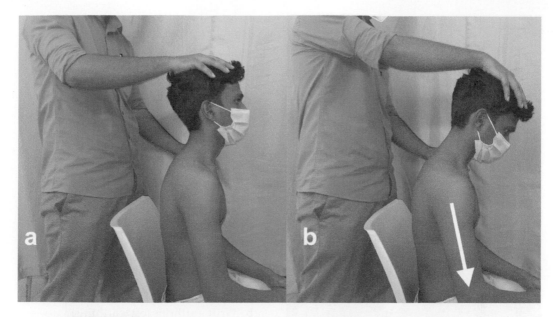

Figure 2.3 Lhermitte's sign. Electric shock sensation occurs when the examined flexes the neck from neutral position. The sensation may radiate down the spine, and some time upper and lower extremities.

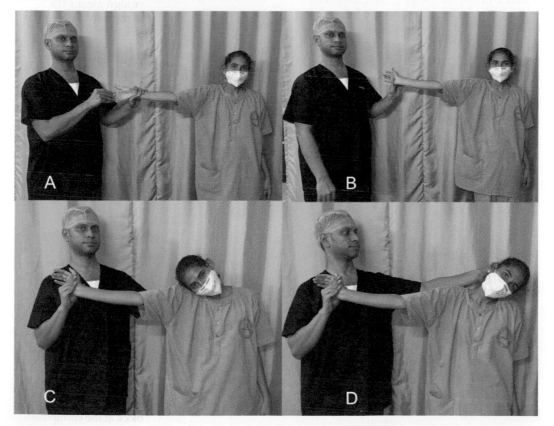

Figure 2.4 Upper limb tension test. (a–d). The head is brought to the affected side. If there is significant pain with just the abduction or wrist extension, the author considers it highly positive. If the patient has pain with the wrist hyperextended and the head away, which is relieved by bringing the head to the affected side, this is also very positive. This test is suggestive of thoracic outlet syndrome.

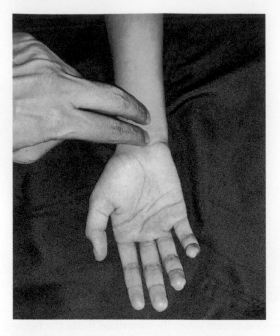

Figure 2.5 Tinel's sign. It is performed by lightly tapping (percussing) over the nerve to elicit a sensation of tingling or "pins and needles" in the distribution of the nerve.

IS THE PAIN ASSOCIATED WITH EARLY MORNING STIFFNESS, IN BOTH HANDS, LASTS FOR 30 MINUTES, AND GOES AWAY WITH ACTIVITIES?

Rheumatoid arthritis:

1. Rheumatoid hand may present with features of tenosynovitis as pain, dysfunction of tendons and ultimately tendon rupture (Figure 2.6). Treatment can relieve the pain and prevent both deformity and loss of function. Median nerve compression may be associated with permanent pain, numbness and thenar muscle loss.

2. Sudden loss of finger extension or flexion (most commonly seen as painless rupture following trivial trauma with extensor tendon of the little, ring and middle fingers are involved).

3. Discrete nodules and finger trigger are commonly associated with rheumatoid hand.

Homework

Learn to differentiate extensor tendon rupture from MCP joint dislocation and posterior interosseous nerve palsy.

What Are the Aggravating and Alleviating Factors of Pain?

1. Pain aggravated by activity and relieved with rest and immobilization.
   a. Wrist level – avascular necrosis (lunate or scaphoid)
   b. Wrist – arthritis (osteoarthritis)

How Does it Affect Daily Activities?

Drummers do repetitive movements while playing in the orchestra. This irritates the extensor pollicis longus tendon over the Lister's tubercle and may cause triggering or EPL tendinitis. This is called as "Drummers Palsy."

Nocturnal Pain and Disturbances

Numbness in the hand more often in the night disturbing the sleep (carpal tunnel syndrome). The patient often flaps or flicks the hands to get relief.

Location of Pain?

Always try with single palpating finger to find the point tenderness and note the underlying joints, bones, soft tissues, tendons and structures for its relevance (Table 2.7).

Table 2.5: Physical Findings Associated with Myelopathy

Finding hyperreflexia	Hypertonia, clonus of ankle, knee or wrist Pathological reflexes or signs: 1. Babinski 2. Hoffmann's sign: Flexion and adduction of the thumb when the examiner flexes the terminal phalanx of the middle finger 3. Lhermitte's sign: A sensation of electrical shock radiating down the spine, precipitated by neck flexion
Clinical gradings Mild	Sensory symptoms Subjective weakness Babinski/Hoffmann's positive or negative No functional impairment
Moderate	Objective motor or sensory signs (a score of >4 on MRC motor grade). No or minimal functional impairment (mild slowing of gait).
Severe	Objective motor or sensory signs with functional impairment (hand weakness, unsteady gait, sphincter disturbances).

Table 2.6: Differential Diagnosis for Pain in the Upper Limb [4]

Thoracic outlet syndrome	Pain in the shoulder and arm aggravated by the use of the arm. Intermittent paraesthesia mostly C8–T1. Reproduction of symptoms by provocative tests. Roo's test: Rapid flexion and extension of fingers while the arms are abducted at 90° and extended at 90°. Normal neurological examination and EMG/NCV. Radial pulse decreased in case of vascular compression.
Parsonage–Tuner syndrome (acute brachial plexus neuritis/neuralgic amyotrophy)	Severe pain starts in the neck, shoulder, and arm, followed within days to weeks by marked arm weakness, typically in C5-6 regions as the pain recedes. (Cervical radiculopathy has pain and neurological findings co-occurring simultaneously.)
Herpes Zoster	Neuropathic pain in a dermatome distribution followed, within several days, by the appearance of the typical vesical rash.
Pancoast syndrome	Pain in the shoulder and arm due to compression of the brachial plexus, paraesthesia and weakness in the C8 -T1 region (intrinsic hand muscles), ipsilateral ptosis, myosis, and anhidrosis (Horner's syndrome).
Rotator cuff disorders shoulder	Pain in the shoulder or lateral arm region that rarely radiates below the elbow is aggravated by active and resisted shoulder movements rather than by neck movements; normal sensation and reflexes.
Carpal tunnel syndrome	Hypoesthesia and weakness in the distribution of the entrapped median nerve-thumb, index, middle finger and radial half of ring finger. Tinel's sign positive. Durkan's test/Phalen's test positive. Normal reflexes. Abnormalities in NCV study.
Cubital tunnel syndrome/ Guyon's canal entrapment	Hypoesthesia and weakness in the distribution of the entrapped ulnar nerve – ulnar ½ of ring finger and little finger (Guyon's canal), dorso-ulnar aspect of the wrist (cubital tunnel syndrome). Tinel's sign positive. Elbow flexion test positive. Normal reflexes.
Complex regional pain syndrome (CRPS)	Diffuse pain, burning and tenderness of the arm and hand, often out of proportion with examination findings, accompanied by skin changes, hyperesthesia, allodynia, vasomotor fluctuations (temperature and colour) or dysthermia; symptoms often occur after a precipitating event. Neurological examination is usually normal.

Homework for Nerve Examination in Wrist and Hand

1. Describe the typical distribution of sensory loss in hand and upper limb (carpal/cubital tunnel syndrome, Guyon's canal).

2. State which nerves to palpate for identifying hypertrophic neuropathy.

3. Describe Tinel's "tapping the nerve" sign.

4. Check the muscles innervated by the median nerve/ulnar nerve.

5. Perform important muscle to test in carpal tunnel syndrome and demonstrate how to test it.

6. Demonstrate Phalen's sign/Durken's test.

7. Look at the usual site of entrapment of the ulnar nerve.

8. Check for muscles in the hand that can be readily tested for weakness from an ulnar neuropathy.

CONDITIONS WITH ACUTE PAIN AND THE SIGNIFICANCE

A famous quote says, "As it takes two to quarrel, so it takes two to make a disease, the microbe and the host." The success of defeating infection is based on the location, infecting organism, timing of surgery, adequacy of surgical drainage, efficacy of antibiotics, health status and immunocompetence of the host (Table 2.8) (Figure 2.7).

Note:

A specific type of staphylococcal infection is staphylococcal-scalded skin syndrome, primarily a disease of young children that results from an exfoliative toxin-producing staphylococcal organism. A high index of suspicion and early differentiation of this process from other skin conditions is important to the treatment outcome. Although this syndrome is extremely rare in adults, it is associated with a high mortality rate, usually because of serious underlying illnesses, such as kidney failure or immunosuppression [5].

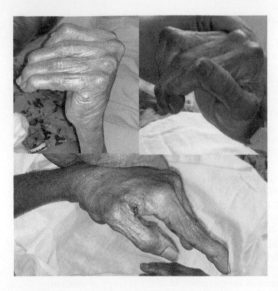

Figure 2.6 Pictures of rheumatoid hand (swan neck deformity and boutonniere deformity).

CONDITIONS WITH CHRONIC INFECTIONS PRESENTING WITH ACUTE PAIN AND THEIR SIGNIFICANCE

Chronic infections of the hand and upper extremity are rare indeed and are primarily a problem of diagnosis. They often are not considered in the differential diagnosis of hand lesions. The involvement may be:

1. Skin: Chronic cutaneous lesions, subcutaneous swellings (lipoma, sebaceous cysts), abscess, fistula, ulcers

2. Tenosynovial

3. Nerve: Schwannoma, nerve and nerve sheath tumours

4. Bone and joint: Benign and malignant tumours

Many surgeons encounter their first case by surprise unless an unusual diagnosis is considered in the presence of unusual symptoms and signs. One must consider infection in any chronic lesion of the hand. In an immunocompromised patient, infection must always be included in the differential diagnosis. Biopsy and cultures should be considered as part of a diagnostic workup for atypical lesions [6] (Table 2.9).

"Culture a tumour and biopsy an infection," is an adage to apply when an unusual lesion is encountered. The four common laboratory tests

used for the identification of the bacteria and mycobacteria are:

1. Direct visualization of the organism by staining

2. Detection of pathogenic-specific antigens and antibodies

3. Cultures in growth media

4. Nucleic acid (DNA and RNA) amplification techniques

Additional evaluation includes a serological test, special stains (methenamine silver stains for fungus), culture at specific temperatures (mycobacterium), presence of CO_2 media (*A. actinomycetemcomitans*), aerobic and anaerobic media (*Actinomyces* spp. and *Nocardia* spp.).

CHRONIC BACTERIAL INFECTIONS AND MANIFESTATIONS
Fungal Infections

Fungal infections have been increasing throughout the world parallel to immunocompromised patients, immunosuppression therapy in organ transplantation, cytotoxic chemotherapy in cancers, corticosteroid therapy and overuse of antibacterial antibiotics. The presentations are cutaneous, subcutaneous and deep infections. The cutaneous and subcutaneous infections cause serious morbidity, whereas deep infections are fatal. The infections are caused by exogenous (not a part of normal human flora, e.g., coccidioidomycosis) and endogenous flora (normal human flora – e.g., *Candida, Aspergillus*). Opportunistic fungi cause serious infections when the host immunity is compromised and lowered (Table 2.20). The commonly seen cutaneous infections are:

1. Cutaneous fungal lesions

Fungi infects and metabolizes keratin causing infections in skin, hair and nails. They do not invade the skin. Clinical manifestations are consequence of host reaction to fungal metabolic products. *Candida albicans* and dermatophytes (*Trichophyton, Microsporum* and *Epidermophyton*) are the cause of the majority of chronic cutaneous, interdigital spaces and nail infections. Chronic cutaneous *C. albicans* infection occurs in the moist palms and webs. The dorsum of the wrist may have typical rings (ring worm) with the lesion and "wristwatch ringworm" occurs in moist skin under a watch or its strap.

2. Chronic paronychia (subcutaneous fungal lesions)

Table 2.7: The Pain and Provisional Diagnosis

Physical Findings (Point Tenderness)		Corroborative History	Provisional Diagnosis
Tenderness is the soft depression between the flexor carpi ulnaris (FCU) tendon, ulnar styloid and triquetrum.	Central tears (central tear of the articular disk has pain over the distal ulna. It can be aggravated by hyper pronation and supination of the wrist).	Fall on an outstretched hand with wrist in extension and pronation bearing the entire axial load.	Triangular fibro cartilage complex injury (TFCC).
	Peripheral tears (ulnar side wrist pain, grip weakness, clicking sensation with forearm rotation).	Sports activities-related injuries – rapid twisting and loading to ulnar side of the wrist (tennis, golf).	
		Manual drilling activities – patients experience forearm torquing or traction when the drilling stops.	
Dorsal subluxation of ulna head.	Foveal tears.		
Tenderness over the extensor carpi ulnaris (ECU).			ECU tendinitis/ tendinopathy/ tenosynovial hypertrophy.
Tenderness over the flexor carpi ulnaris (FCU).			FCU tendinitis/ tendinopathy/ tenosynovial hypertrophy.
Tenderness/joint effusion seen in ulnocarpal joint, radioulnar joint.			Degenerative arthritis (osteoarthritis). Inflammatory arthritis (rheumatoid).
Ulnar-sided wrist pain and noticing a clicking sensation on the ulnar side of the wrist, which developed after playing tennis/shuttle.			Extensor carpi ulnaris instability.
Tender anatomical snuff box.		Fall on an outstretched wrist.	Scaphoid fracture/ nonunion.
This triangle snuff box is formed by APL and EPB. The apex lies over the 1st CMC joint; base radial styloid process; content-scaphoid waist.		Thumb pain.	First CMC. Arthritis
		Pain in thumb movements.	De Quervain's tenosynovitis.
Tender over the lunate, reduced grip strength, joint effusion, reduced wrist movements.		Hyperextension injury; pain aggravated by activity and relieved by rest.	AVN of Lunate-Keinbock's disease.

Chronic paronychia is commonly seen in women, chefs, washerman, bartenders and fishmongers and who work constantly in washing (Figures 2.8 and 2.9). A chronically indurated, retracted and rounded eponychium is the hallmark of diagnosis. Also, the nail is deformed, thickened and has transverse groove because of recurrent inflammatory episodes. Long-standing chronic paronychia has disfigured skin thickening. Smears and skin scraping usually reveals *Candida albicans*. In case of negative, fungal cultures are confirmatory.

3. Sporotrichosis (rose thorn disease)

It is the most common cutaneous and lymphatic fungal infection in North America. The infecting organism is a dimorphic fungus and is termed *Sporothrix* (or *Sporotrichum*) *schenckii*. The infection is seen in rose growers, gardeners, farmers, florists and nursery workers. The infection follows a linear marching nodule on the forearm and arm spreading through lymphatic channels. The clinical presentations are unilateral or bilateral painless ulcers, paronychia with regional lymph node enlargement.

Diagnosis of Fungal Infections

Biopsy gives faster diagnosis than cultures. Most of cutaneous fungi are easily identified on wet KOH preparations. They grow hyphae (Greek hyphos, "a web") readily on a Sabouraud medium. Periodic acid–Schiff or

Table 2.8: Hand Infections

Conditions	Presentation	Clinical History	Check For	Organism	Radiology and Imaging
Acute paronychia (nailbed infection).	Pain, swelling and pus point in the fingertip.	Erythema, swelling, and tenderness immediately adjacent to the nail. If untreated abscess may form along the nail fold. The abscess may extend below the nail plate, either partially or completely or can track into pulp space.	Malnutrition, Diabetes Mellitus, alcoholism, autoimmune diseases, chronic corticosteroid use, hepatitis and human immunodeficiency virus (HIV) infection.	Staphylococcus, Streptococcus, Staphylococcus aureus.	Radiographs to rule out foreign bodies, osteomyelitis.
Chronic paronychia.	Frequent water immersion of hand, repeated episodes of acute paronychia.		Female: male ratio 4:1. Housewives, bartenders, dishwashers, nurses, swimmers and children who suck their fingers.	Gram-positive cocci, gram-negative rods, Candida, and mycobacterial species.	Radiographs to rule out foreign bodies, lytic lesions osteomyelitis.
Cellulitis.	Pain (dolor), Fever.	Increased temperature, with or without erythema (rubor), and tenderness. Temperature note: Elevation is inconsistent.	Abnormalities of the white blood cell (WBC) count and C-reactive protein (CRP) level.	Staphylococcus aureus or β-hemolytic Streptococcus.	
Felon.	Severe throbbing pain, tension, and swelling of the entire distal phalangeal pulp.	Subcutaneous abscess of the distal pulp of a finger or thumb, tender pulp, does not extend DIP joint flexion crease.	Wood splinter, glass sliver or minor cut, "finger-stick felons" can be seen in diabetics during sugar check up with prick.		Radiographs to rule out foreign bodies, lytic lesions osteomyelitis, sequestration of distal phalanx.
Pyogenic flexor tenosynovitis (closed-space infection of the flexor tendon sheath of the fingers or thumb).	Open injury to fingertip.	Kanavel's sign 1. A semiflexed position of the finger. 2. Symmetric enlargement of the whole digit (fusiform swelling). 3. Excessive tenderness limited to the course of the flexor tendon sheath. 4. Excruciating pain on passively extending the finger; the pain should be experienced along the flexor sheath and not localized to a particular joint or abscess.	Immunocompromised patients, who can yield positive cultures for E. corrodens, Listeria monocytogenes, and mixed gram-positive and gram negative infections.	Staphylococcus, S. aureus, anaerobes, β-hemolytic Streptococcus.	Radiographs to rule out foreign bodies, fracture, lytic lesions osteomyelitis, distal phalanx.

(Continued)

Table 2.8 (Continued): Hand Infections

Conditions	Presentation	Clinical History	Check For	Organism	Radiology and Imaging
Human bite (patient strikes the mouth of another person.)	Innocuous-appearing wound on the dorsum of the hand around the MP joint.	Localized swelling, erythema, tender, pus, extensor function loss.	Rapidly spreading up to the forearm and arm. Most common involved site: Third and fourth metacarpal heads of the dominant hand.	*Staphylococcus, Streptococcus, Eikenella corrodens,* Anaerobes.	Radiographs to rule out tooth, foreign bodies, fracture, osteomyelitis.
Diabetic hand infections.	Minor trauma, pinpricks.	1. Superficial (cellulitis, localized abscess). 2. Deep infections (tendons, bones, deep palmar spaces).	Necrotizing fasciitis occurs with greater frequency in diabetics and has been associated with a higher mortality rate.	*S. aureus.* Gram-negative organisms (73%).	
Necrotizing fasciitis (rapidly advancing necrotizing infection affecting the skin, subcutaneous tissue, and fascia).	Minor trauma or puncture Wound.	1. Nonpitting oedema. 2. Swollen erythematous area of exquisite tenderness. 3. Tenderness beyond the area of erythema. 4. Skin: Orange-peel appearance (peau d'orange skin). 5. A probe or finger that dissects easily 6. A thin, watery exudate.	High clinical suspicion in all patients, particularly patients with risk factors, including diabetes, immunocompromise, and intravenous drug abuse.	Streptococcus or polymicrobial infection.	Radiographs frequently demonstrate the presence of gas in the tissues.

41

Coccidioidomycosis and histoplasmosis are asymptomatic or moderate in 75% of the infections (Table 2.22).

Mycobacterial Infections

Tubercle bacillus is the second most common reason for deaths caused by a single infectious agent next to AIDS. With the advent of antitubercular drugs, the new cases and resurgences were decreased steadily in the early 2000s. Unfortunately, multi-drug resistant TB (MDR TB i.e., resistant to more than one agent and at least isoniazid or rifampicin) has emerged as a threat and extensively drug-resistant (XDRTB i.e., resistant to isoniazid and rifampicin, plus resistant to any fluoroquinolone and at least one of three injectable second-line anti-TB drugs) as an imminent dangerous threat.

The most common TB infection of the hand involves the skin. Apart from the skin, it involves subcutaneous tissues, tenosynovium, bursa, joints and bone. *M. tuberculosis* in the past was attributed as the reason for all hand infections. Nontuberculous mycobacterium (NTM) has emerged in recent times with more than 120 species affecting the hand. The clinical presentation of tuberculous and nontuberculous mycobacterium hand infections is identical, and identification of mycobacterium is crucial for treatment.

A positive tuberculin test is not indicative of an active TB infection. The test is positive in patients who had BCG vaccination and negative in debilitated and anergic patients. Acid-fast bacillus (AFB) smear and culture are diagnostic methods to identify the organism. Cultures grow organisms in 1 to 12 weeks on a Lowenstein–Jensen medium.

The three most common *M. tuberculosis* infections of the hand are phalangeal osteomyelitis, flexor tenosynovitis and wrist joint infection. Cold abscess, though rare, may present as mid-palmar space abscess, forearm abscess, compartment syndrome forearm, deltoid, biceps or brachialis abscess. We analyze the tuberculous hand infections based on the involvement, as cutaneous, subcutaneous and deep (Table 2.23).

Spina ventosa: During infancy and childhood, the short tubular bones have a lavish blood supply through a large nutrient artery entering in the middle of the bone. The agent lodges in the centre of the marrow cavity and the interior of the short tubular bone is converted into a virtual granuloma. This leads to a spindle-shaped expansion and inflated shape of the bone. Endosteal resorption of bone is followed by progressive subperiosteal hyperplasia and has been termed as spina ventosa by Dupuytren (Latin spina, "spine," ventosa, "distended with air").

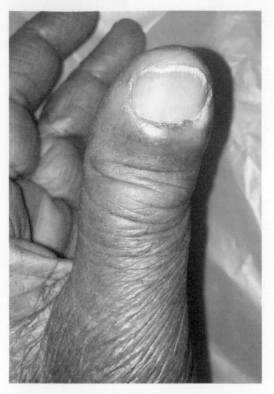

Figure 2.7 Picture of acute paronychia. It is the infection of the skin around a fingernail or toenail. It presents as a localized abscess of the paronychial tissues (pus pointing). Patients with acute paronychia may report localized pain and tenderness of the perionychium. The perionychial area usually appears erythematous and inflamed, and the nail may appear discoloured and even distorted. Fluctuance and local purulence at the nail margin may occur, and infection may extend beneath the nail margin to involve the nail bed.

silver staining will highlight the sporotrichosis as red or black, respectively. Culture is the confirmatory test and if required may be repeated to get results positive in a few days to a month.

Deep Fungal Infections

The deep infections are rare in the hand and upper extremity. If they present, they pose a serious clinical problem with significant morbidity and mortality. The presentations are chronic tenosynovitis, arthritis and osteomyelitis (Table 2.21).

Fungal Osteomyelitis

A high index of suspicion diagnoses mycotic infections developing into osteomyelitis. The three major causes of fungal osteomyelitis are blastomycosis, coccidioidomycosis and histoplasmosis.

Table 2.9: Mycobacterial Infections

Conditions	Presentation	Clinical History	Check For	Organism	Radiology and Imaging
Cutaneous tuberculosis.	Inoculation from an exogenous source through a breach in the skin, inoculation by tattoo needles, by acupuncture needles.	Nontender nodule gradually progresses to single or multiple abscesses that drain clear liquid.	Less common presentations: Erythema, swelling, cellulitis, crusting, verrucous plaque, verrucous nodule, sporotrichoid lesion and ulceration. Cortisone exacerbates the disease.	*M. marinum* (fish tank) *M. bovis* (butcher's wart).	Infections invading phalanges, metacarpals, and ulna. Direct smear examination acid-fast (Ziehl–Neelsen) stain procedure (sensitive 40%).
Subcutaneous tuberculosis.	Non healing ulcer, nodules.	Painless subcutaneous oedema, subcutaneous nodule that secondarily ulcerates with a characteristic undermined edge.	A painless ulcer that has undermined edges and a necrotic centre with hyperpigmented and shiny surrounding skin is pathognomonic of a buruli ulcer.		
Mycobacterial tenosynovitis.	Cold abscess, sausage finger, wrist swelling numbness, tingling sensation over median nerve fingers.	• Flexor tendons of the fingers palm, wrist and forearm are affected more often than extensor tendons. • Inflammatory signs (e.g., erythema, warmth, tenderness) are absent. • Feel rice bodies, millet seeds or melon seeds glide beneath the examining fingers.	Classic presentations 1. Sausage finger, 2. Compound palmar ganglion. 3. Rice body-laden carpal tunnel syndrome. Also look for tendon rupture, sinus, bone and joint infections, ESR elevated.	*M. kansasii* and *M. marinum*.	
Tuberculous Osteomyelitis	Local discomfort, painless, nonsuppurative, and insidious swelling on the fingers.	The proximal phalanx, middle phalanx, distal phalanx, and metacarpals are involved in that order. The second, third and fourth fingers are involved most frequently. A typical fusiform swelling of a finger or a diffuse swelling on the dorsum of the hand. No tenderness or local heat, but the part may appear taut and shiny. The abscess may burst and leave a sinus that drains a cheesy, yellowish exudate.	30% have multifocal tuberculosis. simulate a tumour.	*M. marinum, M. kansasii,* and *M. scrofulaceum.*	Radiographs show endosteal resorption of bone and progressive subperiosteal hyperplasia, periosteal reaction and metaphyseal osteoporosis. Bone destruction with honeycombing. A mixed cystic-sclerotic pattern with a lytic lesion that is surrounded by a sclerotic rim. Bony lytic lesion with bone destruction that resembles bacterial osteomyelitis. A diaphyseal lytic lesion that crosses the epiphyseal plate; this pattern is classic of paediatric tuberculous osteomyelitis. Diagnosis is by biopsy.

(Continued)

Table 2.9 (Continued): Mycobacterial Infections

Conditions	Presentation	Clinical History	Check For	Organism	Radiology and Imaging
Hansen's disease (chronic neurologic and dermatologic disease with immunological overtones). The most common transmission from human to human, primarily as a nasal droplet infection. 15 % by wild armadillos in US.	Nodule, abscess, ulcer, sinus, fistula or a nondescript mass).	1. Ulnar nerve (common). 2. Median. 3. Radial.	The bacteria preferentially infect nerves in the cooler parts of the body. The fine terminal dermal nerves, small subcutaneous nerves and the superficially located large nerve trunks. Sensory loss almost always precedes motor loss because superficial dermal nerve damage precedes deeper nerve trunk damage.	*Mycobacterium leprae* (identified in 1873).	

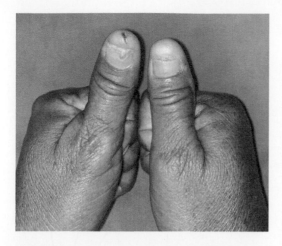

Figure 2.8 Picture of chronic paronychia. Fluctuance is rare, and there is less erythema than is present in acute paronychia. The nail plates become thickened and discoloured, with pronounced transverse ridges. The cuticles and nail folds may separate from the nail plate, forming a space for various microbes, especially Candida albicans, to invade.

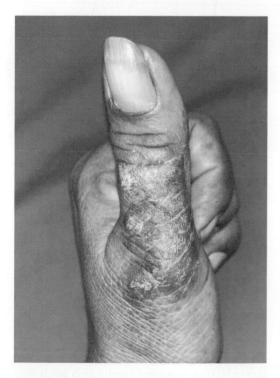

Figure 2.9 Pictures of milker's hand. Hyperpigmented scaly plaque over dorsum of the left thumb.

TUBERCULOUS OSTEOMYELITIS OF ADULT HANDS AND CHILDREN
Hansen's Disease (Leprosy)

Hansen's disease (HD), once called "leprosy," a most ancient, feared and disabling disease in humans, is a neurological and dermatological disease of long duration with 70% of cases involving the ulnar nerve (rarely median and radial nerve) in the upper extremity. *M. lepra*, an acid-fast bacillus infects nerves in the cooler parts of the body, terminal dermal nerves, small subcutaneous nerves, superficially located large nerve trunk (ulnar, common peroneal nerve) and causes sensory loss initially. Deeper nerve trunk damage causes subsequent motor loss. The nerve lesions are the result of immune reactions caused by the lepra infection and the antigens present cause intraneural inflammation and permanent nerve fibrosis. Also, the infected nerves are replaced with hyaline fibrous tissue where the *M. lepra* hides and is not amenable to drugs causing relapses of the disease. Skin lesions (anaesthetic patch) and sensory loss are the common presenting symptoms. About 30% of sensory fibres must be destroyed before sensory impairment becomes evident. The nerve infection is well advanced in a patient with skin patches, and they have palpable, thickened, enlarged adjacent subcutaneous nerves. Apart from skin lesions, the eyes, upper respiratory tract and testis are involved. Untreated cases may have mitten hands and feet because of profound sensory loss and subsequent absorption from damages (Table 2.24).

Antia has described three patterns of sensory loss in HD [7]:

1. Anaesthetic patch from infection of a dermal or subcutaneous nerve

2. Regional loss from infection of a nerve trunk in tuberculoid disease

3. A glove-and-stocking pattern due to confluent involvement of sensory nerves in lepromatous disease

The three main clinical types of HD are tuberculoid (TT, high immunity), lepromatous (LL, low immunity) and borderline (BB, intermediate immunity). Ridley and Jopling divided the borderline cases into three immunologic subsets: BL, BB and BT [8]. Ridley further divided TT and LL into polar (LLp, TTp) and subpolar (LLs, TTs) groups. The World Health Organization (WHO) recommended a simplified, clinical and operational classification of HD into paucibacillary (PB) and multibacillary (MB) for treatment purposes based on the result of slit-skin smears in 1982. When a skin smear is positive, the disease is classified as MB. Most of the indeterminate (I), TT and BT cases are PB, but any of them showing smear positivity are classified as MB for purposes of drug therapy. The smears are positive in LL, BL and usually in BB cases and are classified as multibacillary. When a slit smear is not possible, a patient with more than six skin lesions is classified as MB and with fewer as PB. Again, these skin lesions are clinical manifestations, where a single lesion or multiple lesions may have smear positive or negative and should not be falsely classified.

Cardinal Signs for Diagnosis of Hansen's Disease (WHO Recommendations)

Two of the following three clinical signs are needed for clinical diagnosis:

- A hypopigmented skin patch
- An anaesthetic skin patch
- An enlarged nerve (ulnar nerve at elbow, median nerve at wrist, sensory branch of radial nerve)

The diagnosis must be confirmed by bacteriological examination (fourth sign).

Hypopigmented Anaesthetic Skin Patch

It is the unique sign of HD where the patches are in the distribution of the dermal, cutaneous and the regional distribution of the peripheral nerve trunks (Figure 2.10). A diffuse glove-and-stocking pattern occurs in nerve lesions involving the dermal, subcutaneous and the main nerve trunk.

Thickened Nerve

The ulnar nerve is the first and most commonly affected nerve in the upper extremity with or without skin lesions. Median nerve compression may present as carpal tunnel syndrome in the wrist. These enlarged nerves may be palpable, palpable and visible, or palpable and fluctuant. The nerve may be soft, not rollable, firm or hard. The most common clinical presentation is with numbness or weakness; wasting, deformity and pain/tingling can also be presenting symptoms in a small minority of cases. Sometimes, they present like acute cellulitis with a nerve abscess and caseous granuloma between the nerve fibres (Figure 2.11). The abscess may be fluctuant, non-fluctuant, subcutaneous, deep, painless, painful, collar stud, moderate in size with or without an impending sinus. A longitudinal epineurotomy along the entire enlarge nerve decompresses the extra perineural pressure over the fibrosseous tunnel. Caseous material is drained, and nerve

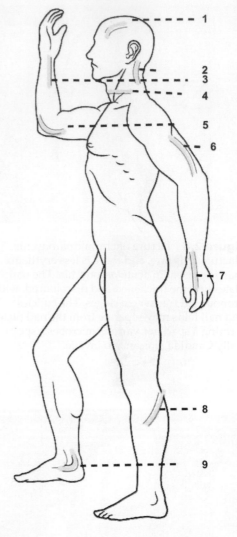

Figure 2.10 Pictures of peripheral nerve involvement in Hansen's disease. M. Lepra infects nerves in the cooler parts of the body. Common sites of the nerve involved shown in the pictures are close to the skin and has colder temperature. 1 - supraorbital, 2 - greater auricular, 3 - median, 4 - cervical, 5 - ulnar, 6 - radial, 7 - radial cutaneous, 8 - common peroneal, 10 - posterior tibial nerves.

fascicles are not disturbed. This relieves pain and prevents further deterioration of the nerve function.

Skin Lesions

The most common and earliest clinical manifestation in HD is a hypopigmented, numb patch of skin. So, the patient's body should be examined in daylight or with light from behind the examiner's shoulders. The skin lesion is symptomless, ill-defined, hypopigmented and anaesthetic. Also,

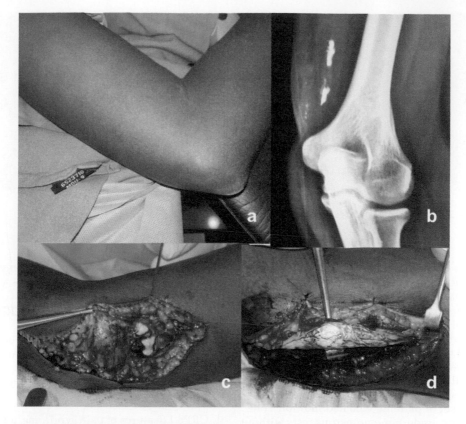

Figure 2.11 a) Swollen and tender medial aspect of the left elbow with superficial to deep fluctuations over the ulnar nerve course. (b) Radiological findings showed calcification along the ulnar nerve. (c) A longitudinal epineurotomy drained the ulnar nerve abscess. (d) Further decompression of the ulnar nerve showed caseous material.

elevation of the margins indicates tuberculoid pole and numerous central elevations of the skin lesion indicate lepromatous pole [8].

DIAGNOSIS

There are various modalities to diagnose HD (Table 2.27):

1. Lepromin test

2. Slit-skin smear

3. Skin biopsy

4. Nerve biopsy

5. Fine needle aspiration technique

6. Electrophysiological studies

7. Imaging (MRI)

The ulnar claw hand is the most common paralytic deformity in HD (Figure 2.12). The second most common deformity is combined median and ulnar nerve paralysis causing a complete claw hand (see Chapter 8 on ulnar nerve palsy for evaluation).

Constitutional symptoms: Constitutional symptoms, rare in solitary skeletal tuberculosis, may be present in multifocal tuberculosis with fever, chills, anorexia and loss of weight. Discharging lesions are more common in multiple lesions than in solitary lesions. Multifocal lesions are more common in immunosuppressed patients, including those with AIDS. Elevated Erythrocyte Sedimentation Rate (ESR) and positive purified protein derivative test (PPD), rare in solitary lesions, may also be present.

Sensory loss always precedes motor loss: Sensory damage and sensory loss lead to gradual and progressive absorption and autoamputation of fingers from recurrent injury and infection; autonomic damage causes loss of protective sudomotor and vasomotor functions, and finally, motor damage causes muscle imbalance, leading to flexible and subsequently fixed deformities (Figure 2.12).

Chronic Pain and its Significance

The most common presentation of patients with long duration of problems, multiple

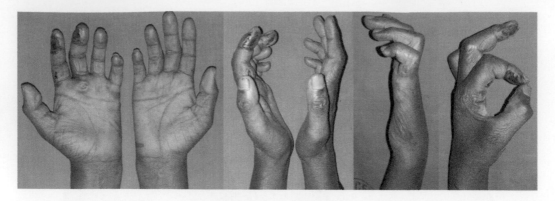

Figure 2.12 Clinical pictures of various presentations of claw hand in Hansen's disease.

visits to doctors and long duration of drugs, psychiatric consultations is chronic pain with or without associated symptoms. This is because the diagnosis is always based on physical examinations, provocative manoeuvres and investigations. There may be certain clinical conditions with chronic pain, which are insidious in onset with highly variable physical findings, negative investigations and poor response to analgesics/opioids. These are the set of patients who had multiple consultations, undergone numerous tests without a definite diagnosis, unremitting symptoms, depression, anger, frustration and despondence who need a multidisciplinary team approach with undue care and proficiency. The very few known reasons could be overlap of symptoms, acute on chronic symptoms, double crush syndromes and when clinicians fail to examine the vital and most important clinical findings in differentiating it from the other.

1. Thoracic outlet syndrome (TOS)

The most common presentation is chronic pain over the shoulder girdle and neck associated with paraesthesia of the upper limb. The paraesthesia (95%) is seen in the median or ulnar nerve distribution making the clinician to detour to the common diagnosis – carpal tunnel syndrome/cubital tunnel syndrome. But then there are few vital symptoms and signs which could narrow the physician to TOS (Figure 2.3). Shoulder pain and fatigue are the classical presentations vital to diagnose TOS [7] (Table 2.10). The vascular and neurogenic are two types of TOS. Further, vascular is divided into arterial and venous subtypes and the neurogenic type has been subdivided into true and disputed

neurogenic (see Chapter 11 on compressive neuropathy).

2. Complex regional pain syndrome (CRPS)

This is one of the interesting topics and very close to the author because of all the controversies, myths and misnomers about CRPS. There are two types of CRPS described in the literature [9].

1. CRPS-I (features of pain syndrome, autonomic dysfunction, functional impairment, trophic changes with NO NERVE involvement)

2. CRPS-II (features of type I with NERVE involvement)

There is compelling evidence to implicate biological pathways that underlie aberrant inflammation, vasomotor dysfunction and maladaptive neuroplasticity in the clinical features of CRPS [9]. Women are three to four times more commonly involved; distal radius fractures have been associated with CRPS in 4–39% of cases. It is rare in children but if involved it occurs in the leg. Trauma, fractures and sprains (60%) with prolonged periods of immobilization are the most common inciting factors. There have been no psychological variables that contribute towards CRPS.

The author has simplified the criteria to the term CRPS. The most commonly used diagnostic criteria are International Association for the Study of Pain (IASP, 1993 – Orlando criteria) and Budapest criteria

1. IASP criteria – mnemonic (CRPS)
C – Continuing pain, allodynia or hyperalgesia where pain is disproportionately high.
R – Rule out other conditions causing pain, trophic changes, autonomic dysfunctions.

Table 2.10: Differences between Thoracic Outlet Syndrome and Carpal/Cubital Tunnel Syndrome

	Thoracic Outlet Syndrome	Carpal Tunnel/Cubital Tunnel Syndrome
Paraesthesia – medial arm, forearm, ulnar two digits/median nerve distribution (lateral 3 ½ fingers).	Same.	Same.
Shoulder pain, neck pain, fatigue in the upper extremity.	Classical findings.	Nil.
Nocturnal symptoms.	Frequent in females. Always prescribed with lots of medicines to sleep (TCA, antidepressant, benzodiazepines).	Carpal tunnel syndrome – hand flags and numbness more in the night.
Psychiatric consultations	Often and more depressions, anger, frustrations, anxiety	Less and rare
CNS symptoms	Migraine headaches, vertigo, syncope, chest pain, eye irritations and face pain and numbness	Nil
Diagnosis	MRI/NCV/EMG	NCV/EMG Local anaesthesia to the carpal and cubital tunnel can reduce the symptoms

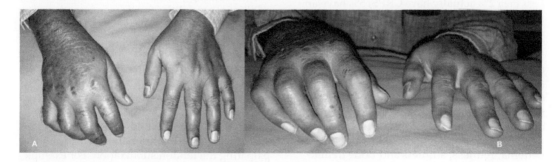

Figure 2.13 Clinical pictures of sudomotor activities seen in CRPS.

Table 2.11: Clinical Findings in CRPS

Category		Remarks
Sensory	Allodynia (to light touch and/or temperature sensation and/or deep somatic pressure and/or joint movement) and/or hyperalgesia (to pinprick)	
Vasomotor	Temperature asymmetry and/or skin colour changes and/or skin colour asymmetry	Temperature asymmetry must be >1°C
Sudomotor/oedema	Oedema and/or sweating changes and/or sweating asymmetry	
Motor/ trophic	Decreased range of motion and/or motor dysfunction (weakness, tremor, dystonia) and/or trophic changes (hair/nail/skin)	

P – Presence of noxious events/prolonged immobilization.

S – Sudomotor activity (skin blood flow increased, oedema, nail changes etc.) (Figure 2.13; Table 2.11).

2. Budapest Criteria

A. The patient has continuing pain which is disproportionate to any inciting event.

B. The patient has at least one sign in two or more of the categories.

C. The patient reports at least one symptom in three or more categories.

Table 2.12: Myths and Misnomers in CRPS

Myth	Rationale	Author's Suggestions
Is there a diagnosis – CRPS?	It is a diagnosis of exclusion.	

CRPS type I exists?	Debatable.	CRPS type I does not exist
		Reason
		  1. No specific etiology.
		  2. No specific signs.
		  3. No specific symptoms.
		  4. Criteria keep changing.

CRPS type II exists?	It does exist. Find out the nerve involvement causing CRPS. Treat it.	Find the cause and treat it.

D. No other diagnosis can better explain the signs and symptoms.

Note: The Budapest criteria have acceptable sensitivity and specificity. Having said that the diagnosis of CRPS does not require diagnostic tests because it is a diagnosis of exclusion. Less than 2% actually have CRPS; 5% have an unspecified type of CRPS; and >50% have a confirmed different diagnosis.

MYTHS AND MISNOMERS IN CRPS

CRPS is compared to a fever of unknown origin. The less we know, the more we resort to CRPS. More and more curiosity and exploration may reduce our simple understanding about CRPS. For an example, if there is an unstable fracture in the distal radius causing oedema, redness, stiffness and bone demineralization, mimicking CRPS, do not fall for it. Always, try and analyze the cause for the development of the symptoms. What could be the rationale in such cases are anatomic reduction and rigid fixation without articular step and may prevent the fractures going to non-union/delayed union, or stiffness there by indirectly halting the progress of nociceptive "pain stimulus" culminating into CRPS. Also, if there is associated carpal tunnel entrapment, adequate surgical release could benefit the patient further (Table 2.12).

There is a definite role of cutaneous neuropeptide signalling with increased cytokines expression which enhances extravasation, limb oedema. Serum concentrations of CGRP, substance P, tumour necrosis factor (TNFα), interleukins (IL-6) are seen high in these patients. The radiograph of the hand (70%) shows diffuse osteopenia, juxta-cortical demineralization and subchondral erosions and cysts.

Tendinopathy

The flexor and the extensor tendons are vulnerable for entrapment during their course of passage and functioning. The tendons' movements produce friction at the rigid retinacular sheath. If it continues over a period of time, swelling occurs and narrows the fibrosseous canal making the symptoms worse and provocative tests positive. Diagnosis is usually clinical findings; ultrasound and MRI are the additional modalities for the confirmation of the entrapment and tenosynovitis [10–13].

EXTENSOR TENDINOPATHY

Extensor Carpi Ulnaris Instability

Extensor carpi ulnaris (ECU) tendinitis may coexist with tendon entrapment making it difficult to diagnosis and treat. The classical presentation of ECU instability is an audible snap, pain during forceful supination activity and palpating the tendon subluxation. For example, while playing tennis or cricket, the player extends their wrist from full pronation to full supination making an audible snap. MRI helps to identify tendon subluxation and differentiates from tenosynovitis shallow ECU groove and anomalous extensor tendons (Table 2.13) (Video 2.1).

Flexor Tendinopathy

The condition typically affects people in their fifth decade and is more often seen in women. It is insidious in onset and repetitive wrist flexion; extension movements cause flexor carpi radialis tendinitis. Pain and swelling over the volar aspect of the forearm is the classic finding aggravated by wrist flexion and radial deviation. Flexor carpi radialis (FCR) tendinitis has to be carefully differentiated from volar ganglion,

 Video 2.1 Videos demonstrating ECU (extensor carpi ulnaris) instability.

www.routledge.com/9780367647162.

Table 2.13: Extensor Tendinopathy

	Age/Gender	Symptoms	Clinical Findings	Remarks
De Quervain's disease "washer-woman's sprain."	5–6th decade, women > men, postpartum and lactating women.	Pain aggravated by thumb movements.	**Eichhoff manoeuvre:** When the thumb is clasped into the palm and wrist force to ulnar flexion, a knife-like pain, tenderness, swelling appreciated 1 to 2 cm proximal to radial styloid. **Finklestein manoeuvre:** Grasp the thumb and abduct the hand ulnar ward, patient experiences excruciating pin over the styloid tip.	Radiographs shows localized osteopenia or spur at the radial styloid.
Intersection syndrome (the entrapment occurs in the area where the muscle bellies of APL and EPB intersect the ECRL and ECRB).	Athletics, rowing, weightlifting and cycling.	Pain, swelling redness, crepitus (severe cases). Note: It may coincide with the findings of de Quervain's disease.	Pinpoint tenderness over the site 4 cm proximal to the wrist.	Controversy exists whether the intersection occurs between EPB and APL or between APL, EPB and ECRL, ECRB. Normal bulge is seen at the same intersection point, 4 cm proximal to the wrist joint which should not be taken into consideration as entrapment. It is the pain and tenderness that confirms the diagnosis.
Extensor pollicis longus (EPL) entrapment.	Colle's fracture, distal radius fracture with plate and screw fixation. The screws may impinge and cause pain, swelling, tendon rupture.	Pain, swelling, crepitus.	Tenderness at lister tubercle. Passive or active flexion of thumb IP joint will have tender and trigger.	It can occur in Colle's fracture with or without tendon rupture because of ischemia at the watershed region just proximal to the Lister's tubercle.
Stenosis of fourth and fifth extensor compartments.	Rheumatoid arthritis, Colle's fracture.		Swelling and tenderness. Provocative tests: Wrist flexion, MP extension, give resistance and look for tenderness at the involved retinacular sheath.	
Extensor carpi ulnaris (ECU) tendinitis – second most common cause of ulnar-sided wrist pain.	Overuse (frequent writing, fixed posture, etc.). Twisting injury.	Nocturnal pain, dysesthesia over the hand.	Very difficult to differentiate from TFCC injury. Deep tenderness, crepitus over ECU tendon.	USG and MRI show tenosynovial thickening, oedema around the ECU tendon.

scaphoid fractures/non-union, de Quervain's disease and degenerative joint diseases. It is seen in degenerative diseases of trapezium, 25% following trapezial excision and suspension-plasty during Carpometacarpal (CMC) arthritis treatment. Applied anatomy of the FCR tendon shows a thin paratenon covering the tendon, encircled trapezium at its attachment and a narrow fibrous sheath making it vulnerable to entrapment (Figure 2.14). The radiographs show diffuse osteoporosis and calcifications over the radial styloid (Figure 2.15).

Differentiating between intersection syndrome and de Quervain's disease (Figure 2.16)

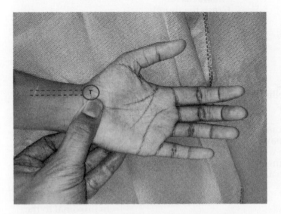

Figure 2.14 FCR musculotendinous tendon is located 8 cm proximal to wrist crease. It is encircled by tubercle of trapezium (T) which constitutes 60 -80% of the wall of the tunnel which is prone for entrapment.

and identification of ulnar styloid process and extensor carpi ulnaris is vital in making diagnosis [10] (Figure 2.17).

Swelling in Hand and the Upper Limb

Ganglions are the most common swelling seen in many sites of the hand and the upper limb. They are cystic swellings and usually painless to start with. Depending upon the location, they have various presentations (Table 2.14).

Dorsal wrist ganglion (Figure 2.18): This is the most common site (60–70%) of hand and wrist ganglions. It is usually located over the scapholunate ligament.

Ganglion cysts are the most common soft tissue lesion of the hand, seen mostly in women between the second and fourth decade of life, containing mucin-filled cysts. They are attached to the underlying joint capsule, tendon or tendon sheath and can arise from almost every joint of the hand and wrist. It is innocuous and patients seek a doctor's attention for the mass, concerned for malignancy, pain because of pressure to the underlying sensory nerves and rarely present with symptoms of Carpal and Guyon's canal syndrome. They can appear quite suddenly or develop over months and may subside with rest or enlarge with activity, rupture or disappear spontaneously. History, clinical examination, cystic consistency and positive trans-illumination are the classical findings and diagnosing features of ganglions. Recurrence (>50%) is alarming if not properly and adequately excised. Pathognomic features of ganglions are:

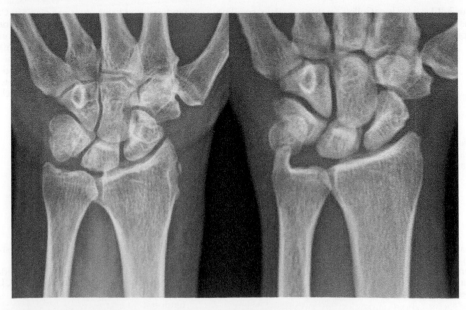

Figure 2.15 Radiographs showing diffuse osteopenia and calcifications at the radial styloidprocess - de Quervain's disease.

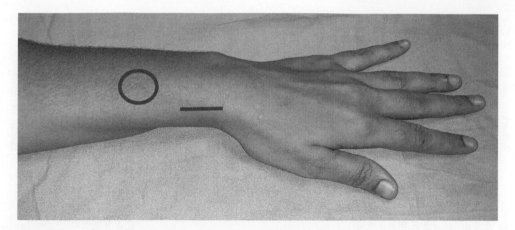

Figure 2.16 Location of intersection syndrome (circle). Location of de Quervain's disease with straight line.

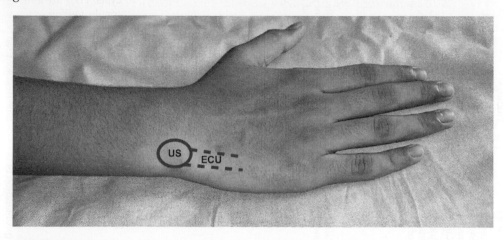

Figure 2.17 The location of ulnar styloid process (US) and the course of extensor carpi ulnaris (ECU). It assumes a linear path in pronation and angulates 30° (approx.) around the ulnar styloid to reach the fifth metacarpal in full supination.

1. Single or multi-loculated cyst.

2. Smooth, white and translucent (trans-illumination positive).

3. Highly viscous clear, sticky, jelly-like mucin made up of glucosamine, albumin, globulin, and high concentration of hyaluronic acid (the reason for injecting hyaluronidase injection into the ganglion cysts).

4. Mucoid degeneration is the widely accepted theory behind the pathogenesis (fibrillation of collagen fibres, accumulation of intra/extra cellular mucin and decreased collagen fibres and stroma cells).

Volar Wrist Ganglion

It is the second most common ganglion (18–20%) of the hand and the wrist, seen directly over the distal edge of the radius (Figure 2.19). It arises from the capsular and ligament fibres of the radiocarpal joint and occurs under the volar wrist crease between the flexor carpi radialis (FCR) and abductor pollicis longus (APL). Sometimes, it can be seen over the scaphoid tubercle with ganglion arising from the capsule of the scaphotrapezial joint. These volar ganglions appear small in size, but they are quite tough and extensive at surgery. The cyst can be very close to the radial artery or sometimes intertwined. It is always important to assess the patency of the radial and ulnar artery with Allen's test. It is preferable to preserve arteries during the surgical excision of the ganglions.

Nodules and Deformity
Dupuytren's Disease

This disease is common in Caucasian men in the fifth to sixth decades of age with blue

Table 2.14: Swelling in Hand and the Upper Limb

	Location	History	Findings	Diagnosis	Remarks
Ganglion cysts.	Nail and nailbed.	Pain, recurrent swelling around the nail, nailbed. Nail deformity.	Ridged nail, ragged nail, grooving, thinning or roughening of nail (pressure).	Cystic swelling, osteophytes of DIP joint	Treatment: Excise osteophyte and drain ganglion. Care not to injure extensor tendon.
	Dorsum wrist.	Pain, swelling sudden/delay onset of mass appearance.	Diffuse swelling, cystic, trans-illumination positive.	USG, MRI and positive arthrogram if the ganglion has communication between wrist joint and the cyst.	Bible hit treatment (hitting a ganglion hard will rupture its cyst wall and cause the intracystic viscous fluid to escape out and get absorbed from the wrist joint through the connection by a univalvular mechanism.
	Volar wrist.	Pain, recurrent swelling.	Second most common site. Cystic or hard consistency. Found between FCR and FPL tendons.		Pedicle may arise from volar SL joint, ST joint, STT joints or first CMC joint.
	Other places. Volar retinacular ganglion (flexor tendon sheath ganglion). Mucous cyst (ganglion of the distal interphalangeal joint). Carpometacarpal boss. Proximal interphalangeal joint. Extensor tendon. First extensor compartment (dorsal retinacular ganglion). Carpal tunnel. Guyon's canal. Intraosseous ganglion.				
	Extensor digitorum brevis manus muscle (EDBM). Anomalous muscle on the dorsum of the hand (3%). It usually arises between index and middle finger metacarpals. It inserts in the extensor hood of index or middle fingers.		Cyst appearance.	It becomes firm when wrist is flexed, and fingers extended.	
Glomus tumour (a tumour arises from the glomus body that regulates temperature and blood flow in the finger).	50% (sub-ungual). Beneath the nailbed.	Exquisite pain (proliferation of angiomatous tissue within confined nailbed- pressure).	Pinpoint tender. Blue discoloration beneath the nail. **Tender to pressure and cold.**	USG, MRI	Surgical excision. Beware of recurrences!

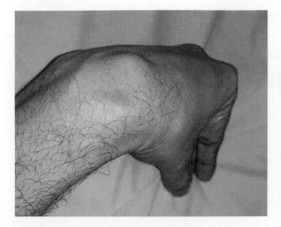

Figure 2.18 Dorsal wrist ganglion.

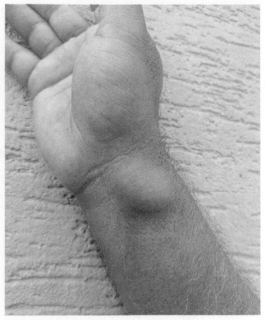

or green eyes, women and family history of the condition. It is uncommon under the age of 40 years. This disease is commonly overlooked and underreported; 50% has bilateral involvement. The ring and little finger are most commonly involved; the first thing to notice is skin crease deformation or dimples. Nodules are commonly seen, and they are usually flat rounded or ovoid areas of subdermal firmness, fixed to the dermis and have no distinct peripheral margins (Figure 2.20).

Figure 2.19 Volar wrist ganglion.

The earliest and classical signs of Dupuytren's disease:

1. Skin tightness (exaggerated blanching with finger extension)

2. Contour changes (skin crease deformation, dimples)

3. Nodules, cords without contractures, or prominence of the palmar monticuli

Dorsal Dupuytren's Nodules (DDN)

It is as common as one in five patients with Dupuytren's disease. These are firm masses on the extensor aspect of the digital joints, commonly in proximal interphalangeal (PIP) joints, but occasionally the distal interphalangeal (DIP), metacarpophalangeal (MCP) or interphalangeal (IP) joint of the thumb called Garrod pads or knuckle pads (Table 2.15).

Nodules may not progress to Dupuytren's contracture, but contractures without nodules are commonly seen in 25% patients.

Differential Diagnosis for Palmar Nodules

1. Fibrosarcoma

2. Fibrous histiocytoma

3. Giant cell tumour

4. Synovial sarcoma

5. Calcifying aponeurotic fibroma

6. Epithelioid sarcoma

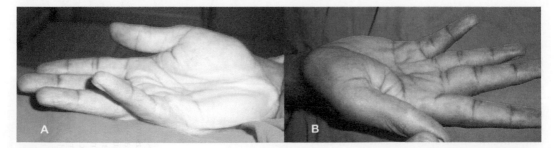

Figure 2.20 A, B nodules, cords with contracture and flexion deformity seen in the ring and little fingers.

Table 2.15: Differences between Dupuytren's Nodules and Others

Dorsal Dupuytren's Nodule	Dorsal Cutaneous Pads	Hyper-Keratosis/Local Dorsal Skin Thickening
Nodules are fixed to the superficial paratenon of the extensor mechanism, subcutaneous tissues and retinacular fibres. They may have tethered depression of the extensor skin creases.	Nonnodular cords, feel firm, well-defined margins and are not fixed to the dermis.	No underlying adherence/ tethering.

Table 2.16: Progression of the Dupuytren's contractures in the Hand

MCP Joint	PIP Joint	DIP Joint	IP Joint
Flexion contracture.	Flexion contracture.	Flexion contracture.	Flexion contracture, radial. Palmar adduction contracture.

Clinical Findings

1. Passive extension deficit due to a contracted cord (MCP and PIP joints of the fingers). (Table 2.16).

2. Nonnodular cords feel firm.

3. Feel for a change from soft to firm as the finger is passively ranged from flexion to extension.

4. Most cords are noted along the lines of mechanical tension produced by passive extension or abduction.

5. Contracture on the ulnar aspect of the palm may produce MCP flexion/abduction contractures mimicking "claw hand."

Note: Patients with aggressive Dupuytren's disease/biology or who have had prior treatment are more likely to vary from these common patterns.

DEFORMITIES

Applied Anatomy

Before understanding the pattern of Dupuytren's disease, let us see the normal anatomy, gradual and progressive changes in palmar fascia, attachments, subcutaneous tissues, dermis and compensatory neurovascular path change.

PALM

The superficial palmar fascia is triangular in shape and lies in the coronal plane of the palm. The apex of the triangle contains the transverse carpal ligament and terminal fibres of the palmaris longus tendon. The apex is confluent, and the base is divergent lying under the transverse retinacular ligament. There are four central bands (pretendinous bands) which originate from the apex and extend distally to each finger except the thumb. The base is wide, and all these four bands are bridged by a superficial transverse palmar ligament. This ligament continues as proximal first webspace ligament along the radial border of the index central band reaching to the radial sesamoid of the thumb MCP joint (Figure 2.21).

The pretendinous bands (central bands) have three branches of different directions (Figure 2.22).

1. Superficial fibres: They lie under the dermis where Dupuytren's nodules commonly arise.

2. Intermediate fibres: The central bands divide into two sections (green colour Figure 2.22) which pass to the lateral borders of the fingers. They are called a spiral band. As the name suggests, they pass close to the neurovascular bundle in spiral

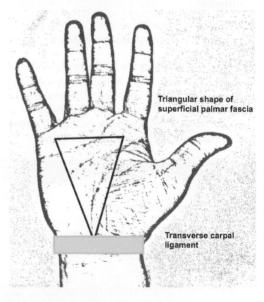

Figure 2.21 Superficial palmar fascia in Dupuytren's disease.

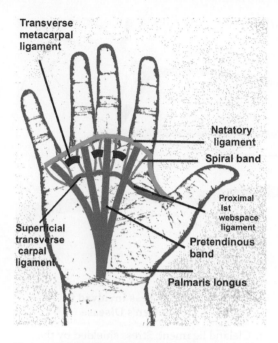

Figure 2.22 Pretendinous bands.

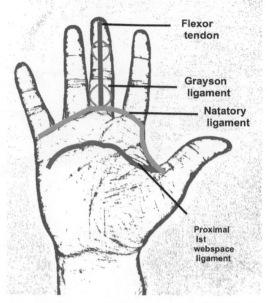

Figure 2.24 Webspace and ligaments involved in Dupuytren's disease.

fashion. Central and superficial proximally and lateral and deep beneath in the distal portion of fingers.

3. Deep fibres: They continue in the dorsal aspect of the hand and finger and merge with sagittal fascia, transverse MP ligament and sagittal bands of the extensor mechanism.

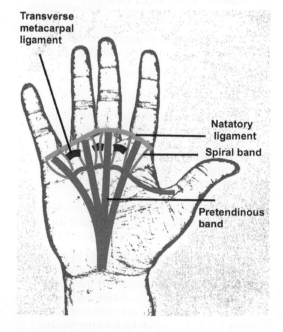

Figure 2.23 Spiral bands.

SPIRAL BAND
Figure 2.23 shows a description of spiral band.

Web Spaces
The natatory ligament is a subdermal fascial layer seen in the periphery of webspace from the little finger to the radial side of the index finger. It continues down as a distal first webspace ligament. It becomes a proximal webspace ligament and reaches the sesamoid bone of the thumb at the MP joint. Fibres from the natatory ligament extend distally along the lateral border of each finger to continue as the Grayson ligament (Figure 2.24).

Digits
Finger dissection to find the ligaments is quite difficult because of the intricate and delicate arrangements of neurovascular structures and their surrounding thin layers of fascia. The ligaments are named based on the location to the neurovascular bundles. Cleland ligaments lie dorsal and Grayson ligaments lie palmar to the neurovascular bundles (Figure 2.25 red – digital artery; yellow – digital nerve).

Both these ligaments have multiple layers of crossing oblique fibres originating in continuance with retinacular ligaments of the fingers, flexor tendon sheath and retinacular fingers attached to the palmar skin.

The little finger has lateral fascial attachments that continue from abductor digiti minimi

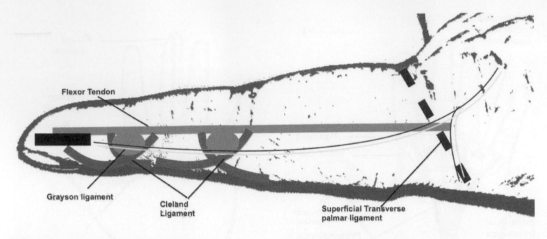

Flexor Tendon

Grayson ligament

Cleland
Ligament

Superficial Transverse
palmar ligament

Figure 2.25 Finger involvement.

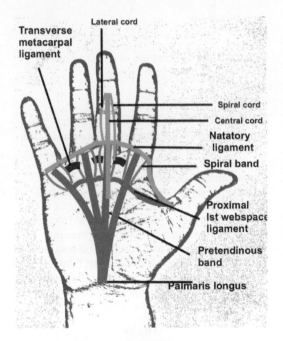

Transverse
metacarpal
ligament

Lateral cord

Spiral cord

Central cord

Natatory
ligament

Spiral band

Proximal
lst webspace
ligament

Pretendinous
band

Palmaris longus

Figure 2.26 Cords pattern.

fascia and tendon to its ulnar border. This diseased lateral retrovascular band is seen in Dupuytren's disease causing one of the most concerns for surgeons because of its location and meticulous identification for complete excision [14].

Pathology Seen in Dupuytren's Disease

1. Nodules on the palmar skin

2. Cords

3. Contractures

Structures Less Involved in Dupuytren's Disease

1. Cleland ligament: Stress shielded by the adjacent phalanx

2. Transverse superficial palmar ligaments: Shielded by transverse metacarpal ligament

3. Septa of Legue and Juvera: Shielded by metacarpal

4. Longitudinal fibres deep to transverse superficial palmar ligaments: Shielded by central bands

COMMON CORD PATTERNS IN DUPUYTREN'S DISEASE

1. Cords confined to palm: central palmar, spiral and proximal first web (Figure 2.26)

2. Cords confined to digits:

   Central, spiral and lateral cords

   Pain and deformity (acute mallet and chronic mallet) – (Table 2.17) (Figure 2.27)

HOW TO DIFFERENTIATE BETWEEN SWAN-NECK DEFORMITY BY MALLET FINGER AND OTHER CAUSES

1. Swan-neck deformity (hyper extension at PIP joint and flexion and DIP joint) due to congenital PIP joint laxity (Figure 2.28(a)).

2. Manually blocking the PIP joint hyperextension will eliminate the DIP joint flexion deformity. This indicates that the entire extensor mechanism is intact, and the PIP joint has congenital hyper-extension since birth (Figure 28.8(b)). Other fingers may have the deformities with variable

Table 2.17: Acute and Chronic Mallet Deformity

	History	Symptoms	Remarks
Acute mallet The flexion deformity or absence of extension at the DIP joint caused by injury to the terminal extensor tendon at DIP joint. Acute injuries may not have compensatory adaptation at the PIP joint, but they soon have swan neck deformity at the PIP joint (hyperextension at PIP joint and flexion at DIP joint). The swan neck deformity is because of the central slip compensating at the PIP joint.	Snagging the extending finger on a pant cuff, bedsheet or solid object. Injury (cricket, basketball). Familial predisposition (maybe).	1. Tendon rupture. 2. Bone avulsion (large fracture of the base of distal phalanx).	Most commonly involved fingers are little finger, ring finger and middle finger.
Chronic mallet (more than four-week-old mallet deformity).	Neglected injury.	Extensor lag >30°. Swan-neck deformity.	-

levels of involvement. This deformity is commonly seen and needs simple intervention by splints blocking the PIP joint hyperextension.

3. Picture of acute mallet little finger with sudden o nset of flexion at the DIP joint (extension lag) (Figure 2.27). The compensatory PIP joint hyperextension is not developed because of its acute onset. Treatment either by splints or surgical intervention gives good results [15].

Reasons for Swan-Neck Deformities Other Than Mallet Injury

1. Overactivity of extrinsic extensor tendons (EDC) or intrinsic extensor mechanism (lumbricals, interossei), for example: Cerebral palsy with spastic upper limb

2. Volar plate injury

3. Flexor digitorum superficialis tendon injury

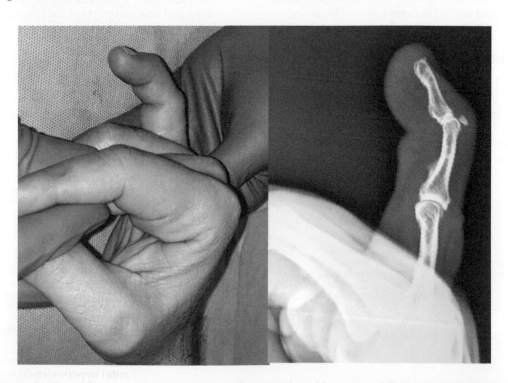

Figure 2.27 (a) Picture of acute mallet little finger with sudden onset of flexion at the DIP joint (extension lag). (b) Radiographs showing mallet fractures and subluxation of the distal phalanx.

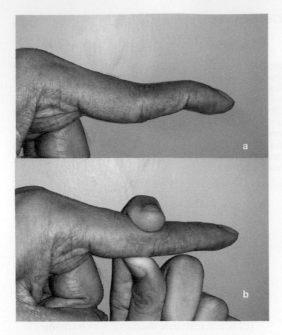

Figure 2.28 (a) Swan-neck deformity. (b) Differentiate in swan-neck deformity due to congenital PIP joint laxity.

MANOEUVRE TO APPRECIATE THE SWAN NECK DEFORMITY

The examiner manually flexes the hyperextended PIP joint and appreciates a pseudo triggering. This is because of the increased tension in central slip and two lateral bands moving away from the PIP joints axis, making flexion resembling a trigger finger. A normal finger has equally distributed tension in the central slip and two lateral bands during the flexion – extension of the PIP joint. Since the lateral bands are away and close to the PIP joint flexion axis, they always cause PIP joint flexion and DIP joint extension distally. Swan neck deformity has more central slip and lateral bands in midline preventing PIP joint flexion and subsequently compensating with DIP joint flexion through the Landsmeer ligament (spiral oblique retinacular ligament). When the extensor tendon (EDC), interossei and lumbricals act with the extensor expansion, it facilitates the MCP joint flexion and IP joint extension (Table 2.18).

Critical Points in Physical Examination

1. Deformities
   a. How does it start (injury, long duration of illness associated with skin patches)?
   b. Is it gradually worsening or improving?
   c. Associated with numbness, temperature changes.

2. Weakness
   a. Sudden onset.
   b. Gradual onset (rheumatoid tenosynovitis can cause pain, dysfunction of the tendons and finally rupture of the tendons by the proliferating synovium).

Table 2.18: Extensor Expansion Mechanism

	Action	PIP Joint Axis	Ligaments Preventing Them from Slipping or Changing Direction	Significance
Central slip	Extension of PIP joint.	Close to the axis (causes extension at PIP joint).	Triangular ligament at PIP joint (keeps both central slip and lateral bands in anatomical position).	Boutonniere deformity (injury of central slip causing radial bands too close to PIP joint flexion axis causing PIP joint flexion). Compensatory DIP joint extension by the lateral band becoming close to the PIP joint axis and exerting its action at the DIP joint by SORL ligament producing DIP joint extension.
Two lateral bands.	Flexion of PIP joint and extension at DIP joint (SORL).	Away from the axis (causes flexion at PIP joint).	Landsmeer ligament (spiral oblique retinacular ligament) at middle phalanx – it originates from the volar flexor sheath and inserts to the lateral aspect of the terminal extensor tendon (DIP joint).	Terminal extensor cut produces mallet finger. When there is discontinuity in the terminal extensor tendon, the extension action by the EDC tendon and intrinsics muscles increase the tension in the central slip. It becomes more active and pulls the lateral bands close to it causing hyperextension deformity. The lateral bands will have no effect in DIP joint extension because of the cut terminal tendon due to injury there.

Video 2.2 Videos showing the swan neck deformities and boutonniere deformities in a rheumatoid hand.

www.routledge.com/9780367647162.

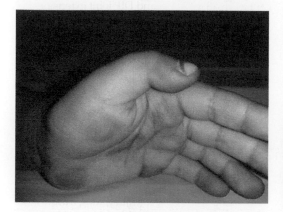

Figure 2.29 Congenital trigger thumb.

c. Current deficit.
d. Which portion of hand/fingers involved?
e. Associated with sensory loss.

3. Finger movement absent/weakness/ deformity
   a. Sudden following injury (cut injury to tendons).

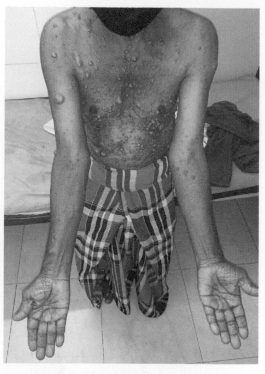

Figure 2.30 Neurofibromatosis I in an elderly man with multiple brownish dome-shaped lesions (neurofibromas) on the entire body.

Table 2.19: Diabetes and Immunocompromised Conditions

Conditions	Associated	Comments
Diabetes mellitus.	Hand infections (acute paronychia). Chronic paronychia.	Diabetes is associated with trigger fingers, joint stiffness, contracture, and amputation.
Leukaemia, aspergillosis, mucormycosis.	Cutaneous, subcutaneous, tenosynovial, nerve, joint or bone lesion (i.e., nodule, abscess, ulcer, sinus, fistula, or a nondescript mass).	Diagnosis is made with drainage, aspirate, punch biopsy, needle biopsy or open biopsy.
Immunodeficiencies (HIV, systemic lupus erythematosus, haematological malignancies, organ transplantation, pancytopenia, anaemia).	Unusual tumours (nonspecific lesions). Fungal infections, atypical and typical mycobacteria and bacterial infections.	Diagnosis is made with serological tests, biochemical tests, drainage, aspirate, punch biopsy, needle biopsy or open biopsy.
Anaerobic infections.	Slow growing organisms (*M. tuberculosis* divides approximately every 24 hours). Few organisms require a specific temperature for growth (e.g., *Sporotrichum schenckii, M. marinum, M. haemophilum, M. chelonae*, and *M. ulcerans* grow at 30°C; *M. xenopi* grows at 42°C). Some organisms do not grow at all unless ideal growth medium is provided (i.e., *M. haemophilum* requires haemoglobin).	Improper collection and/or delay in transportation of specimens may impair growth of organism and results in delayed treatment.

Table 2.20: Bacterial Infections in the Hand

Bacterial Infections	Causative Organism	Type	Mechanism of Infection	Clinical Finding	Investigations	Diagnosis
Actinobacillosis.	*Actinobacillus actinomycetemcomitans.*	Gram negative bacillus.	Fist injury.	Tenosynovitis extensor tendons and finger flexors. Abscess, recurrent draining sinus.	X-ray- osteitis.	CO_2 media culture
Actinomycosis.	*Actinomyces israelii.*	Gram positive.	Human bites, fist injury.	Painful nodule, sinus, abscess.	X-ray- sclerosis / lytic changes.	"Yellow sulphur granules" from sinus or pus culture (25% positive) biopsy are confirmative.
Anthrax (black eschar)	*Bacillus anthracis.*	Gram positive, encapsulated, spore-forming bacillus.	Infected herbivores, contaminated meat, wool, leather, accidental inoculation in the laboratory, weaponized spores of bioterrorism.	Painless necrotic black ulcer (95%), vesicles, lymphadenopathy, eschar.	Pulmonary anthrax (CT scan).	Gram staining.
Botryomycosis (granular bacteriosis).	*Staphylococcus aureus, Pseudomonas vesicularis, Moraxella nonliquefasciens,* and tuberculosis.			Soft tissue infection hand with clumps of bacteria resembling "grains."		Histology – "bunch of grapes."
Brucellosis.	*B. abortus.*	Gram-negative coccobacilli.	Direct or indirect contact with cattle. Skin cuts, inhalation of aerosols, ingestion of unpasteurized milk.	Osteomyelitis, septic arthritis, tendinitis, dactylitis.	X-ray-osteitis.	Blood culture, bone needle aspirate, chocolate agar.

(Continued)

Table 2.20 (Continued): Bacterial Infections in the Hand

Bacterial Infections	Causative Organism	Type	Mechanism of Infection	Clinical Finding	Investigations	Diagnosis
Mycetoma (actinomycetoma) Triad 1. Tumificatoin (woody and indurated swelling). 2. Draining sinus. 3. Granules in the discharging pus.	Actinomycetoma (bacteria)	Large filamentous bacteria.	Traumatic implantation from soil, wood splinters, thorn prick into the bare hand.	Slow growing, painless, progressive, destructive granuloma. Both bacterial and fungal mycetoma clinically look the same. Patients of 30–60 years affected. Finger, palm, dorsum of hand and wrist, forearm and upper arm can be affected.		Haematoxylin and eosin stain is adequate to detect the grains (actinomyces spp.). Grains (0.2 to 5.0 mm) contain clusters of organisms. Deep wedge biopsy is better than collecting superficial exudate and grains. Acid–Schiff stain for fungi.
	Nocardia spp.	Gram-positive, aerobic, acid-fast, and filamentous bacteria.		Nocardia (3 types) 1. Acute infection- cellulitis or abscess. 2. Lymphocutaneous infection. 3. Actinemycetoma with nodules.		
	Eumycetoma (Fungi-Maduramycosis, Madura foot).			Mycetoma stage Stage I (nodular): 2–3 months. Stage II (sinusoidal) 4–12 months. Stage III (skeletal) osteomyelitis. Stage IV (skeletal) deformity (1 year).		
Syphilis.	Treponema pallidum.	Gram negative.		Congenital syphilis: Bilateral dactylitis, metacarpitis. Clinical findings: Oedema of hand and fusiform swelling (resembles tuberculous spina ventosa). Pathological metacarpal fractures. Painless, large epitrochlear and axillary nodes. Non-healing ulcers. Secondary syphilis (paraonychia, ulcers in hand/wrist). Tertiary syphilis: Gummas (nonspecific, chronic granulomatous lesions that may involve tissues from skin to bone).	X-rays: New bone formation (reactive sclerosis) in phalanges and metacarpal. Bone destruction (patchy rarefaction). Periosteal new bone formation. Infantile osteomyelitis.	Dark-field microscopic examination of ulcer exudate shows spirochetes. VDRL, fluorescent treponemal antibody absorption (FTA-ABS) test, and the rapid plasma reagin (RPR) test is presumptive because of false positive (yaws).
Yaws (bacterial zoonosis).	Treponema pallidum ssp. pertenue (T. p. pertenue).	Gram negative,	Poor hygiene and overcrowded places, Direct skin contact,	Children <15 years (75%). Multiple, bilateral nodules/papillomas. Ulcers.	Periostitis, sclerosis, thickened, enlarged and widened cortex.	Morphological and serological tests are identical to syphilis.

Table 2.21: Fungal Infections in the Hand

Fungal Infections	Organism	Mechanism of infection	Clinical Presentation	Diagnosis
Aspergillosis.	*A. fumigatus.*	Immunocompromised patients infect blood vessels and cause tissue necrosis. Burns, puncture wounds after IV or catheter insertion, leukaemia patients and organ transplants.	Dermal nodules. Necrotic ulcers in finger, hand and forearm.	Biopsy, Wet KOH preparation.
Blastomycosis.	*Blastomyces Dermatitidis.*	Soil, direct contamination, traumatic infestations in veterinarians.	Plaque, ulcer, nodules (single/multiple). Cutaneous nodules, abscess, fistulas, ulcers, tenosynovitis, osteomyelitis, dactylitis and septic arthritis.	Biopsy, PAS (periodic acid Schiff) or silver stain.
Candidiasis.	*C. albicans, C. tropicalis, C. glabrata* and *C. parapsilosis.*	Interdigital ulcer (C. albicans). Local and systemic spread. Association with HIV.	Flexor/extensor tenosynovitis, septic arthritis and osteomyelitis. Joint implant infections and prosthetic valve infections.	Joint infection aspiration KOH stain and culture.
Coccidioidomycosis	*Coccidioides immitis* (dimorphic fungus).	Trauma. Local and systemic spread.	Tenosynovitis (extensor rupture may mimic rheumatoid arthritis) joint infection, osteomyelitis (may mimic enchondroma).	Biopsy.
Cryptococcosis.	*Cryptococcus neoformans.*	Immunocompromised patients. Pigeons' droppings, avian habitats.	Papules, pustules, plaques, cellulitis, abscesses, nodules, sinuses, and ulcers phalanx osteomyelitis.	India ink stain, cryptococcal antigen titer and growth of the fungus from biopsy specimens.
Histoplasmosis.	*Histoplasma capsulatum.*	Lungs.	Cutaneous infection, tenosynovitis, tendon ruptures, carpal tunnel syndrome, arthritis and in severe burns of the upper extremity with fatal necrotizing myofascitis.	Grocott silver stain. Biopsy, complement fixation test
Mucormycosis	*Rhizopus Mucor hiemalis*	Vascular invasion. Hematogenous dissemination. Soil contamination in open wounds. Thorn prick. Catheter, surgical dressings. Trauma (50%), high energy motorcycle accidents and agricultural injuries (*Mucor*). Immunocompromised (50%). Organ transplants, kidney failures, leukaemia and diabetes.	A triad of rapid cutaneous and subcutaneous gangrenous destruction, diabetes, and blood vessel thrombosis (i.e., arterial or venous). Enlarging black skin eschars and gangrene should lead one to consideration of advanced mucormycosis, both in immunocompetent and immunocompromised hosts.	Biopsy and histopathologic examination.
Sporotrichosis.	*Sporothrix schenckii*	Lungs.	Bones, joints, or tenosynovium in the hand. Joint infection with sinus. Extensor tenosynovitis (extensor tendon rupture). Sporotrichal flexor tenosynovitis (carpal tunnel syndrome or ulnar nerve entrapment). Olecranon bursitis, osteomyelitis and joint infections.	Histologic examination (cigar-shaped yeasts). Culture.

Table 2.22: Fungal Infections in Bones

Fungus	Presentation	Radiological Findings	Diagnosis
Blastomycosis	Carpal bones	Sharp, well-defined destruction	Complement fixation test biopsy
Coccidioidomycosis	Wrist and elbow joints, sinus	Sharply demarcated cystic lesions discrete osteolytic lesion surrounded by a zone of dense bone	Skin and serologic tests complement fixation test biopsy
Mucormycosis	Osteomyelitis		Complement fixation test biopsy

b. Slow progression with deviation of fingers (rheumatoid hand) (Video 2.2).
c. Associated with palm nodules (Dupuytren's contracture) [14].

4. Trigger symptoms
a. Since birth/duration: Congenital trigger is always noticed by the parents between one and three years of age. The thumb function and opposition develop by nine months of age. So, they get to notice that the child keeps the thumb flexed and initially could be corrected passively. They always present with fixed flexion deformity in the interphalangeal joint (IP joint) thumb. Most of the time, it is fixed and cannot be extended (Figure 2.29).

HISTORY

- Age, sex
- Hand dominance
- Occupation
- Previous hand injury
- Pre-existing impairment or conditions that may affect function
- Multiple skin/nerve nodules (Figure 2.30)

Occupational infections (Table 2.25)
Viral infections (Tables 2.20–2.27)
Treatment history

- Drug history (Hansen's disease/tuberculosis/rheumatoid arthritis (DMARDS)/immunosuppressants, etc.)
- Previous surgery details
- Previous medicine intake (leprosy and tuberculosis, very common in India)
- Long duration of corticosteroids may reactivate tuberculosis

Comorbid Conditions (Table 2.19)
Trauma history
When the injury/condition occurred

- Mechanism of injury
- Pattern of symptoms
- Handedness
- Patient's attitude towards injury/condition
- Level of discomfort

Social Information

Work status: Barbers have association to develop interdigital sinuses. Immigrants are prone to develop reactivation of tuberculosis, food contaminations with pork ingestion and developing helminth infections.
Home status

Hobbies

Mental state

Travel Information

A recent travel history (national and international)

Read. At Leisure

The McGill Pain Questionnaire

Overview: The McGill Pain Questionnaire can be used to evaluate a person experiencing significant pain. It can be used to monitor the pain over time and to determine the effectiveness of any intervention. It was developed by Dr Melzack at McGill University in Montreal, Canada, and has been translated into several languages.
Sections:

1. What Does Your Pain Feel Like?

2. How Does Your Pain Change with Time?

3. How Strong is Your Pain?

Table 2.23: Tuberculosis Infections in the Hand

Tuberculosis Infections	Organisms	Spread	Clinical Presentations	Diagnosis	Differential Diagnosis
Cutaneous.	M. marinum (M. balnei).	Skin. Hematogenous. Pulmonary or extrapulmonary. Fish tank exposure.	Paronychia. Butcher's wart (M. bovis). Nodules, abscess, ulcer or plague lesion in fingers, hand or forearm.	Mycobacterial detection by PCR AFB and culture may not show organisms.	Sporotrichosis (multiple, marching, linear lesions may be seen along the lymphatics on the hand, wrist, and forearm) blastomycosis, histoplasmosis, syphilis, and yaws.
Subcutaneous.	Mycobacterium ulcerans (Buruli ulcer).	Skin trauma.	Subcutaneous oedema, nodule, ulcers. Buruli ulcer: Painless ulcers with undermined edges and a necrotic centre with hyperpigmented and shiny surrounding skin.	Direct smear examination (sensitivity —40%) Culture (sensitivity – 20–60%) PCR (sensitivity –98%) Histopathology (sensitivity –90%) FNAC (nodular cases only).	Sarcoidosis (poorly or non-caseating granuloma).
Deep 1. Tenosynovitis. 2. Tuberculous bursitis. 3. Tuberculous arthritis.	M. marinum M. kansasii. Ratio of M. kansasii and M. marinum is 1:5. M. avium-intracellulare complex.		4 to 7 decades of age. Digital flexor tenosynovitis (examine by palpating rice bodies, millet seeds, or melon seeds glide beneath the examining fingers). Sausage finger. Compound palmar ganglion. Rice-body laden carpal tunnel syndrome. No cold abscess.	ESR (increased). Hand tuberculosis are paucibacillary (smear and cultures are negative). MRI (tenosynovitis, wrist infection). PCR.	
	M. tuberculosis.		Subdeltoid bursa, olecranon bursa bicipitoradial bursa.	Bursa calcifications. USG. Incision and drainage, histopathological evaluation.	
	M. tuberculosis	Blood-borne untreated flexor tenosynovitis. Extra-pulmonary TB.	Wrist pain, swelling, limitation of joint movements monoarticular.	X-ray – Phemister triad (findings – juxtaarticular osteoporosis, subchondral cysts, and gradual narrowing of the cartilage space). Phase-I: Periarticular osteoporosis. Phase-II: Subchondral cysts (pannus). Phase-III: Gross reduction, deformity, dislocation or ankylosis. Diagnosis is made with biopsy and culture.	Rheumatoid arthritis.
	M. bovis (children)	Extra-pulmonary: TB (20%) AIDS (70%),	Painless, not warm, nonsuppurative, and insidious swelling on the fingers (phalangeal infection) or the hand (metacarpal infection). Typical fusiform swelling of a finger or a diffuse swelling on the dorsum of the hand. Abscess, multiple draining sinus (cheesy yellowish exudate).	X-rays – endosteal resorption of bone and progressive subperiosteal hyperplasia. Joint effusion, periarticular osteopenia, joint space narrowing, endosteal thinning with cortical irregularity, lytic lesions, periosteal new bone formation and advanced epiphyseal maturity. AFB stain. Biopsy.	Tumour.

Table 2.24: Tuberculosis Infections in Adults and Children

	Children	Adult
Order of involvement.	The proximal phalanx, middle phalanx distal phalanx and metacarpal. The index, middle and ring fingers are involved most frequently.	The proximal, middle and distal phalanx. Middle and ring fingers more common than index and little fingers
Tuberculosis.	Multifocal (30%). Tuberculous dactylitis. Metaphyseal tuberculous osteomyelitis.	Multifocal (immunosuppressed). Discharging lesions. Tuberculous dactylitis. Associated with extrapulmonary TB (e.g., cervix). Solitary.
Radiographs.	X-rays – endosteal resorption of bone and progressive subperiosteal hyperplasia. Joint effusion, periarticular osteopenia, joint space narrowing, endosteal thinning with cortical irregularity, lytic lesions, periosteal new bone formation and advanced epiphyseal maturity.	1. Soft tissue swelling (early) followed by periosteal reaction and metaphyseal osteoporosis. This is followed by a well-defined cystic lesion that simulates a bone cyst. 2. Bone destruction with honeycombing (mimics a GCT when it is near the metaphysis). 3. A mixed cystic-sclerotic pattern with a lytic lesion that is surrounded by a sclerotic rim. 4. A diaphyseal lytic lesion that crosses the epiphyseal plate; this pattern is classic of paediatric tuberculous osteomyelitis. 5. Spina ventosa. 6. Bony lytic lesion with bone destruction that resembles bacterial osteomyelitis (Al-Qattan).
Diagnosis.	Biopsy.	Biopsy.
Differential diagnosis.	Subacute osteomyelitis of pyogenic origin.	Yaws, syphilis, leishmaniasis, brucellosis, blastomycosis, leprosy, and blistering distal dactylitis. Non-infectious causes of dactylitis are sarcoidosis, sickle cell anaemia and celiac disease.

Table 2.25: Occupational Infections

Infections	Cause	Prevalence	Clinical Findings	Diagnosis
Barber's interdigital pilonodal sinus.	Foreign body hair granuloma.	Male barbers and hairdressers.	Pit or sinus in the interdigital web space. Cyst, abscess or a nonspecific granuloma. Third webspace commonly involved second and fourth webspace (less common).	Several loose hairs protrude from the sinus.
Shearer's disease.	Sheep shearers and the wool.	Male.	Small tufts protrude from the sinus.	Recurrent pilonodular sinus, chronic osteomyelitis of phalanx.
Milker's interdigital granuloma.	Cattle hair, foreign body reaction.	Male.	Painful, red, granulating, discharging, vegetating lesion. Pea size to nut size second and third interdigital webspace (common location).	Foreign body reaction under the skin of milker's hand due to cattle hair penetration.
Slaughterer's interdigital granuloma.	Slaughtered animals' hair.			

Table 2.26: Viral Infections

Infections	Virus	Cause	Clinical Findings	Diagnosis
AIDS.	HIV-1. HIV-2.	Intravenous drug users.	Patients with AIDS have fingers red with painless erythema, periungual telangiectasia, blue nails with clubbing and frequent surgical debridement scars.	Grading of AIDS based on CD4+ lymphocyte counts.
Herpes simplex virus.	Herpes simplex virus type 2.	HIV. Immunosuppression.	Multiple vesicular lesions on an erythematous base. Chronic infections, finger necrosis or gangrene (overt HIV).	Direct immunofluorescent antibody, indirect immunoperoxidase. Staining. Viral culture (gold standard).
Bacillary angiomatosis.	*Bartonella henselae* and *Bartonella quintana.*	Transmitted by cats, ticks, fleas and lice.	Infectious, cutaneous, vascular, tumour-like disorder found almost exclusively in HIV-positive individuals.	Fine-needle aspiration Warthin-Starry stains show perivascular accumulations of bacilli. Electron microscopy. Culture *Bartonella* DNA by polymerase chain reaction.
Kaposi sarcoma.	Human herpes virus type 8.	Sexual transmission.	Solitary or multiple nodules. Plaques, painless pruritic, firm tumours. Regional lymph node and mucocutaneous lymph node enlargement.	Biopsy (punch/open).
Warts.	Human papillomaviruses (HPVs).	Direct inoculation, veterinary surgeons, butcher's meat packers, fowl handlers, poultry processors, fish handlers.	1. Verrucated warts: Painless, cauliflower-like, raised, demarcated, and greyish mass, with an irregular surface traversed by many projections. 2. Flat warts. 3. Multiple warts.	Electron microscopy. Viral culture.
Human orf (milkers') nodule, ecthyma contagiosum, contagious pustular dermatitis),	A large paravaccinia DNA virus that belongs to the subgroup of pox viruses,	Direct contact with infected sheep and goats or with products or objects that come into contact with sheep and goats, shepherds, butchers, veterinary surgeons, "Haji" pilgrims exposed to sheep slaughtering.	The lesion has an umbilicated red centre, a white middle and a peripheral violaceous halo. The lesion may be bulbous and affect multiple fingers.	electron microscopy
Milkers' nodules (manual milking).	Paravaccinia virus, pseudocowpox.	Manual milking from cows or buffaloes. Veterinarians.	Multiple nodules in the fingers involved in manual milking.	Electron microscopy.

Table 2.27: Diagnostic Tests

Test	Significance of Test	Positive	Negative	Remarks
Lepromin test.	It essentially indicates the host resistance (immunity) of the patient.	Subclinical infection, healthy individuals in endemic areas, tuberculoid type.	Lepromatous type.	This test differentiates mononeuritis types and determine PB or MB status.
Slit-skin smear.	Gold standard for diagnosis of HD.	AFB positive – MB.	AFB negative –PB.	Diagnose HD and classify PB and MB based on the test results.
Skin biopsy.	When a slit-skin smear is negative, a skin biopsy may be considered if the clinical diagnosis is in doubt.			The biopsy must include full depth of the dermis together with a portion of subcutaneous fat to include a dermal nerve.
Nerve biopsy.	Primary neuritic HD (neuritic pain with an enlarged nerve and without a skin lesion).			A thickened pure sensory nerve with minimal functional deficit (e.g., sural, radial sensory, supraclavicular) is preferable.
Fine needle aspiration technique.	The direction of the needle is always kept parallel to the length of the nerve.			Hematoxylin and eosin and AFB staining are done.
Electrophysiological studies.	EMG/NCV assess the site of compression neuropathy before surgery and in assessing the extent of nerve damage.			
Imaging (MRI).	Ulnar abscess and calcification.			

REFERENCES

1. Eubanks JD. Cervical radiculopathy: Nonoperative management of neck pain and radicular symptoms. *Am Fam Physician*. 2010; 81(1):33–40.

2. Caridi JM, Pumberger M and Hughes AP. Cervical radiculopathy: A review. *HSS J*. 2011; 7(3): 265–272.

3. Durkan JA. A new diagnostic test for carpal tunnel syndrome. *JBJS*. 1991; 73(4): 535–538.

4. Carette S and Fehlings MG. Clinical practice. Cervical radiculopathy. *N Engl J Med*. 2005; 353(4):392–399. doi:10.1056/NEJMcp043887

5. Li MY, Hua Y, Wei GH, et al. Staphylococcal scalded skin syndrome in neonates: An 8-year retrospective study in a single institution. *Pediatr Dermatol*. 2014; 31(1):43–47.

6. Huang JI, Seeger LL and Jones NF. Coccidioidomycosis fungal infection in the hand mimicking a metacarpal enchondroma. *J Hand Surg*. 2000; 25B:475.

7. Antia NH, Enna CD and Daver BM. *The Surgical Management of Deformities in Leprosy*. Mumbai: Oxford University Press, 1992.

8. Jopling WH and McDougall AC. *Handbook of Leprosy*. New Delhi: CBS. Publishers, 1996.

9. Koman LA, Smith BP and Smith TL. *A Practical Guide for Complex Regional Pain Syndrome in the Acute Stage and Late Stage*, 7th edition. Green's Operative Hand Surgery, Philadelphia, PA: Elsevier, 2015, p. 1797.

10. Wolfe S. *Tendinopathy*, 7th edition. Green's Operative Hand Surgery, Philadelphia, PA: Elsevier, 2015, p. 1904.

11. Weiss AP, Akelman E and Tabatabai M. Treatment of de Quervain's disease. *J Hand Surg [Am]* 1994; 19(4):595–598.

12. Finklestein H. Stenosing tendovaginitis at the radial styloid process. *J Bone Joint Surg Am.* 1930; 12:509–540.

13. Grundberg AB and Reagan DS. Pathologic anatomy of the forearm: intersection syndrome. *J Hand Surg [Am].* 1985; 10(2):299–302.

14. Eaton C. *Dupuytren Disease,* 7th edition. Green's Operative Hand Surgery, Philadelphia, PA: Elsevier, 2015, p. 128.

15. Jerome J Terrence Jose and Malshikare Vijay A. Fragment specific dorsal Kirschner wire extension block pinning in mallet fractures—A retrospective study of 20 cases. *Orthoplastic Surg.* 2021; 4:1–5. doi: 10.1016/j.orthop.2021.02.001

3 Physical Examination of the Hand

J Terrence Jose Jerome

CONTENTS

Clinical examination of the hand and upper limb always precedes a detailed history and significant observations. The dominant hand, function of the whole upper limb and contra-lateral upper limb, professional and recreation activities and the psychological state are noted. These factors influence the potential for recovery and rehabilitation. Also, the age, aerobic activity level, sports and leisure activities, an extensive medical record and a list of medications with particular attention to conditions that might affect bone mass or bone quality, including endocrine disorders, inflammatory diseases, renal disease, steroid use and other factors are essential for clinical diagnosis. The clinical examination of the hand must provide a basis for understanding, both objective and subjective. All clinical assessments should be reproducible with reliable and relevant methods or tests. The chapter discusses the examination as:

DOI: 10.1201/9781003125938-3

1. Inspection

2. Palpation

3. Vascular examination

INSPECTION

Tenderness

Inspection and palpation maximal tenderness is one of the most useful tools in the diagnosis of hand pathology, especially in patients with chronic dysfunctions. In acute trauma or dislocations, because of extensive soft tissue damage, tenderness is seldom elicited at specific points, but rather in a diffuse manner. Nonetheless, palpation should always be performed in a methodical way (Table 3.1).

Examination of the Skin

Inspection of the skin includes, assessing the suppleness, thickness and callouses in the palmar, dorsal and the interdigital webspace (Figure 3.1). A manual labourer has calloused, thick and less mobile skin which implies reduced cutaneous sensation and cautions surgical repair and wound dehiscence. Long-term steroid therapy is associated with skin atrophy, shiny appearance, loss of elasticity, stellate pseudoscars, reduced thickness and persistence of skin creases is associated with poor skin healing. The presence of vasculitis suggests active rheumatoid disease. Scaly patches, plaques and nail changes are seen in psoriatic arthritis. Kober's phenomenon is the development of psoriatic patches along the length of the scar engendered by surgery. Skin abrasions, contusions, or ecchymosed areas may be helpful in determining the mechanism of injury and the potential areas of damage.

Acute Hand Burns

The hand is involved in more than 80% of all severe burns, severely limiting the function and developing devastating contractures if left untreated. Also, the social stigma and psychological stress for an injured individual is more worrisome where meticulous planning and treatment can get back the social and professional life. The physical examination includes the extent and probable depth of the burn, associated injuries and general health of the patient.

All injuries should be documented carefully to create a solid foundation for further decisions and a baseline for follow-up and evaluation of outcome during the treatment.

Photographic documentation is highly recommended, especially in view of potential medicolegal issues. The status of perfusion, capillary refill, skin colour, and other characteristics have to be documented to facilitate decisions about escharotomy, compartment release or acute eschar excision.

Classification of Burns

Scald burns are seen in younger patients which are mixed-depth patterns involving the palm and have high capacity for spontaneous recovery. Flame burns are the most serious types of burns (deep partial thickness or full thickness) and often require surgical intervention. The dorsal skin is thin, flexible and lies on a thin layer of subcutaneous fatty tissue. This arrangement offers maximum tendon excursion and joint mobility but little mechanical protection. The skin wrinkles over the Metacarpophalangeal (MCP), proximal interphalangeal (PIP) and distal interphalangeal (DIP) joints, stretches with finger flexion and deepens in extension. The dorsal skin contains large superficial veins, hair follicles and sebaceous glands, but contains no sweat glands. The skin is especially thin over the PIP joints, where the extensor tendons are at risk (Table 3.2).

The palmar skin resembles the plantar skin of the foot. The thick subcutaneous fatty layer has a honeycomb-like structure that has shock-absorbing properties and provides grip stability by means of numerous fibrous septa that connect the skin with the deep fascia. Thick epidermal layers are found in the areas of greatest mechanical stress. In the finger, the Cleland ligament (dorsal to the neurovascular bundle) and Grayson ligament (palmar to the neurovascular bundle) provide stability. Common postburn hand deformities are shown in Figure 3.2 (a–e):

1. First web adduction contractures, thumb (IP) joint contractures (Figure 3.2(a))

2. Web space contractures (Figure 3.2(a))

3. Dorsal skin contractures, with associated finger deformities (Figure 3.2(e))

4. Digital flexion contractures (varying angles of contractures in fingers depending upon the injury pattern) (Figure 3.2(c, d))

5. Boutonnière deformity (can be associated with swan-neck deformities in other fingers) (Figure 3.2(b))

Table 3.1: **Tenderness and Specific Locations**

Location	Tenderness	Significance	Remarks
Flexing the wrist and palpate the dorsum of the capsule distal to the Lister's tubercle	Sharp pain	Scapholunate joint (SL) injury	Scaphoid shift test determines the abnormal scaphoid subluxation
Resisted finger extension test Extend the index and middle finger fully against resistance with wrist partially flexed	Sharp pain in SL area	Synovitis at the radio scaphoid joint	Sensitive Not specific
SL ballottement test The lunate is firmly stabilized with the thumb and index finger of one hand, while the scaphoid, held with the other hand (i.e., thumb on the palmar tuberosity and index on the dorsal proximal pole) is displaced dorsally and palmarly	Pain, crepitus, and excessive mobility of the scaphoid.	Scapholunate (SL) joint injury	
LT ballottement test The lunate is firmly stabilized with the thumb and index finger of one hand, while the triquetrum and pisiform are displaced dorsally and palmarly with the other hand	Pain, crepitus, and abnormal displacement of the LT joint	Lunotriquetral (LT) joint injury	"Shear test" described by Kleinman is a variation of the ballottement test that can be done with a single hand: By stabilizing the dorsal aspect of the lunate with the index finger, the pisiform is loaded by the thumb in a dorsal direction, creating a shear force at the LT joint that causes pain
Midcarpal shift test The test reproduces the painful clunk by passive palmar translation and ulnar inclination of the wrist in pronation	Painful clunk	A manoeuvre to determine the amount of midcarpal joint laxity	Based on how much force is necessary to maintain the wrist palmarly subluxed in ulnar inclination, wrists are classified into five grades. In grade I, the palmar midcarpal ligaments are so tight that the distal row can hardly be displaced palmarly. Grades II and III can still be found in normal individuals and represent increasing levels of midcarpal laxity allowing the palmar sag to be obtained in ulnar inclination, although it reduces when the applied force is removed. In grade IV, subluxation is easily achieved, and the wrist remains subluxed after removal of the external force. Grade V instability occurs when the patient can actively reproduce and maintain the palmar sag in ulnar inclination without assistance from the examiner
Tenderness in the soft depression between the flexor carpi ulnaris (FCU) tendon, ulnar styloid, and triquetrum ("Ulnar Fovea Sign")		Foveal disruption and ulnotriquetral (UT) ligament injuries	The ulnar fovea sign is positive when there is exquisite tenderness compared with the contralateral side. This tenderness must replicate the patient's complaint of pain in terms of character and location. The patient with a positive ulnar fovea sign often demonstrates facial winces during the maneuver.

(Continued)

Table 3.1 (Continued): Tenderness and Specific Locations

Location	Tenderness	Significance	Remarks
Tenderness and or crepitus of the ECU and FCU tendons		Tenosynovial hypertrophy or tendinopathy	ECU tendinitis and lunotriquetral ligament tears can mimic DRUJ symptoms
Palpating the pisotriquetral interval and press the pisiform	Pain	Pisotriquetral arthritis	
Piano key sign This describes the relative hypermobility of the ulnar head with the forearm in full pronation.	Pain elicited following release of the ulnar head after transient palmar depression	DRUJ instability	
DRUJ ballottement test Increased anteroposterior translation of the radius on the ulna during passive manipulation is evidence of DRUJ instability.	pain elicited during translation	DRUJ instability	Because joint translation varies with forearm position and among individuals, the test should be done in all forearm positions and should be compared with the opposite side
Ulnocarpal stress test The patient's forearm is positioned vertically on the examination table and the examiner grasp the hand and applies an axial load through the wrist. The wrist is moved passively through radial and ulnar deviation while being moved through an arc of pronation and supination	Pain	Ulnocarpal instability caused by disk tears or ulnocarpal degeneration.	
Press test The patient grasps the arm of a chair and pushes up toward a standing position	Pain and instability	DRUJ instability	Dynamic loading of the ulnocarpal joint by the patient is done using the press test
"Snuffbox tenderness"	Pain	70% of scaphoid waist fractures	Sensitive and low specificity (74–80%)
Tenderness over lunate The lunate lies just distal to the distal radius dorsal lip in line with the third ray. Some patients will provide a history of recent hyperextension injury	Patients frequently describe an insidious onset of dull pain centred over the radiolunate joint	AVN lunate	Patients complain of pain aggravated by activity and relieved with rest and immobilization
Medial humeral epicondyle tenderness	Pain (at 70–120°) This is the position of late cocking and early acceleration of throwing, characteristically occurs in medial collateral ligament insufficiency	Chronic elbow medial instability	**Valgus stress elbow** The examiner stabilizes the forearm and supports the proximal arm at the axilla. The elbow is flexed past 30° and a valgus stress is applied across the elbow joint. **The "milking" manoeuvre** It consists of static traction placed on the thumb with the elbow flexed beyond 90° and the shoulder externally rotated **The moving valgus stress test** It involves a similar load applied to the elbow while the joint is taken through a range of motion

(Continued)

Table 3.1 (Continued): Tenderness and Specific Locations

Location	Tenderness	Significance	Remarks
Lateral epicondylitis (tennis elbow) Tenderness localized to the lateral epicondyle and at the ECRB origin, just slightly distal and anterior to the lateral epicondyle	The pain is exacerbated by resisted wrist extension, forearm pronated and elbow fully extended	Lateral epicondylitis	
Resisted supination with the wrist flexed	Pain at lateral epicondyle	Lateral epicondylitis	
The "chair test" Patient is asked to lift a chair with the arm in forearm pronation and wrist flexion	Pain at lateral epicondyle	Lateral epicondylitis	There is an overlap with radial tunnel syndrome in patient complaints and physical findings with use of provocative tests (chair test, resisted supination test)
Monoarticular tenderness and swelling (Figure 3.5)	Pain over the lateral condyle, head of the radius, restricted pronation and supination movements	Rheumatoid elbow	

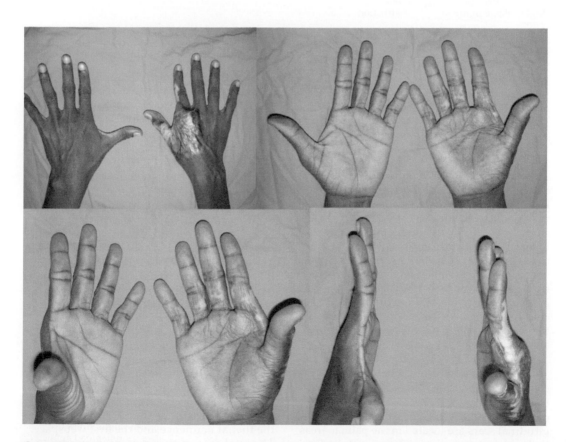

Figure 3.1 Physical appearance of postburn contractures with unsightly scars, reduced web-space and hypo/hyperpigmented skin lesions.

Table 3.2: Classifications of Burns

Degree	Characters	Pain	Potential to Heal	Scar Formation
Superficial, first-degree burns (e.g., sunburn)	Erythematous epidermis without blistering	Moderately painful	Yes	Nil
Superficial partial-thickness second-degree burns	Erythema Blisters Pink	Most painful (sensitive nerve endings are not damaged)	Heal by virtue of regeneration from the living epidermal elements remaining in the dermis (sweat or sebaceous glands and hair follicles)	Scar formation is directly dependent on the depth of injury and the quality of the regenerated skin is inversely proportional
Deep partial-thickness second-degree burns	Blisters Patchy white/pink appearance	Less pain (nerve endings are still present)		
Full-thickness third-degree burns	White Veins thrombosed Leathery skin	No pain (destroyed nerve endings)	Cannot heal by epithelial regeneration	
Fourth-degree injury (contact burns or high-voltage injuries)	Charred Deep destruction			

6. Dorsal skin deficiency

7. Digital loss secondary to ischemia

8. Median and ulnar nerve compression syndrome

Trophic Changes and Sweating

The examiner should examine the skin, nails, dorsal hairs, soft tissue thickness and pulp to look for trophic changes which are caused by vasomotor and neurological factors. Skin colour changes, sweating and distribution of sweating provide information about the vasomotor changes such as in complex regional pain syndrome (CRPS). Peripheral nerve lesions have localized difference in sweat secretions (Figure 3.3). Assessment of nails and the atrophic changes helps us in diagnosing and differentiating from systemic illness such as chronic anaemia.

Scar and Skin Contractures

Careful examination of the scar and skin contractures is essential for assessing the mobility of the wrist and fingers. The most common longitudinal scars are located in the palmar areas that run across the flexion creases interfering with extension of the fingers. Also, dorsal scars create adhesions reducing the flexion and the extensibility (elasticity) of the skin. Webspace

scars invade the palmar interdigital systems producing wide separation of the fingers and flexion at the metacarpophalangeal joint (Figures 3.1 and 3.2).

PALPATION

Examination of the Aponeurotic Lesions

Dupuytren's disease has palmar nodules or bands seen in the mid-palmar aponeurosis, first webspace and fingers producing various degrees of flexion contractures (Figure 3.4). The knuckle pad on the dorsum of the PIP joints causes extension contractures in the fingers. The objective evaluation of the nodules allows accurate assessment of the deformity and improvement needed and achieved by surgery.

The hand is divided into five segments. Each segment involves a finger with palmar zone, pretendinous band of the palmar aponeurosis and adjacent segment of the palmar aponeurosis for index, middle, ring and little fingers. The thumb has a fascia of the thenar eminence and the first webspace. The total deformity is measured by adding together the individual flexion deformity (deficiency of extension) of the three joints – the metacarpophalangeal (MCP), proximal

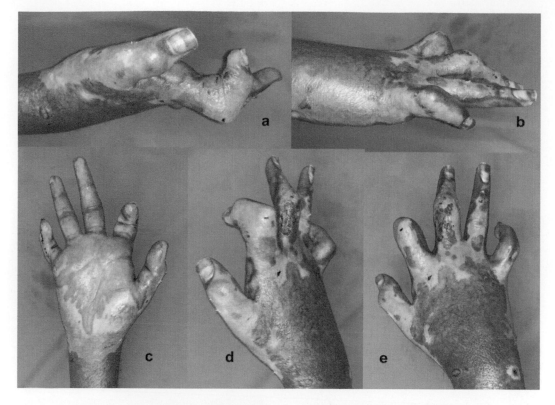

Figure 3.2 Postburn contracture of the right hand with severe flexion contracture of the index finger (a, c), boutonnière deformity of middle finger (b, d), and swan-neck deformity (e).

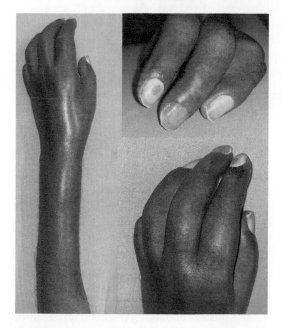

Figure 3.3 Hand pictures of CRPS with nail, hair and skin changes. The hair is atrophic, nail is brittle, skin is shiny, stretched mottled, oedematous and associated with finger stiffness (autonomic dysfunction).

interphalangeal (PIP) and distal interphalangeal (DIP) joints.

The MCP and interphalangeal (IP) joint contractures and first webspace contractures are assessed for thumb deformity. Also, the first webspace contracture is measured by the angle formed by the line joining the axes of the first and second metacarpal where they intersect in the sagittal plane (normal value = 45°).

Earliest signs of Dupuytren's disease:

1. Skin tightness (exaggerated blanching with finger extension)

2. Contour changes (skin crease deformation, dimples)

3. Nodules

4. Cords with contractures, or prominence of the palmar monticuli

TENOSYNOVITIS

1. Dorsum of the wrist

Usually seen in rheumatoid arthritis as a double swelling caused by the common

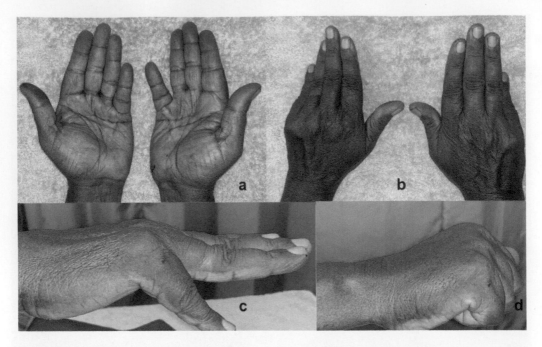

Figure 3.4 Dupuytren's contracture with progressive tightening of the bands of fibrous tissue (called nodules) inside the palms, causing a curling in of the fingers that eventually can result in a claw-like hand.

extensor tendon and extensor carpi ulnaris synovitis. Swelling may also be seen on the radio dorsal aspect of the wrist due to extensor carpi radialis tendons and thumb extensors synovitis.

DE QUERVAIN'S TENOSYNOVITIS

Synovitis and degeneration around the first dorsal extensor compartment produce pain and tenderness 1–2 cm proximal to the radial styloid process. The first compartment tendons (abductor pollicis longus, extensor pollicis brevis) pass through an unyielding osteoligamentous tunnel formed by a shallow groove in the radial styloid process (Figure 3.5). The tunnel is covered by a tough overlying roof composed of transverse fibres of the dorsal ligament and bordered by vertical septa between the retinaculum and radius. De Quervain's disease is also known as "washerwomen's sprain" where frequent abduction of the thumb and simultaneous wrist ulnar deviation produces friction at the rigid retinaculum, swelling or narrowing of the fibrosseous canal produces localized pain in the radial side of the wrist aggravated by thumb movements. The average age is during the fifth and sixth decades and is six times more common in women. Recently, postpartum and lactating women reported this disease. Finkelstein's test and the Eichhoff manoeuvre are specific for diagnosing the disease.

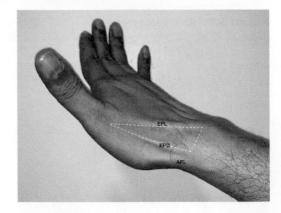

Figure 3.5 The triangle in the picture depicts the anatomical snuff box, where extensor pollicis longus (EPL) and extensor pollicis brevis (EPB) mark the boundary.

1. Finkelstein's test: Harry Finklestein subsequently described the pathognomonic examination manoeuvre that bears his name: "On grasping the patient's thumb and quickly abducting the hand ulnar ward, the pain over the styloid tip is excruciating" (Video 3.1).

2. Eichhoff manoeuvre: Passive flexion of the wrist in ulnar deviation with thumb held in the palm causes tension on the abductor

Video 3.1 Demonstration of the Finklestein test.

www.routledge.com/9780367647162.

 Video 3.2 Demonstration of the Finklestein test and Eichhoff's test.

www.routledge.com/9780367647162.

 Video 3.3 Demonstration of Grinding test for thumb CMC arthritis. The examiner rests the patient's hand on an examining table, stabilizes the wrist with one hand and applies an axial load to the thumb axis. Pain may be elicited as well as crepitus as the degenerative articular surfaces are compressed. The CMC subluxation test is done in a similar fashion, although the objective is to gently force the CMC joint to sublux; the examiner determines whether this elicits a pain response. Crepitus may also be apparent.

www.routledge.com/9780367647162.

pollicis longus and extensor pollicis brevis and reproduction of classical symptoms (knifelike pain) (Video 3.2).

Both tests should be performed in patients with suspected de Quervain's disease (Video 3.3). Occasionally, radiographs show localized osteopenia or spurring at the radial styloid. This tenosynovitis has to be differentiated from radial sensory nerve compression (Wartenberg syndrome). Patients with de Quervain's disease demonstrate normal sensory testing in the dorsal radial aspect of the hand, in contrast to radial sensory nerve compression where Tinel's sign is positive with symptoms (paraesthesia, pain or numbness) along the nerve distribution.

 Video 3.4 Videos of trigger thumb.

www.routledge.com/9780367647162.

In addition, patients with de Quervain's disease have pain on percussion over the first extensor compartment. Finkelstein's test can also be positive in Wartenberg syndrome.

DIFFERENTIAL DIAGNOSIS

(a) Intersection syndrome: Pain, swelling and in severe cases, crepitus, is found over the second dorsal compartment tendons more proximally. The condition has also been confused with trigger thumb, and this may be related to the presence of a separate fibroosseous tunnel and "pseudotriggering" of the extensor pollicis brevis (EPB) tendon.

(b) Thumb carpometacarpal (CMC) or scaphotrapezial-trapezoid joints (or both): Patients with CMC arthritis present with varied complaints of localized pain, or vague complaints such as throbbing or burning in the radial aspect of the hand. Advanced osteoarthritis often has adduction contracture thumb and a compensatory MCP joint hyperextension. These patients may show laxity of the joint in hyperextension. A grinding test and joint subluxation test evaluate thumb carpometacarpal joint arthritis.

a) Grinding test: The examiner faces the patient and rests his/her hand on the examination table. Once the wrist is stabilized with the other hand, an axial load is applied to the thumb axis to elicit pain as well as crepitus seen in degenerative arthritis (Video 3.4).

b) CMC subluxation test: The test is similar to the grinding test where the examiner gently forces the CMC joint to subluxate and note the pain and crepitus.

In addition, pinch strength, two-point key pinch or three-point cuck pinch test increases the force across the CMC joint by a

 Video 3.5 Winging of scapula. The medial and inferior borders come closer to the spine and lifted superiorly when compared to the normal side. Scapular winging can be accentuated when the patient is asked to forward flex his arms to the horizontal and/or push on a wall in a push-up motion. In this position, the vertebral border of the scapula lifts further from the thoracic wall due to the loss of serratus anterior scapular protraction.

www.routledge.com/9780367647162.

factor of 12. This helps in comparing the values with the contralateral side. Radiography and physical examination assist in differentiating from de Quervain's disease and carpal tunnel syndrome (30%) from arthritis, although these lesions may coexist because of their similar demographics.

(c) Scaphoid fracture and arthrosis involving the radiocarpal or intercarpal joints: Anatomical snuff box tenderness (Figure 3.5) radiographic study with scaphoid fractures and radiocarpal joint space reduction, cyst resorption, bone resorptive changes and narrowing or pointing of the radial styloid excludes de Quervain's disease.

2. Flexor tenosynovitis

Synovitis of the flexor tendons in the distal forearm has diffuse swelling. In the fingers the synovial sheaths lie along the flexor tendons, with their "cul-de-sac" at the level of the distal palmar crease. Infection causes pain or pressure along the radial three fingers (Video 3.5). The thumb and the little finger have flexor sheaths proximal to the proximal wrist crease. So, pressure over the proximal wrist crease produces pain in the thumb and little finger.

Rheumatoid synovitis presents with discrete swelling, is less painful and associated with incomplete flexion and triggering of the fingers.

POSTURE OF THE HAND/ ATTITUDE OF THE UPPER LIMB

Each extremity should be evaluated separately. Of the most important is the attitude of the upper limb which helps us in diagnosing the disease and making swift decisions.

1. Spastic deformities (cerebral palsy)

Most of the deformities present with shoulder internal rotation, elbow flexion, forearm pronation, wrist flexion, finger flexion, intrinsic spasticity and thumb-in-palm deformity (Figure 3.6). In addition to the attitude, certain activities such as overhead lifting, supination and pronation, opening and closing the hand and a range of movements assist in the clinical diagnosis.

The spastic deformities should be differentiated from muscle contractures. In a relaxed patient with spastic deformity, the passive range of movements are full and normal at the affected joint. Muscle or joint contracture has restricted passive movements in the affected joints. Spasticity is classically classified by the number of limbs involved: Monoplegia (one

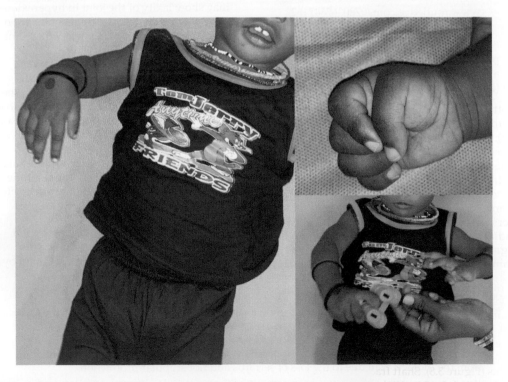

Figure 3.6 Spastic upper limb presents with shoulder internal rotation, elbow flexion, forearm pronation, wrist flexion, finger flexion, intrinsic spasticity and thumb-in-palm deformity.

extremity), hemiplegia (one arm, one leg), diplegia (two legs), triplegia (two legs, one arm) and quadriplegia (all four extremities). Motor function is also classified as spastic, flaccid and athetoid. Many patients have a combination of movement patterns (Table 3.3).

2. Hand fractures

Hand fractures have robust healing potential and remodelling capacity in most of the injuries involving children and adults. The greatest remodelling is seen in fracture displacement in the plane of the adjacent joint motion. Rotational deformity and radioulnar angulation remodelling are not possible in children and adults because of poor remodelling, potential and radioulnar joint movements.

The examiner should watch for swelling, ecchymosis and restricted range of movements, which will guide to the injured or pathological site. The tenodesis effect or gentle pressure applied to the more proximal muscle bellies of the forearm helps in assessment of both tendon integrity and angular or rotational deformity.

a) Malrotation

Malrotation can be assessed by clinical examination of the nailbeds of adjacent digits in extension. A rotation >10° out of the plane of adjacent nail plates indicates rotational malalignment. Rotational deformity can be better evaluated by assessing the digital alignment with finger flexion (Figure 3.7). Normally, the index, middle and little fingers point to the scaphoid tubercle in flexion, parallel in alignment. A few patients may have underlap such as little finger beneath the ring finger. Always one should examine the contralateral hand for baseline alignments. In patients who are anxious or unable to flex their fingers, the tenodesis effect assess the rotational alignment.

b) Angulation

Various authors have suggested acceptable angulation for metacarpal neck and shaft fractures with wide variations. Most authorities agree up to 30° of sagittal plane deformity is acceptable in physeal fractures, particularly in young patients with remaining growth potential. Also, 20–45° of apex dorsal angulation is acceptable in metacarpal neck fractures, with greater deformity allowable in the more ulnar digits (Figure 3.8). Shaft fractures tolerate 10–15° of angular deformity in the index and middle fingers; 30–40° in the ring and little fingers.

3. Complex regional pain syndrome (CRPS)

The physical examination of suspected CRPS should include history about an initiating event, post injury response, patient adaptability, time, detailed examination of the extremity (skin, nails), neurological assessment and cervical and thoracic spine evaluation (Table 3.4). Before diagnosing as CRPS, the examiner should follow essential steps:

i. Cervical spine and shoulder range of movements.

ii. Vascular or neurogenic claudication causing thoracic outlet syndrome should be ruled out.

iii. Adhesive capsulitis or frozen shoulder should be evaluated.

iv. Grip and pinch strength, motor function, sensation, oedema, vasomotor tone of the upper limb should be assessed.

v. Neurological examination, brachial plexus evaluation, Tinel's sign should be looked at in brief:

4. Position of fingers

a) Trigger fingers/thumb

The most common cause of pain and disability is tendon entrapment in the fingers and thumb. The patient presents with painful catching or popping of the involved flexor tendon during digits flexion and extension (Video 3.6). In lesser occasions, the patients present with digits locked in flexion and require passive assistance to extend the digits. It is unusual to see digits blocked in extension. Over the time, patients become reluctant to flex the fingers because of pain and develop PIP joint contractures.

There are 22 extrinsic tendons crossing the wrist to provide power and dexterity to the hand. Each tendon passes through a series of tight fibroosseous tunnel designed to adjust the balance between the movements and production of force very close to the joint or the joint that it controls.

Division, attenuation or rupture of a critical retinacular ligament, or pulley, will allow the tendon to drift away from the joint's centre of rotation and consequently increase its moment arm for production of force and lead to tendon imbalance and

 Video 3.6 Elson test for boutonnière deformity.

www.routledge.com/9780367647162.

Table 3.3: Key Points for Physical Examination of Spastic Disorders

Region	Position at Rest	Reason for Spastic Contracture	Articular Changes	Secondary Deformity	Specific Clinical Findings
Shoulder	Internal rotation and adduction	Subscapularis and pectoralis major muscles	Glenohumeral dysplasia, capsular contracture, and thickening of the surrounding fascia	Severe internal rotation and adduction posture of the shoulder occurs secondary to spasticity or contracture of the rotator cuff muscles	Patient's ability to position the hand in space restricted
Elbow	Flexion	Elbow flexors (biceps, brachialis, brachioradialis)	Soft tissue and joint contractures	Severe hyperflexion with antecubital skin breakdown and intertriginous infections	
Forearm	Pronation	Pronator teres	Contracture of the interosseous membrane or disruption of the radioulnar joint(s) radial head dislocation (2%) distal radioulnar joint dislocation	Severe spasticity, force patients to assume a reverse grasp posture, using the ulnar aspect of the hand to grasp objects (because they are unable to present the radial aspect of the hand)	Examine the distal and proximal radioulnar joint for dislocation, subluxation, or instability. Palpate for the radial head in supination and pronation and determine radial head alignment
Wrist and fingers	Flexion contracture	Spastic wrist flexors	Volar wrist capsular contracture of the wrist flexors or even the radiocarpal joint		Measure Volkmann angle to assess the flexor tendon tightness (Figure 3.5)
Thumb	Thumb in palm deformity	Adduction and flexion contracture Assess the adductor pollicis brevis (APB), flexor pollicis brevis (FPB), first dorsal interosseous, flexor pollicis longus (FPL), abductor pollicis longus (APL), extensor pollicis brevis (EPB), and extensor pollicis longus (EPL)	Hyperextension at the MP joint and volar plate laxity	First webspace contracture and poor ability to grasp or open the hand for holding the objects	Measure the adequacy of the first web space with measurements of the passive and active web space angle

flexion contracture. Clinical diagnosis of a hard tender nodule over the MCP joints confirms the trigger. Pulley disruption also effectively lengthens the tendon and limits its excursion.

The phenomenon of trigger finger is due to mechanical impingement of the digital flexor tendons as they pass through a narrowed retinacular pulley at the level of the metacarpal head [1].

Middle-aged women have been found predominant in association with trigger digits. The involvement of multiple digits is not unusual.

The thumb is most commonly involved, followed by the ring, long, little and index fingers [2]. Insulin-dependent diabetes mellitus has 10% incidence of trigger digits when compared to 2% of non-diabetes [3]. Various other diseases such as gout, rheumatoid arthritis, renal disease and other seronegative rheumatoid diseases are associated with trigger digits.

David Green has modified the Quinnell classification of trigger digits to provide the clinician a way to record the disease [4]:

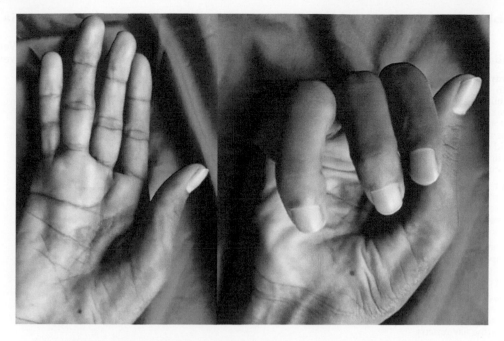

Figure 3.7 Clinical picture of finger scissoring (overlapping of the ring finger over little finger) suggests malrotation.

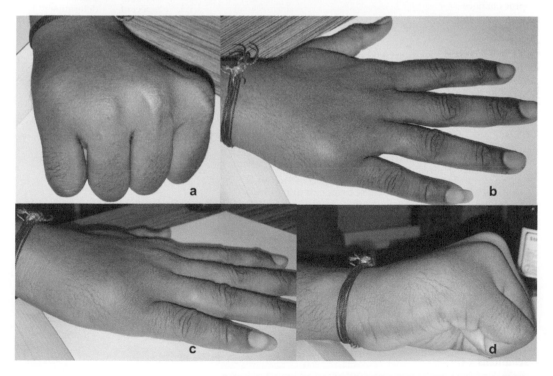

Figure 3.8 Metacarpal malunion results in apex dorsal angulation in the sagittal plane. Failure to correct dorsal angulation may not be associated with functional disability.

Table 3.4: Rating Subjective Symptoms According to the Budapest Criteria

Budapest Criteria	0, None	1, Mild	2, Moderate	3, Severe	4, Very Severe

Symptoms
Pain
Swelling
Weakness
Deformity
Discoloration
Cold sensitivity
Radiculopathy
Dystonia (movement)

Pain
Pain "out of proportion"
Sensory: Hyperaesthesia
Sensory: Hyperpathia
Sensory: Allodynia

Vasomotor Function
Temperature asymmetry
Skin colour changes
Skin colour asymmetry

Pseudomotor function
Oedema
Sweating changes
Sweating asymmetry
Other

Motor or trophic abnormality
Stiffness
Decreased range of motion
Trophic changes
Weakness
Tremor
Dystonia
Functional impairment

Proposed Refinement of Original Budapest Clinical Diagnostic Criteria for CRPS

1. Continuing pain that is disproportionate to any inciting event
2. Must report at least one symptom in three of the four following categories:
   • Sensory: report of hyperesthesia and/or allodynia
   • Vasomotor: reports of temperature asymmetry and/or skin color changes and/or skin color asymmetry
   • Sudomotor/edema: reports of edema and/or sweating changes and/or sweating asymmetry
   • Motor/trophic: reports of decreased range of motion and/or motor dysfunction (weaknesses, tremor, dystonia) and/or trophic changes (hair, nails, skin)
3. Must display at least one sign at time of evaluation in two or more of the following categories:
   • Sensory: evidence of hyperalgesia (to pinprick) and/or allodynia (to light touch and/or deep somatic pressure and/or joint movement)
   • Vasomotor: evidence of temperature asymmetry and/or skin color changes and/or asymmetry
   • Sudomotor/edema: evidence of edema and/or sweating changes and/or sweating asymmetry
   • Motor/trophic: evidence of decreased range of motion and/or motor dysfunction (weakness, tremor, systonia) and/or trophic changes (hair, nails, skin)
4. There is no other diagnosis that better explains the signs and symptoms

Grade 1 (pretriggering) – Pain, history of catching, but not demonstrable on physical examination, tenderness over the A1 pulley

Grade II (active) – Demonstrable catching, but the patient can actively extend the digit

Grade III (passive) – Demonstrable catching requiring passive extension (grade IIIA) or inability to actively flex (grade IIIB)

Grade IV (contracture) – Demonstrable catching with a fixed flexion contracture of the PIP joint

b. Congenital trigger thumb

The common cause of abnormal thumb posture in flexion or extension is termed as congenital trigger thumb. It is rare to see trigger in children, contrary to adults where they present with catch or popping. The incidence of unilateral congenital trigger thumb is 0.5% and bilateral is 25–33%. Though termed congenital, many authors reported that trigger thumb is overlooked at least during the first six months of age because of characteristic flexion posturing of the thumb in newborns.

MUSCLE WEAKNESS/WASTING

The examiner should assess the muscle wasting seen in the peripheral nerve injury or lesions (Table 3.5). Median nerve injury has thenar muscle wasting (abductor pollicis brevis and opponens) with resultant depression seen in the thenar eminence. Ape thumb deformity is seen, and the first metacarpal is seen on the radial aspect of the hand along the plane of radius (Figure 3.9).

Table 3.5: Muscle Grading System of the British Medical Research Council

Grade	Description
0	No contraction
1	Flicker or trace of contraction
2	Active movement with gravity eliminated
3	Active movement against gravity
4	Active movement against gravity and resistance
5	Normal power

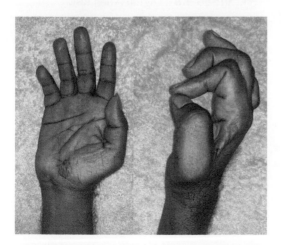

Figure 3.9 A case of low median nerve palsy with thenar atrophy and absent thumb abduction and opposition. The thumb extrinsic muscles (EPL, EPB) hyperextend the MCP joint and FPL causes IP joint flexion.

Ulnar nerve palsy has interossei wasting, depression of dorsum of the first webspace and dorsal wasting between metacarpals (Figure 3.10). Hypothenar atrophy is seen on the ulnar aspect of the palm.

Pain, weakness in flexion and supination with ecchymoses in the antecubital fossa or abnormal contour of the biceps suggest distal biceps rupture.

Hook Test (described by O'Driscoll and colleagues)

A test to assess intact biceps tendon by "hooking" the examiner's finger around biceps with elbow at 90° and in supination (Figure 3.11). The examiner can feel the tight distal biceps tendon. In case of rupture or avulsion, the hook test will not feel the tight tendon.

SWINGING OF SCAPULA

The patient is asked to flex their shoulders forward while raising their arms above their head. Scapular position and movement are noted with the movement and at end range of motion. As the arms are slowly lowered, the examiner looks for any winging of the scapula to evaluate for serratus anterior strength (Video 3.7).

TRAPEZIUS STRENGTH

The patient is asked to shrug the shoulders against resistance to check the degree and symmetry of muscle power. Also, feel the vertebral, clavicular and spinal portion of the muscle (Video 3.8).

EXAMINATION OF MUSCULOTENDINOUS UNITS

The extensor tendons are accessible to inspection and palpation because of the superficial location and thin dorsal skin on the hand. The examiner should inspect and palpate the tendons from radial to ulnar directions.

1. The abductor pollicis longus (APL) and extensor pollicis brevis (EPB) are seen between the radial styloid and the base of the first metacarpal (Figure 3.5).

2. The extensor pollicis longus (EPL) is seen running from the radial styloid to the ulnar base of the first metacarpal and attaches with the distal phalanx.

3. The extensor digitorum communis (EDC) and extensor indices proprius (EIP) lie in the axis of each metacarpal and can be felt up to the level of proximal phalanx.

4. The extensor carpi radialis longus (ECRL) and brevis (ECRB) are palpable for a short distance over the dorsum of the resisted extended wrist at the base of the second and third metacarpal.

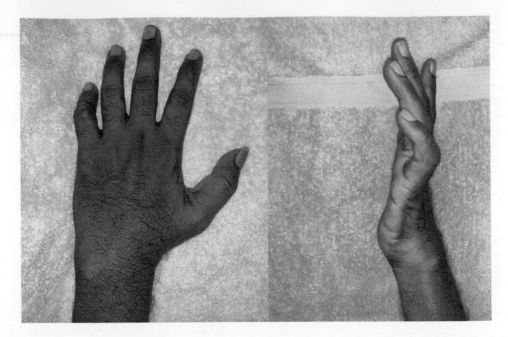

Figure 3.10 Claw hand with interossei wasting on the dorsum of the hand. Also, note hyperextension at MCP joint and flexion at the IP joints in fingers due to intrinsic paralysis.

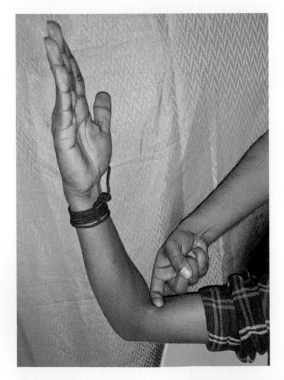

Figure 3.11 O'Driscoll and colleagues described the Hook test which involves assessment for intact biceps tendon by "hooking" the examiner's finger around the biceps with the elbow at 90°s and in supination.

Video 3.7   Allen test performed at the wrist level.

www.routledge.com/9780367647162.

Video 3.8   Digital Allen test.

www.routledge.com/9780367647162.

5. The extensor carpi ulnaris (ECU) is palpable during resisted extension and ulnar deviation of the wrist immediately distal to the ulnar styloid up to the fifth metacarpal.

6. The flexor carpi ulnaris and radialis (FCU, FCR) are felt on the ulnar and the radial aspect of the actively flexed and resisted wrist.

Physical examination includes manual muscle charting (Table 3.1). In addition to manual muscle charting, the examiner should evaluate joint movements (passive and active range of movements).

JOINT RANGE OF MOTION

A goniometer evaluates the active and passive range of motion in the hand and upper limb. It should not touch the digit or hand during active movements so as to prevent errors made

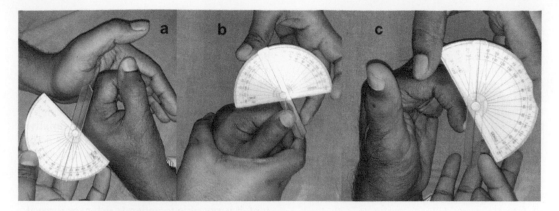

Figure 3.12 Methods to measure range of motion using goniometer.

by goniometer assistance. The limbs of the geometer should be short enough not to impede movements. Always place the goniometer on the dorsum of the fingers to measure the range of movements (Figure 3.12). The examiner should record active and passive movements for the involved digits/hand.

TOTAL ACTIVE AND PASSIVE MOTION (TAM)

The American Society for Surgery of the Hand (1976) set up a committee to recommend a formula for measuring total active and passive movements (Figure 3.12).

Total passive mobility = total passive flexion (MP + PIP + DIP) − lack of passive extension (metacarpophalangeal + proximal interphalangeal + distal interphalangeal).

Total active mobility = total active flexion (MP + PIP + DIP) − lack of active extension.

$$(MP + PIP + DIP).$$

BUCK–GRAMCKO'S METHOD

In 1976, Buck–Gramcko proposed a method involving composite flexion, extension deficit, total active motion and flexion deficit (Table 3.6). He preferred that examination should be done in slight wrist extension and no support.

a) Composite flexion: The sum of the angular measurement of flexion of all three joints.

b) Extension deficit: The sum of the angular measurements of loss of extension of all three joints.

c) Total active motion: The difference between the composite flexion and extension deficits.

d) Flexion deficit: The distance between the finger and the distal palmar crease.

DEFORMITIES

Examination of individual joints and associated deformities is an essential part of physical examination:

1. Boutonnière deformity

The boutonnière deformity is caused by a lesion in the central slip tendon producing flexion at the proximal interphalangeal joint (PIP) and hyperextension at the distal interphalangeal joint (DIP). The etiologies include traumatic rupture, division or degeneration due to rheumatoid arthritis of the central slip of the extensor apparatus on the dorsum of the PIP joint.

Table 3.6: Buck–Gramcko's Method

Distance finger pulp	0–2.5 cm	≥200°	6 points
Distal composite flexion crease	2.5–4 cm	≥180°	4 points
	4–6 cm	≥150°	2 points
	>6 cm	<150°	6 points
Extension deficit		0–30°	3 points
			2 points
		51–70°	1 point
		>70°	0 points
Total active motion		≥160°	6 points
		≥140°	4 points
		≥120°	2 points
		<120°	0 points

Classification
Excellent: 14–15 points
Good: 11–13 points
Satisfactory: 7–10 points
Poor: 0–6 points

Because of the central slip injury, the proximal phalanx head buttonholes through the gap in the extensor apparatus. The lateral bands of the extensor apparatus dislocate to the volar side causing flexion of the PIP joint. Also, the flexion is exaggerated by the pull of the long flexor tendons. The extension force required to extend the PIP joint is diverted to the lateral bands which lie volar to the PIP joint axis and attached finally in the dorsum of the distal phalanx, thus hyperextending the DIP joint.

ELSON TEST

When the PIP joint is passively flexed completely, the central slip insertion is pulled distally along with its proximal attachments,

and "slack" is created between the lateral band insertions on the terminal tendon and the lateral connections of the central slip to the lateral band (Figure 3.13) [4]. This slack can be easily appreciated by manually assessing the resistance to passive flexion of the DIP joint with the PIP joint fully extended versus fully flexed. This elegant mechanism permits full flexion of the DIP joint when the PIP joint is maximally flexed (Figure 3.13(a)). A corollary is that active extension of the DIP joint becomes impossible when the PIP joint is fully flexed because of the slack in the lateral bands (see Figure 3.13(b)).

When the central slip is injured or incompetent, it is possible to generate extensor force at the DIP joint with maximal passive PIP joint

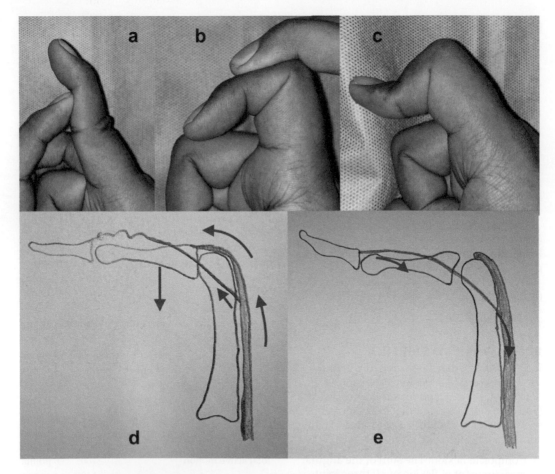

Figure 3.13 (a) The examiner keeps passive PIP joint extension in maximum which prohibits full DIP joint flexion by normal tension in lateral bands. (b) The examiner keeps the PIP joint flexion in full which allows slack in the lateral bands and permits full DIP joint flexion. (c) In a central slip injury, DIP joint can be actively extended with maximum PIP joint flexion. (d) Schematic diagram shows maximal passive flexion of PIP joint induce slack in the lateral bands via proximal interconnections, resulting in loss of power of active DIP joint extension and increased DIP joint flexion. (e) Schematic diagram shows injury to central slip, eliminates the slack in the lateral bands produced by passive PIP joint flexion and allows extensor tension to be generated at DIP joint. This is the basis for the Elson test.

Video 3.9 Demonstration of flexor tenosynovitis.

www.routledge.com/9780367647162.

flexion, which is the basis of the Elson test for detecting acute central slip rupture. As described by Elson, the examiner passively flexes the PIP joint 90° to the tabletop and asks the patient to attempt active extension of the PIP joint while the examiner resists PIP joint extension. When acute rupture of the central slip occurs, no extension power is felt at the PIP joint but significant extension power, or hyperextension, is produced at the DIP joint. This test has been found to be the most sensitive physical examination test to detect acute central slip rupture (Video 3.9).

2. Swan-neck deformity

Hyper extension at the PIP joint with flexion at the DIP joint is termed as swan-neck deformity. One of the common pathologies seen here is excessive traction on the central slip insertion at the middle phalanx base and dorsal translation of the lateral bands (Figure 3.14). Because of the excessive traction of the central slip and dorsal translation of the lateral bands, the extension effect on the distal phalanx diminishes, thus flexing the DIP joint.

To begin with, the swan-neck deformity is reducible, but the deformity becomes fixed if neglected or untreated. Various factors contribute to the swan-neck deformities:

a) Articular: Fractures, dislocations at the PIP joints.

b) Interosseous muscle contractures (volar subluxation of the proximal phalanx brings the interosseous tendons dorsal to the MCP joint axis directing the extensor force to the extensor apparatus culminating in a swan-neck deformity).

c) Chronic flexion wrist deformity.

d) Extensor digitorum communis (EDC) injury proximal to MCP joint.

3. Ulnar deviation of the fingers

Normal extension of the fingers has normal and physiological ulnar deviation. When the ligaments and capsules rupture, divide or degenerate due to rheumatoid arthritis, pathological ulnar deviation occurs. Ulnar deviation of the EDC tendon is seen on the ulnar side of the MCP joint.

4. Extensor-plus syndrome

Shortening of the extensor tendon, adherence, postburn contractures proximal to the MCP joint cause inability to flex the MCP and PIP joint simultaneously. Individually, the MCP and PIP joint can be flexed but not together.

5. Mallet finger

Injury, rupture, avulsion or chronic elongation (inflammatory) of the terminal extensor tendon produces mallet finger with loss of active DIP joint extension (Figure 3.15).

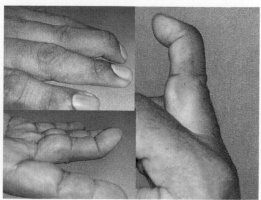

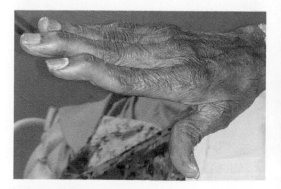

Figure 3.14 Swan-neck deformity (hyperextension of the PIP joint with flexion at the DIP joint) seen in a woman with rheumatoid arthritis.

Figure 3.15 Mallet finger is characterized by discontinuity of the terminal extensor tendon resulting in an extensor lag at the DIP joint with or without compensatory hyperextension at the PIP joint.

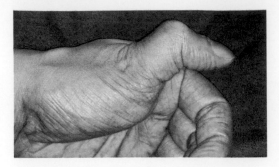

Figure 3.16 Z-deformity of the thumb. Flexion at the CMC joint, hyperextension at the MCP joint and IP joint flexion. Weak or ruptured dorsal stabilizing ligament at the CMC joint causes dorsal subluxation, overstretched volar plate at the MCP joint with taught flexor pollicis longus causes the deformity.

6. Ulnar claw hand

Hyperextension of the MCP joint and flexion at the interphalangeal (IP) joints produces claw hand and it is usually appreciated in the ring and the little finger. This is seen in low ulnar nerve palsy because of loss of interosseous muscle function and active long flexors flexing the IP joints. High ulnar nerve palsy has minimal claw deformity because of the absent long flexor function. The index and middle fingers have lumbricals innervated by the median nerve which does the function of the interosseous muscle, thus exhibiting no claw deformity. There are specific tests to elicit ulnar and median nerve palsy (described in the ulnar nerve palsy chapter (Chapter 8C) and median nerve palsy chapter (Chapter 8B)).

7. Z-deformity of the thumb

Hyper extension of the IP joint of the thumb with lack of active extension of the MCP joint produces Z-deformity of the thumb. Trauma, rupture, interruption, volar dislocation of the extensor pollicis brevis and rheumatoid arthritis are the well-known reasons for this deformity (Figure 3.16).

8. Adducted thumb

Contracture of adductor pollicis and first dorsal interosseous muscle produces first web space narrowing and adducted thumb. In addition, the thumb has a compensatory MP joint hyperextension causing a boutonnière deformity. First CMC joint arthritis (inflammatory or degenerative) is a classic example for adducted thumb deformity.

9. Thumb-in-palm deformity

Flexion and adduction of the thumb at the MCP joint with extension at the IP joint is thumb-in-palm deformity (Figure 3.17). It is the most complex problem of the upper extremity, seen especially in cerebral palsy with multilevel joint involvement (CMC, MCP and IP joints). This deformity will interfere with grasp and all thumb activities. Five key elements have to be considered in this deformity:

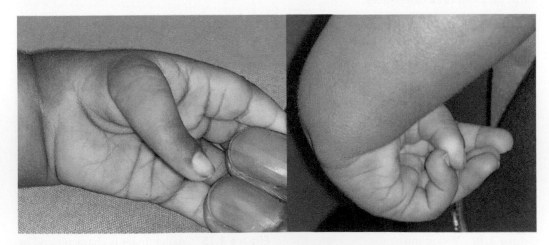

Figure 3.17 Thumb-in-palm deformity: Clinical picture showing thumb flexed at MCP joint and IP joints extended and adducted into the palm with first webspace contracture. The examiner appreciates the deformity better done in wrist flexion and extension. This deformity prevents grasp and manipulation of objects.

a) Spastic flexors and adductors.

b) Flaccid extensors and abductors.

c) Hypermobile MCP joint.

d) Webspace skin contracture.

e) Volkmann's angle (Figure 3.18) – the angle indicates severity and degrees of spasticity and shortening. This angle may help us to choose the type of technique necessary to achieve flexor lengthening.

The spasticity between the flexor digitorum superficialis and flexor digitorum profundus tendons at each finger should be differentiated. This is best done by placing the wrist in maximum extension and passively extending the proximal and distal inter-phalangeal joints. Limited passive extension of the proximal and distal inter-phalangeal joints indicates flexor digitorum superficialis and profundus spasticity, respectively.

VASCULAR EXAMINATION
Circulation

Clinical examination of the patient is not complete without vascular examination. Physical examination is the clinical and primary method to evaluate patients with vascular diseases. It is vital to look for radial pulse in both upper extremities. The radial artery lies more superficial

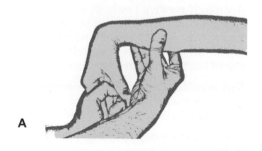

A

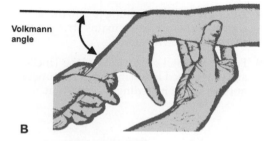

Volkmann angle

B

Figure 3.18 Volkmann angle: The examiner brings the wrist from maximum palmar flexion to extension with the fingers extended. The angle at which the digits go into a flexed posture is called the Volkmann angle.

in the forearm running under the anterior aspect of the brachioradialis. It crosses the supinator to enter the anterior and radial aspect of the forearm. We can palpate the radial pulse between the brachioradialis and flexor carpi radialis at the wrist. In 10% of individuals, a persistent median artery is felt along the course of the median nerve. The persistent median artery contributes to form the superficial arch and passes deep to the transverse carpal ligament.

Assessment of the Vascularity

1. Colour: The examiner should note whether the skin or the fingers are pale, red or cyanosed. Also, look for evidence of gangrene or ulcerations. Feel the warmth of the hand to rule out sympathetic overactivity in the presence of nerve compression.

2. Distal arterial flow: The examiner should measure the time taken for the colour to return to the nailbed after pressure. The digital–brachial index, which is the ratio of the blood pressure as measured in the brachial artery and the finger, can be measured with small blood pressure cuffs. This is similar to the ankle–brachial index, and in the upper extremity any value below 0.7 is felt to designate a significant occlusive problem somewhere in the forearm or hand.

3. Pulse:
   a) Radial pulse: The radial artery pulse is felt at the radial wrist groove, anatomical snuff box, proximal part of the dorsal first webspace.
   b) Ulnar pulse: The ulnar pulse is felt at the entry to the Guyon's canal.
   c) Digital pulse: The collateral digital arteries are felt at the base of the finger just anterior to the dorsopalmar cutaneous line.

4. Arterial territories: An Allen test assists in deciding whether the radial or ulnar artery is responsible for the major artery supply to the hand. An Allen test (Figures 3.19 and 3.20) (Videos 3.10 and 3.11) manoeuvre is performed at the wrist level and repeated to look for the predominant blood supply. Usually, radial artery remains the predominant artery supply for the hand.

5. Venous return: The venous return or insufficiency is difficult to measure. Oedema is the common feature of abnormal venous return. Localized cyanosis is a sign of venous stasis.

6. Oedema hand: Dorsal hand oedema is obvious with fullness in the hand. Minimal oedema is seen around the metacarpal

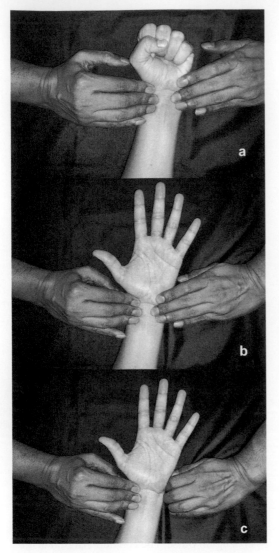

contours. Also, there is disappearance of shallow transverse furrows which are otherwise seen in normal dorsal skin. Palmar hand oedema has fullness and obliteration of the concavity between the thenar and hypothenar eminence. In addition, oedema limits finger flexion.

TINEL'S SIGN

Tinel's sign is one of the most valuable indicators in medicine and if properly elicited and interpreted, permits the clinician to understand the level and the severity of a nerve lesion and, in later examinations, to show whether regeneration is occurring. Tinel's sign is detectable on the day of injury. The sign is of supreme importance in the urgent analysis of a closed-traction lesion of the brachial plexus or peripheral nerve injuries.

METHOD

The examiner's finger taps (percussion) along the course of the affected nerve in distal-to-proximal direction and evokes strong, indeed painful, sensory symptoms distally over the nerve's cutaneous distribution (Table 3.7). When the finger percusses over the zone of regenerating fibres, the patient feels a sensation of pins and needles, which may be quite painful, in the cutaneous distribution of the nerve. The clinical significance of the Tinel's sign can be summarized as follows:

1. A strongly positive Tinel's sign over a lesion soon after injury indicates rupture of the axons. This sign has been found regularly on the day of injury, most especially with a closed traction rupture.

2. Regeneration of axons, either spontaneous or after repair of the nerve, can be confirmed when the Tinel's sign is centrifugally moving.

Tinel's sign is persistently stronger than that at the suture line.

■ After a repair that is going to fail, the Tinel's sign at the suture line remains stronger than that at the growing point.

■ Failure of distal progression of the Tinel's sign in a closed lesion indicates rupture or another lesion impeding regeneration.

Figure 3.19 Allen test: The patient is asked to raise and clench his hand to squeeze the blood out of the cutaneous vascular bed. (a) The examiner compresses the radial artery in the radial groove and the ulnar artery in the Guyon's canal. (b) The patient opens his hand without hyperextending his fingers. The palm appears exsanguinated. (c) The examiner releases one compression and notes the time taken for the palm to recover its normal pink colour. The manoeuvre is repeated to test the ulnar artery.

 Video 3.10 Demonstration of the Finklestein test. Finkelstein's test: The examiner rests the patient hand over a support and asks them to ulnar deviate the wrist. Slight traction of the thumb and flexing it causes severe and excruciating pain.

www.routledge.com/9780367647162.

Video 3.11 Demonstration of the Eichhoff's test. Eichhoff's test: The examiner instructs the patient to grip the thumb in the palm by the other fingers and passively ulnar deviate their wrist. The patient experiences severe and excruciating pain proximal to styloid process of the wrist. Stretching the tendons and sheath of the first dorsal compartment cause pain in de Quervain's tenosynovitis. Eichhoff's manoeuvre produces a greater degree of ulnar deviation of the wrist, because the patient's entire hand is abducted ulnarward by the examiner rather than just the thumb in Finkelstein's test.

www.routledge.com/9780367647162.

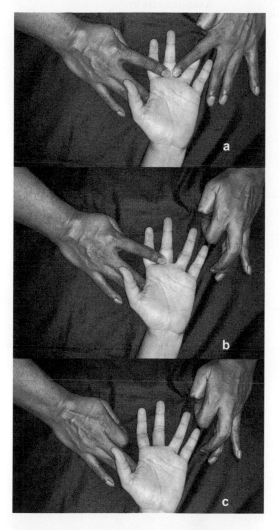

Figure 3.20 Digital Allen test: (a) The test is performed at the base of the finger similar to the Allen test at the wrist level. (b, c) Release of one digital artery at a time may reveal a unilateral occlusion. This test is useful to diagnose digital artery thrombosis.

■ The Tinel's sign advances more swiftly in cases of axonotmesis (i.e., ~2 mm/day) than it does after nerve repair. It is also faster in

the proximal segment of the limb than in the distal. In the axilla, rates of progress of 3 mm/day are not unusual.

FUNCTIONAL ANATOMY OF THE HAND
Dorsum of the Hand

The dorsum of the hand is one cutaneous unit which extends from the wrist to the proximal interphalangeal (PIP) joints and the interphalangeal joint of the thumb. Excess dorsal skin is seen over the interphalangeal joints to promote mobility and excursion. The dorsal aspect of the middle phalanx is fine and tight. The nailbed with its matrix over the distal phalanx is integument with the distal phalanx.

PALMAR SURFACE OF THE HAND

The palm extends from the distal transverse crease of the wrist to the transverse crease at the base of the digits. The palmar skin is divided into two separate zones by the oppositional thumb crease. The radial skin is well vascularized, covering the thenar eminence and the external part of the mobile aspect of the palm. The ulnar skin and the distal portion cover the hypothenar eminence which is less mobile. The distal part of the palm beyond the distal transverse crease is the true hinge and lies at the level of the MCP joint. The central triangular portion of the palm is fixed and poorly vascular. This covers the superficial palmar aponeurosis.

WHY SKIN INCISIONS IN THE HAND ARE ZIGZAG (BRUNNER'S)

Littler (1974) explains the area of contact in the flexed and extended digits. The integument of the palmar skin is divided into phalangeal units [5]. The phalangeal units are separated by three digital flexion folds in the fingers and two flexion folds in the thumb allowing coordinated flexion movements. The contact region is a diamond shape in finger extension and the sides of the diamond do not undergo variations in the length during the flexion and extension

Table 3.7: Tinel's Sign

Tinel Percussion	Painful Sensory Symptoms	Nerve Involved	Remarks
Posterior triangle of the neck	As far as elbow	C5	85% sensitive
Posterior triangle of the neck	radial aspect of the forearm and to the thumb	C6	90% sensitive
Posterior triangle of the neck	Dorsum of the hand	C7	90% sensitive

Depth of Nerve Injury		
	Conduction Block	Axonotmesis or Neurotmesis
Etiology	Compression Low-energy transfer of long bone fracture	Open injuries High-energy fractures and dislocations
Loss of sensory modalities	Some preserved, usually pinprick (sharp/dull)	All modalities absent
Muscle power	Paralysis sometimes patchy and incomplete	Complete paralysis
Sympathetic function	Usually preserved	Sympathetic paralysis (injured part is warm and dry)
Tinel's sign	Absent	Present

movements of the fingers (Figure 3.21). This is the reason we prefer Brunner's incision in the fingers which will not undergo retraction or contraction during the finger movements. Also, Brunner's incision gives excellent exposure for all flexor, neurovascular and bone surgeries.

In order to minimize hypertrophic scars, the incision should not be vertical and should not cross the flexion crease.

WEBSPACE

The webspace is formed by the two (dorsal and palmar) non-symmetrical cutaneous surfaces. The dorsal slope has a gradual incline and supple skin not adhered to the adjacent regions. The palmar surface is flat, precipitously interrupted and densely adhered to the commissural skeleton. The interdigital palmar (natatory) ligament between the fingers and distal transverse ligament at the level of the thumb forms the commissural skeleton. Surgeons should take into account the contour of these cutaneous features and webspace anatomy (Figure 3.22).

PULP

The pulp is a highly specialized tissue for the fingertip made up of integrated fibrofatty septa, sweat glands and sensory organs. The pulp is essential for prehensile function, grasp and papillary crest ensuring good adhesions. The subcutaneous tissue is thick, malleable and is

formed by the fatty tissues separated by fibrous septa. These septa create small fibrous fat-filled compartments providing a union between the dermis and the periosteum limiting the pulp skin glide over the distal phalanx. The pulp is

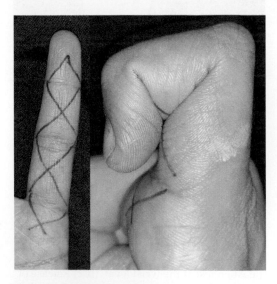

Figure 3.21 The areas of cutaneous contact in fingers. These contact regions are diamond shaped when the digit is extended. The sides of the diamond undergo little variation in length during flexion-extension movements, and any incision made along their lines will not retract.

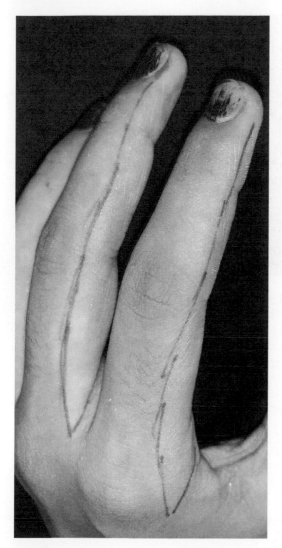

Figure 3.22 Dorsal view of the first and second commissures. The dorsum of the web slopes gently and the skin is supple and non-adherent.

fixed against the distal phalanx and nail providing support for the fingertip (Figure 3.23).

FINGERNAILS

The nail on the distal phalanx provides support to the pulp allowing precise grip to pick small objects and enhances the pulp sensibility. The fingernail is composed of nomenclatures such as perionychium, paronychium, eponychium, nail plate, nailfold, nailbed, cuticle, lunula and hyponychium (Figure 3.24). The perionychium is formed by the nailbed and the tissue around the sides and base of the nail. The sides and base of the nail are called the paronychium. The proximal end of the nail is enfolded into a depression on the finger called the nailfold. The skin over the dorsum of the nailfold is the nail wall. The eponychium is a thin membrane extending from the nail wall to the dorsum of the nail. The nail cuticle or vest is a stratified and cornified material seen between the eponychium and the nail (Figure 3.25).

The lunula is a convex white area seen at the nail base. The nail plate separates the dorsal roof from the ventral roof of the nailfold. The nail bed has two portions namely germinal matrix and sterile matrix. The hyponychium is the keratinized skin between the distal nail and fingertip. The anastomosis between the lateral arteries of the finger forms two arterial arch, runs above the periosteum of the distal phalanx and supply nailbed.

PALMAR CREASES

The palmar creases are "flexion creases" corresponding to the lines along which the skin is folded when the hand is closed. The exception is the opposition crease which forms the boundary of the thenar eminence. Distal and proximal creases are seen in the palm marking the dermal termination of numerous longitudinal fibres of the palmar fascia. The distal palmar crease lies in the ulnar half of the palm and runs proximal to the medial metacarpophalangeal joint. The proximal crease lies in the radial half and well above these joints. The central portion of the palm (poorly vascularized) is in shape and fixed to the underlying skin and covers the entire superficial palmar aponeurosis.

SIGNIFICANCE OF PALMAR CREASES

Closing your fingers involves the sequence where in the metacarpophalangeal joints is flexed first and subsequently the proximal on the distal interphalangeal joints flexed. Any disturbances in this sequence will make closing of fingers, grasping or fist impossible. Also, the amplitude of flexion, strength with which objects are held, range of mobility of flexors tendons, suppleness of joints, flexion power and soft tissue pliability are appreciated in terms of distal palmar crease (Figure 3.25).

In cases of severe flexion deficit, the pulp fails to reach the palm and the overall flexion deficit is measured as palm-pulp distance (Figure 3.26). The surgical incision should never cross a flexion crease vertically but should be broken by an angled or Z-plasty. This prevents hypertrophic scar formation.

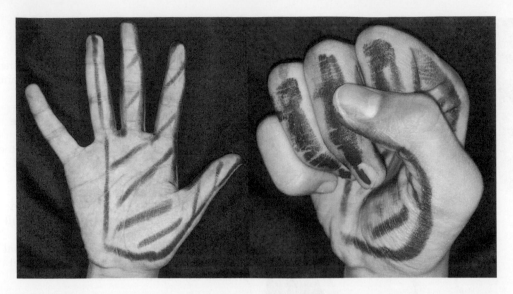

Figure 3.23 The median nerve supplies lateral 3½ volar aspect of the hand and fingertips of the index, middle and ring fingers. During a fist, the thumb approximates with index and middle finger which are all innervated by median nerve.

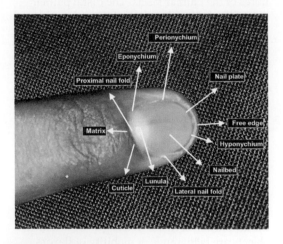

Figure 3.24 Fingernail complex.

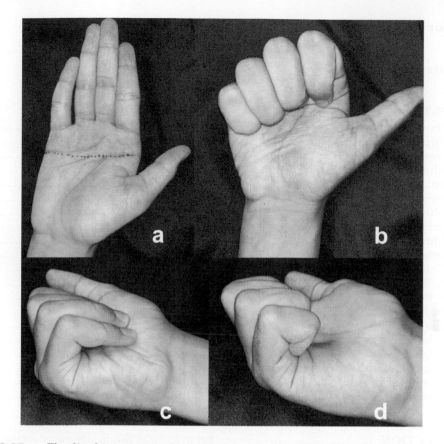

Figure 3.25 a. The distal transverse palmar crease is defined as a transverse line joining the ulnar end of the distal palmar crease to the radial end of the proximal crease. b. Four fingertips (pulp) can be actively brought into contact with the palm along this transverse line in a normal hand. c. Patience with isolated interphalangeal joint stiffness manage their digital pulps to touch proximal to the palmar crease. This is because of the compensation happened by hyper flexing the metacarpophalangeal joints. d. In an isolated metacarpophalangeal joints stiffness, the pulps touch the palm distal to the palmar crease, because of the compensatory hyper flexion at the interphalangeal joints.

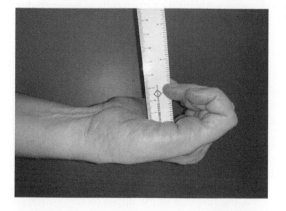

Figure 3.26 The palm-pulp distance is measured in centimetres when the fingers cannot reach the palm (finger stiffness, flexor adhesions, etc.).

REFERENCES

1. Sampson SP, Badalamente MA, Hurst LC, et al. Pathobiology of the human A1 pulley in trigger finger. *J Hand Surg [Am]* 16(4):714–721, 1991.

2. Fahey JJ and Bollinger JA. Trigger-finger in adults and children. *J Bone Joint Surg Am* 36(6):1200–1218, 1954.

3. Patel MR and Bassini L. Trigger fingers and thumb: When to splint, inject, or operate. *J Hand Surg [Am]* 17(1):110–113, 1992.

4. Elson RA. Rupture of the central slip of the extensor hood of the finger. A test for early diagnosis. *J Bone Joint Surg Br* 68:229–231, 1986.

5. Littler JW. Hand, wrist and forearm incisions. In: Littler JW, Cramer LM and Smith JW, eds, *Symposium on Reconstructive Hand Surgery*, St Louis: CV Mosby, 1974.

4 Motor Neurological Examination of the Hand and Upper Limb

G Karthikeyan

CONTENTS

INTRODUCTION

For any machine to move, a power source or motor is needed, a transmission agent that links or conveys the power to the machine is essential, and the actual machine itself which can move to do the work must be available.

When we compare this analogy to the hand, the muscle is the motor, the tendons and soft tissues form the transmission agent and the actual moving parts are the joints of the hand and upper limb.

When considering the motor system of the hand, we are actually studying the muscles, their ability to function and the intactness of the nerves supplying them. It is not just the contraction of the muscle fibres that is important, but also the capability of the muscle to relax and stretch when needed.

This ability of the muscles to function, based on their neurological supply, can be compromised in two situations: Upper motor neuron lesions and the lower motor neuron lesions. The upper motor neuron lesion involves any part of the upper motor neuronal pathway and the lower motor neuron lesion involves any part of the lower motor neuronal pathway.

The Upper Motor Neuronal Pathway

There is an elaborate pathway (Figure 4.1) to control the function of the muscles. The signals begin in the opposite side motor cortex, travel down through the internal capsule, then the brain stem, consisting of the crus cerebri in the mid-brain, pons and pyramids in the medulla, and then most of the fibres (about 85%) decussate at the pyramidal level and then descend in the lateral corticospinal tract to the anterior horn cells of the corresponding segment of the spinal cord. These upper motor neurons synapse with anterior horn cells of lower motor neurons, usually via interneurons.

Some fibres do not decussate at the pyramids (15%) but continue down the spinal cord on the same side, forming the ventral spinothalamic tract to the corresponding segment of the spinal cord. Only here do they decussate to reach the anterior horn cells of the opposite side.

Both these corticospinal tracts are referred to as the pyramidal tracts. Within these corticospinal tracts the fibres to the cervical upper motor neurons are located centrally and the motor neurons to the lumbar and sacral region are located peripherally.

So, the function of the upper motor neurons is to transmit information from the brain to the spinal cord. Lesions can occur in the brain or the spinal cord and affect this upper motor neuron tract.

When such lesions occur in the upper motor neuron system, the clinical manifestations seen

DOI: 10.1201/9781003125938-4

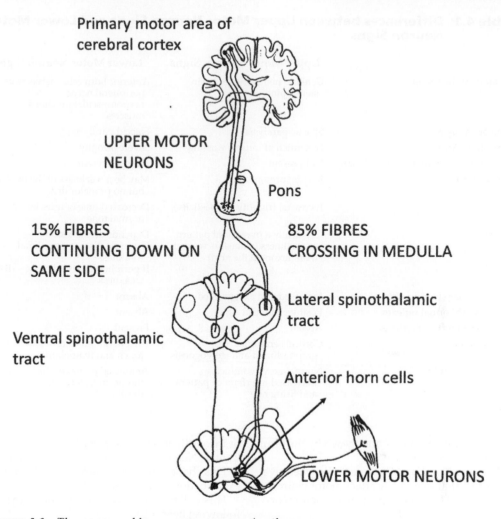

Figure 4.1 The upper and lower motor neuronal pathways.

can be muscle weakness and decreased control of active movement, particularly slowness and spasticity.

Stroke, multiple sclerosis, Friedrich ataxia, traumatic brain injury, cerebral palsy, atypical Parkinsonisms, multiple system atrophy and amyotrophic lateral sclerosis are some of the lesions that can cause upper motor neuron disruption.

The Lower Motor Neuronal Pathway

Once the upper motor neurons reach the spinal cord and synapse at the anterior horn cells, the lower motor neuron pathway begins (Figure 4.1). The cell body of these neurons are the anterior horn cells, and these neurons leave in the ventral root of the spinal nerve. After they are joined by the dorsal root, they form the proper spinal nerve and leave the spinal canal via the intervertebral foramen.

From here, they combine with other spinal nerves to form the brachial plexus, and ultimately reach the neuromuscular junction of the designated muscles.

The lower motor neurons are of different types, based on the type of muscle fibre they innervate [1]. They are discussed in detail in the segment on "reflexes."

Damage to any part of the lower motor neuron tract can cause lower motor neuron lesions (LMNL). They usually manifest as muscle wasting (atrophy), decreased strength and decreased reflexes in affected areas.

A summary of differences between upper motor neuron lesions and lower motor neuron lesions can be seen in Table 4.1.

Apart from the characteristic upper and lower motor neuron lesions that we have seen above, there may be some presentations with findings of both. These lesions with a finding

Table 4.1: Differences between Upper Motor Neuron Signs and Lower Motor Neuron Signs

	Upper Motor Neuron Signs	Lower Motor Neuron Signs
Location of the lesion	Cerebral hemispheres, brain stem, spinal cord	Anterior horn cells, nerve roots, peripheral nerves, neuromuscular junctions, muscles
Type of paralysis	Spastic paralysis	Flaccid paralysis
Inspection: Atrophy	Not much of muscle wasting	Severe atrophy
Inspection: Fasciculation/fibrillation	Not present	May be present
Pronator drift	May be present	May be a weakness of the muscles, but no pronator drift
Tone	Increased (rigidity or spasticity)	Decreased tone of muscles or normal tone
Power	Classically a pyramidal pattern of weakness (extensors weaker than flexors in the arm)	Depends on the lesion: If muscle disease – proximal weakness If peripheral nerve disease – distal weakness
Reflexes: Deep tendon reflexes	Increased and exaggerated	Absent
Reflexes: Abnormal reflexes	Positive Babinski sign	Absent
Reflexes: Superficial reflexes	Absent	Present
Sensory loss	Cortical sensations, like graphesthesia and stereognosis	Peripheral sensations, like pain, touch and temperature
Electromyography	Normal nerve conduction, decreased interference pattern and firing rate	Abnormal nerve conduction, large motor units, fasciculations and fibrillations

of both UMN and LMN are known by the term "motor neurone disease."

These are a group of rare neurodegenerative disorders that selectively affect motor neurons, which could be either upper motor neuron or lower motor neuron [2].

The conditions that can cause motor neurone disease (MND) could be amyotrophic lateral sclerosis (ALS), progressive bulbar palsy (PBP), pseudobulbar palsy, progressive muscular atrophy (PMA), primary lateral sclerosis (PLS) and monomelic amyotrophy (MMA), as well as some rarer variants resembling ALS.

The clinical findings in such patients with MND could include some UMNL features and some LMNL features. There can be lower motor neuron findings (e.g., muscle wasting, muscle twitching), upper motor neuron findings (e.g., brisk reflexes, Babinski reflex, Hoffmann's reflex, increased muscle tone) or both [3].

For example, in ALS, features will denote both upper motor and lower motor involvement, in PLS there will be features suggesting involvement of the upper motor neurons, and in PMA, lower motor neuron symptoms will predominate.

So only a good and structured clinical examination will help to make a clear clinical diagnosis. This will be required in any patient presenting with weakness, imbalance or incoordination, or as part of generalized Central Nervous System (CNS) examination.

This chapter deals specifically with the motor examination of the upper limb.

This will be discussed in detail under the following headings:

- Inspection
- Tone
- Power
- Co-ordination
- Reflexes
- Special considerations in children

Before the motor examination begins, preparation needs to be made and the procedure of the examination understood.

Procedure

Remember the mnemonic "WINE gives PEP"

Wash your hands, and don PPE

Introduce yourself

Name of patient to be confirmed and if necessary, the date of birth

Explain the procedure

Permission and consent to examine the motor system must be obtained

Expose adequately for examination of the upper limb

Position: Comfortably sitting on edge of couch or lying on the couch in 45° recline and make sure that they do not have any pain.

Then begins the examination.

INSPECTION

The first step of any clinical examination is inspection. There are several findings that can be made out in a very thorough inspection of the patient and the upper limb.

In order not to miss out any inspection finding, the features to be examined are the following, in the same order:

A. General appearance

B. Abnormal movements

C. Scars

D. Muscle bulk

A. **General appearance:** The general appearance of the patient who is being examined, must be noted, for two important reasons:
   i. He must be capable of comprehending the test that is being done.
   ii. Any alteration of the general condition may point to a lesion that is contributing to the clinical condition.

   In assessing the general condition, the following features must be noted and recorded.

   - The level of consciousness

   - The attention from the patient to the proceedings

   - The orientation with respect to space and time

   - The fluency and ability to comprehend the language that is supposed to be comfortable for the patient

   - Memory for events – recent and old

   - Intellectual function and mood

B. **Abnormal movements:** There are some abnormal movements that should be checked for. Here is a description of the abnormal movements that can occur and the significance of the movements:
   1. **Tremors**: These are rhythmic, oscillatory movements of the limbs or trunk. They can occur due to lesions of the cerebellum, sensory system, motor system or even the basal ganglia. Tremors are the most commonly seen abnormal movements in clinical practice.

   Tremors may present as:

   - Rhythmic shaking in the hands, arms, head, legs or torso

   - Shaky voice

   - Difficulty writing or drawing

   - Problems holding and controlling utensils, such as a spoon

Some tremors may be triggered by or become worse during times of stress or strong emotion, when an individual is physically exhausted, or when a person is in certain postures or makes certain movements.

There are different types of tremors and understanding the types is the basis of understanding the control of the motor system of the body.

   Basically, there are two types of tremors: Resting tremors and action tremors.
   a. **Resting tremors** occur when the muscle is relaxed, like when the hands are resting on the lap and the person's hands may shake even when they are in this position of rest. The tremor only affects the hand or the fingers. This type of tremor is usually seen in people with Parkinson's disease (PD) and is called a "pillrolling" tremor because the circular finger and hand movements resemble rolling of small objects or pills in the hand. The frequency of this tremor is about 3–6 Hz (oscillations per second). These tremors are classified as slow tremors.
   b. **Action tremors** occur with the voluntary movement of a muscle. Most of the types of tremor fall under this category.
      i. **Postural tremor** occurs when a person maintains a position against gravity, such as holding the arms outstretched. These tremors are usually in the range of 5–9 Hz (intermediate tremors).
      ii. **Kinetic tremor** is associated with any voluntary

movement, such as moving the wrists up and down or closing and opening the eyes.

   iii. **Intention tremor** is produced with purposeful movement toward a target, such as lifting a finger to touch the nose. This type of tremor will become worse as an individual gets closer to their target.

   iv. **Task-specific tremor** only appears when performing highly skilled, goal-oriented tasks such as handwriting or speaking.

   v. **Isometric tremor** occurs during a voluntary muscle contraction that is not accompanied by any movement such as holding a heavy book or a dumbbell in the same position.

Action tremors are usually seen with lesions of the cerebellum or the sensory system and may also be idiopathic (benign familial tremor or senile tremor). Action tremors may also be rapid tremors (3 to 10 Hz).

2. **Fasciculations**: The second most common type of abnormal movement that is seen in practice are fasciculations. They are worm-like contractions of muscle due to random discharge of an entire motor unit, which refers to all of the muscle fibres attached to a single motor neuron. These can be felt and often seen. They are random and involuntary occurrences and do not result in movement of a joint. These can be seen in the following situations:

   i. Anterior horn cell disorders: Associated with frequent fasciculations in conditions like ALS.

   ii. LMN lesions: In such situations, fasciculations are accompanied by weakness, decreased tone and after some time, loss of muscle bulk.

   iii. Normal individuals: Fasciculations are sometimes seen with simple muscle fatigue following exercise and are of no clinical consequence. These will not be associated with any weakness or other motor system abnormalities.

3. **Myoclonus**: This refers to brief, involuntary, irregular twitching of a muscle or group of muscles that move an entire limb across a joint. All individuals experience benign myoclonus on occasion (e.g., whilst falling asleep); however, persistent widespread myoclonus is associated with several specific forms of epilepsy (e.g., juvenile myoclonic epilepsy). Myoclonus is also frequently seen with metabolic or hereditary neurologic disorders.

4. **Chorea, athetosis and hemiballism**: Brief, irregular, asymmetric writhing movements of basal ganglia origin.

   i. Chorea is a rapid, fleeting, random and non-stereotyped movement which is worsened by anxiety, and which can be suppressed for short periods by conscious effort. It occurs due to lesions of the basal ganglia. This may be due to causes like a type of cerebral palsy, post infectious (Sydenham's chorea), hereditary (Huntington's chorea), metabolic (Wilson's disease) or cerebrovascular.

   ii. Athetosis is a slow, writhing, snakelike movement of body part or parts more proximally.

   iii. Dystonia is a sustained twisting of the body, usually the trunk or neck.

   iv. Hemiballism is a flinging motion of one side of the body, potentially resulting in falls.

5. **Other abnormal movements**:

   i. Pseudoathetosis:abnormalwrithing movements (typically affecting the fingers) caused by a failure of proprioception and indicates disruption of the proprioceptive pathway, from nerve to parietal cortex.

   ii. Hemipseudoaothetosis refers to pseudoathetosis on one side of the body, usually the upper limb and is most commonly caused by a lesion affecting the cuneate tract or cuneate nucleus in the cervical spine or lower brainstem (medulla), respectively. It may be mistaken for choreoathetosis; however, these abnormal movements are relatively constant irrespective of whether the eyes are open or closed and occur in the absence of proprioceptive loss.

   iii. Tardive dyskinesia: Involuntary, repetitive body movements which can include protrusion of the tongue, lip-smacking and grimacing. This condition can develop secondary to treatment with neuroleptic medications including antipsychotics and antiemetics.

iv. Hypomimia: A reduced degree of facial expression associated with Parkinson's disease.

v. Ptosis and frontal balding: Typically associated with myotonic dystrophy.

vi. Ophthalmoplegia: Weakness or paralysis of one or more extraocular muscles responsible for eye movements. Ophthalmoplegia can be caused by a wide range of neurological disorders including multiple sclerosis and myasthenia gravis.

Pronator Drift or Pyramidal Drift

The pronator drift or pyramidal drift is a pathologic sign seen during inspection. It was first described by Jean Alexandre Barré and hence the sign is sometimes referred to as the Barré test or sign. Checking for pronator drift is a useful way of assessing for mild upper limb weakness and spasticity.

Method of performing the test:

1. The patient is asked to hold their arms out in front of them at 90° if in a standing/sitting posture or 45° if in a reclined position, with their palms facing upwards. Normally, a person will be able to hold their upper limbs in the said position for about one minute without any change. In upper motor neurone disease conditions, the affected side forearm will start pronating. The examiner must observe for 20–30 seconds to detect signs of pronation.

2. If no pronation occurs, the patient is asked to close their eyes and observe once again for pronation (this typically accentuates the effect due to the reliance on proprioception alone).

3. If there is still no pronation, the patient is asked to move their head back and forth while doing the test and the examiner looks for any pronation occurring. The examiner can also tap gently on the palms of the patient to hasten up the reaction.

Responses that can occur:

■ Normal response:
  a. Palm will remain flat, supine, elbows straight and the limbs horizontal.

  b. Symmetrical deviation on both sides from this position and both forearms may go in for pronation, but the dominant hand may pronate slightly more than the non-dominant hand.

■ Positive pronator drift:

  If the forearm pronates, with or without downward movement, the patient is said to have a pronator drift.

Interpretation of the result:

  The inability of the forearm to stay in a supinated position, and pronation of the forearm of the affected arm, indicates a lesion in contralateral side, involving the contralateral pyramidal tract. Pronation occurs because, in the context of an upper motor neuron lesion, the supinator muscles of the forearm are typically weaker than the pronator muscles.

C. **Scars:** The presence of scars may provide clues regarding previous spinal, axillary or upper limb surgery either to the nerves or the skeletal system (Figure 4.2).

D. **Muscle Bulk:** In general, the bulk of the muscle should be symmetric throughout the limbs, when comparing the left and right sides, and proximal and distal portions.

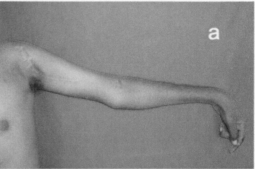

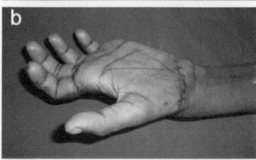

Figure 4.2 (a) Scar on upper arm showing radial nerve palsy. (b) Scar on wrist showing total claw due to median nerve and ulnar nerve palsy.

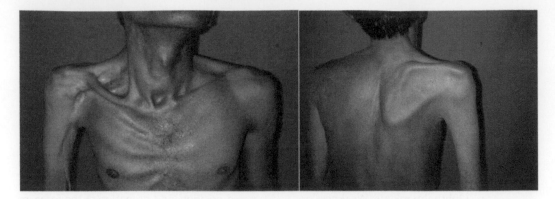

Figure 4.3 Brachial plexus injury on the right side with muscle atrophy.

Loss of muscle bulk is known as atrophy, and is seen in two pathologic conditions:

- Denervation atrophy: Seen when there is a lower motor neuron lesion. In such a situation, there is severe loss of bulk, which usually begins at least a week after acute injury and gets progressively worse with time (unless reinnervation takes place) (Figure 4.3).

- Disuse atrophy: This is a milder form of atrophy that can be seen when the muscle is not being used, as in conditions like upper MND, corticosteroid use, collagen vascular disorders and with musculoskeletal problems like bed rest, cast. There is little overall change in strength.

The methods of assessing muscle bulk are by:

1. Inspection:
   i. Generalized loss of muscle bulk, known as cachexia, could be due to systemic diseases like neoplasia or even conditions like starvation.
   ii. Symmetry is important, with consideration given to handedness and overall body habitus. Some areas can be adequately evaluated by inspection alone, such as the thenar and hypothenar regions or the shoulder contour.

2. Measurement:

   Some areas like the arm, forearm, thigh and leg can be best evaluated for loss of bulk by measurement.

The measurement needs to be done at particular points to avoid wrong values. For the arm and forearm, the measurement needs to be done twelve centimetres above elbow and ten centimetres below elbow, respectively, and always compared to the opposite side.

TESTING MUSCLE TONE

Muscle tone refers to the tension within the muscle – irrespective of whether the muscle is in a state of active contraction or not. The muscle tone is defined as the resistance to passive motion due to the inherent attributes of muscles – viscosity, elasticity and extensibility. This resting muscle tone is greatest in anti-gravity muscles that maintain the body in an erect posture.

When checking the tone of the muscles, there are four different conditions that can occur:

1. Increased tone
   a. Spasticity
   b. Rigidity

2. Decreased tone or flaccid state

3. Paratonia

4. Myotonia

1. **Increased tone of the muscles:** There are two types of increased tone – spasticity and rigidity. Spasticity and rigidity both involve increased tone, so it is important to understand how to differentiate them clinically.

   Spasticity is associated with pyramidal tract lesions (e.g., stroke) which are a type of upper motor neuron lesions (UMNL). Spasticity is "velocity-dependent," meaning the faster the limb is moved, the more the spasticity.

   There is typically increased tone in the initial part of the movement which then suddenly reduces past a certain point, it is known as "clasp knife spasticity." This initial resistance gives way and then there is less resistance over the remaining range of motion. Spasticity is also accompanied by weakness of the muscle being tested.

   This can be detected by the pronator catch test. The examiner grasps the hand of the patient, as if he were shaking hands, and quickly flicks the forearm from prone to supine. If spasticity is present, the examiner will feel a brief "catch" in the movement as he rotates the forearm before it releases to let the movement proceed. This is called a "pronator catch," a "supinator catch" or just a "spastic catch."

Rigidity is associated with extrapyramidal tract lesions (e.g., Parkinson's disease). Rigidity is "velocity independent," meaning it feels the same whether the limb is moved rapidly or slowly. The increased tone is seen throughout the range of movements. There are two main sub-types of rigidity:

a. **Lead pipe rigidity** involves uniformly increased tone throughout the movement of the muscle. This subtype of rigidity is typically associated with neuroleptic malignant syndrome.

b. **Cogwheel rigidity** involves a tremor superimposed on the hypertonia, resulting in intermittent increases in tone during movement of the limb. This subtype of rigidity is associated with Parkinson's disease (PD).

2. **Decreased tone of the muscles:** This refers to flaccid paralysis of the muscles as occurs in lower motor neuron lesions.

3. **Paratonia**: Many elderly individuals have a motor finding, called "paratonia." This is a phenomenon in which the patient is essentially unable to relax during passive movements. The resistance is usually irregular and generally greatest when there is a change in the pattern of movement. Most of these individuals have apparently normal tone when you test them in a standing position and move their shoulders about.

Extreme paratonia is common in patients with cognitive impairment or mental disorders, particularly in relation to frontal lobe dysfunction.

There are two types of paratonia: Oppositional and facilitatory.

- Oppositional paratonia ("gegenhalten" – the German word meaning "to resist or hold against") occurs when subjects involuntarily resist the passive movements attempted by the examiner.

- Facilitatory paratonia ("mitgehen" – the German word meaning "to go along") occurs when subjects involuntarily assist passive movements by the examiner.

4. **Myotonia**: Myotonia refers to a slowness of relaxation of muscles after a voluntary contraction or a contraction provoked by muscle percussion. This can affect any muscle group. Repeated effort will be needed to relax the muscle, although the condition usually improves after the muscles have warmed up.

As a result of this condition, individuals may have trouble releasing their grip on objects or may have difficulty rising from a seated position. They may walk with a stiff, awkward gait, because of the inability of the contracting muscles to relax after every step in the process of walking. Myotonia may also be triggered by exposure to cold.

Myotonia is caused by a problem in striated muscle and not due to an abnormality of innervation. It is seen in conditions such as myotonic dystrophy, congenital myotonia (a disorder of ion channels) or even metabolic diseases of the muscle (such as hypothyroidism). Myotonia can be easily observed by asking the individual to reverse a muscle action quickly (i.e., trying to rapidly open a tightly clenched fist) or by tapping on a muscle belly (such as the thenar muscles).

Method of Assessing Tone of Muscles

Assess tone in the muscle groups of the shoulder, elbow and wrist on each arm, comparing each side as you go:

1. Support the patient's arm by holding their hand and elbow.

2. Ask the patient to relax and allow you to fully control the movement of their arm.

3. Move the muscle groups of the shoulder (circumduction), elbow (flexion/extension) and wrist (circumduction) through their full range of movements.

4. Feel for abnormalities of tone as you assess each joint (e.g., spasticity, rigidity, cogwheeling, hypotonia).

- Hold hand, support elbow, bend up and down.

- Support wrist, bend up and down.

- Support elbow, alternate pronation and supination fast.

TESTING MUSCLE POWER
Strength
The ultimate goal of strength testing is to decide:

- Whether there is true "neurogenic" weakness.

- To determine which muscles/movements are affected.

- To determine the particular part of the nervous system that is at fault to produce this weakness, which can be done after the complete motor examination.

Probably the most important decision is whether the weakness is due to damage to the upper or lower motor neurons (UMN or LMN). This has been discussed earlier.

Upper motor neuron weakness is due to damage to the descending motor tracts (especially corticospinal) anywhere in its course from the cerebral cortex through the brain stem and spinal cord. It is typically characterized by two features, increased reflexes and a spastic type of increased tone.

LMN weakness is due to damage of the anterior horn cells or their axons (found in the peripheral nerves and nerve roots). This type of lesion is also associated with two characteristic features: Decreased stretch reflexes in the affected muscles and decreased muscle tone.

To determine that the muscles are weak, can be done by a systematic examination of the strength of the muscles. When testing the muscles we need to remember the root value of the muscles to be tested and in a particular order.

This assessment can be made with greater precision when there is a normal side with which to compare it.

The method of testing the strength of muscles in the upper limb:

1. Ask the patient to hold their arms horizontally out in front with the palms up and eyes closed.

   - Diffuse weakness of the upper limb often produces a "pronator drift," i.e., downward drift of the weak limb with the hand pronating (turning in).

   - If the limb drifts straight down, without pronation, this is not suggestive of physiologic weakness and the patient may have a conversion disorder or malingering.

   - Erratic drift of the limb can be seen with proprioceptive sensory loss (confirmed by testing of proprioception).

2. When assessing the strength of the muscles, it is important to understand that to get the patient to contract the tested muscle, they must make the effort. So, assessment of the effort should also be made. Poor effort is usually reflected as good initial contraction, followed by a collapse (often termed "breakaway" or "collapsing" weakness). This is not seen in true neurologic injury where the strength is typically inadequate but usually constant. This "collapsing" weakness can be detected if the examiner applies varying force during the muscle test. With true neurologic weakness, the maximum force that the patient applies does not vary appreciably.

There are several potential causes of "collapsing" weakness, ranging from pain to the conscious embellishment of symptoms.

When this pattern is seen, examination of the strength of the motor system may not reveal the true problem, and other more objective elements of the examination (such as reflex testing) become more important.

3. Basic principles of testing the strength of muscles:

   - Each instruction to test a muscle should be clearly communicated to the patient. Demonstrating the position that will be tested will also help in clear understanding by the patient.

   - Each relevant joint must be stabilized and isolated for each assessment, to ensure correct measurement of the strength.

   - Only one side should be assessed at a time.

   - After every single assessment of a muscle, the corresponding muscle must be tested on the opposite normal side.

   - The MRC muscle power assessment scale (Table 4.2) should be used for scoring muscle strength.

4. A particular sequence should be followed in testing the muscles of the upper limb (Table 4.3), to ensure that all the muscles are tested and no muscles are left untested (Video 4.1).

Simple sequence of performing the tests:

Table 4.2: MRC Power Assessment Scale

Score	Description
0	No contraction
1	Flicker or trace of contraction
2	Active movement, with gravity eliminated
3	Active movement against gravity
4	Active movement against gravity and resistance
5	Normal power

Table 4.3: Sequence of Testing the Muscles of the Upper Limb

Joint Tested	Movement Tested	Myotome Assessed (Nerve)	Muscles Assessed	Method of Testing
Shoulder	Shoulder abduction	C5 (axillary nerve)	Deltoid (primary) and other shoulder abductors	1. Ask the patient to flex their elbows and abduct their shoulders to 90°: "Bend your elbows and bring your arms out to the sides like a chicken." 2. Apply downward resistance on the lateral side of the upper arm whilst asking the patient to maintain their arm's position: "Don't let me push your shoulder down."
	Shoulder adduction	C6/7 (thoracodorsal nerve)	Teres major, latissimus dorsi and pectoralis major	1. Ask the patient to adduct their shoulders to 45° bringing their elbows closer to their body: "Now bring your elbows a little closer to your sides." 2. Apply upward resistance on the medial side of the upper arm whilst asking the patient to maintain their arm's position: "Don't let me pull your arms away from your sides."
Elbow	Elbow flexion	C5/6 (musculocutaneous and radial nerve)	Biceps brachii, coracobrachialis and brachialis	1. Ask the patient to flex their elbow: "Put your hands up like a boxer." 2. Apply resistance by pulling the forearm whilst stabilizing the shoulder joint: "Don't let me pull your arm away from you."
	Elbow extension	C7 (radial nerve)	Triceps brachii	1. With the patient's elbows still in the flexed position, apply resistance by pushing the forearm towards the patient whilst stabilizing the shoulder joint: "Don't let me push your arm towards you."
Wrist	Wrist extension	C7 (radial nerve)	Extensors of the wrist	1. Ask the patient to hold their arms out in front of them with their palms facing downwards: "Hold your arms out in front of you, with your palms facing the ground." 2. Ask the patient to make a fist and extend their wrist joints, keeping their wrists in this position whilst you apply resistance: "Make a fist, cock your wrists back and don't let me pull them downwards."
	Wrist flexion	C6/7 (median nerve)	Flexors of the wrist	With the patient still holding their arms out in front of them, now ask them to flex their wrist joints and keep them in this position whilst you apply resistance: "Ok, now point your wrists downwards and don't let me pull them up."
Fingers	Finger extension	C7 (radial nerve)	Extensor digitorum	Ask the patient to hold their fingers out straight whilst you apply downwards resistance: "Hold your fingers out straight and don't let me push them down."

(Continued)

Table 4.3 (Continued): Sequence of Testing the Muscles of the Upper Limb

Joint Tested	Movement Tested	Myotome Assessed (Nerve)	Muscles Assessed	Method of Testing
	Finger flexion	C8 (median and alnar nerves)	Flexor digitorum superficialis and profundus	Ask the patient to make a tight fist: "Curl up the fingers and don't let me uncurl them."
	Finger Abduction	T1 (ulnar nerve)	• First dorsal interosseous (FDI) • Abductor digiti minimi (ADM)	Ask the patient to abduct their fingers against resistance. "Splay your fingers outwards and don't let me push them together."
	Finger adduction	C8 (ulnar nerve)	Palmar interossei	Ask the patient to hold the fingers straight and grip a piece of paper between the fingers, whilst you also grip the paper between the same fingers on your hand that the patient is using. "Don't allow me to pull the paper away from between your fingers."
Thumb	Thumb abduction	T1 (median nerve)	Abductor pollicis brevis	Ask the patient to turn their hand over so their palm is facing upwards and to position their thumb over the midline of the palm. Advise them to keep it in this position whilst you apply downward resistance with your own thumb: "Point your thumbs to the ceiling and don't let me push them down."
	Thumb adduction	T1 (ulnar nerve)	Adductor pollicis	Ask the patient to hold a piece of paper between the side of the thumb and fingers, whilst you also grip the paper between the same fingers on your hand that the patient is using: "Don't allow me to pull the paper away from between your thumb and fingers."

a. Push up arms like wings – shoulder abduction

b. Push the arms down – shoulder adduction

c. Bring arms to front

d. Pull me towards you – elbow flexion

e. Push me away – elbow extension

f. Extend elbows

g. Cock up wrists – wrist extension

h. Wrist flexion

i. Finger extension - push against my finger

j. Finger flexion – hold my index and middle fingers

k. Finger abduction – push fingers apart

l. Finger adduction – hold fingers together and grasp a paper – must be demonstrated first by using the same paper grasped between the same fingers on the opposite hand

m. Thumb adduction – hold paper between thumb and fingers

n. Thumb abduction – lift thumb to ceiling

TESTING COORDINATION

The part of the brain that helps in the coordination of voluntary, automatic and reflex movement is the cerebellum. So, we need to test the coordination if we are to assess the integrity of the cerebellum.

Though the cerebellum is the primary centre in the brain for coordination for movement and the ability to execute smooth accurate motor response, other systems are also involved. The vestibular system, motor system, the pliability

Video 4.1 Motor examination of the upper limb.

www.routledge.com/9780367647162.

of the joints and the musculoskeletal system, deep sensations and vision also play a role in achieving coordination in movements.

The definition of coordination is the ability to execute smooth, accurate, controlled motor responses.

- Coordination is the ability to select the right muscle at the right time with proper intensity to achieve proper action.

- Coordinated movement is characterized by appropriate speed, distance, direction, timing and muscular tension.

It is the process that results in activation of motor units of multiple muscles with simultaneous inhibition of all other muscles in order to carry out a desired activity.

There are three different types of skills for motor coordination:

1. Fine motor skills: These are coordinated movements of small muscles like those of the hands and face. Examples of these fine motor skills include writing, drawing or buttoning a shirt.

2. Gross motor skills: These are coordinated movements of large muscles or groups of muscles like those of the trunk or extremities. Examples include walking, running and lifting activities.

3. Hand-eye skills: These skills refer to the ability of the visual system to coordinate the visual information received and then control or direct the hands in the accomplishment of a task. Examples include catching a ball, sewing and a surgeon using a laparoscope.

Causes of coordination Impairments:

Uncoordinated movement or coordination impairment is known as ataxia. The causes of ataxia range from chronic conditions to sudden onset, and most of these conditions will relate to damage or degeneration of the cerebellum.

Some of the diseases and injuries that can lead to ataxia include traumatic brain injury, alcoholism, infection, neuropathies, spinal cord injuries, Parkinson's, multiple sclerosis, cerebral palsy and brain tumours.

Coordinated movements are dependent on many individual but connected processes.

1. Volition: This is the ability to initiate, maintain or stop an activity or motion. In other words, the voluntary control of the movements.

2. Perception: This is very important to integrate motor impulses and the sensory feedback. If the patient is not able to perceive or feel where his joint is, he may not be able to perform the required movement. When proprioception is affected, it is usually compensated with visual feedback.

3. Engram: This refers to a postulated physical or biochemical change in neural tissue that represents a memory. High repetitions of precise performance must be performed in order to develop an engram. This is seen in complicated dance movements, where repeated performance will ensure perfection.

So, these tests will be valid only if the power and tone are normal. Hence testing the power and tone must precede the testing of cerebellar function through tests of coordination.

The testing of coordination is done by assessing a part of a sequence of movements.

- Past pointing
  - Finger/finger test
  - Finger/nose test

- Rapidly alternating movements (dysdiadochokinesis)

- Intentional tremor

- Rebound phenomenon

Tests that are done:

1. a. Finger-to-nose test – the shoulder is abducted to 90° with the elbow extended, the patient is asked to bring tip of the index finger to the tip of nose. The patient should keep their eyes open.

   Hold one of your fingertips up in front of, and at a short distance (about 30–40 cm) from, the patient.

   Ask the patient to touch the tip of their nose and then to touch your fingertip alternately and repeatedly. You can continuously change your fingertip position to make the test more difficult.

   You can then test for sensory ataxia by asking the patient to close their eyes and to touch the tip of their nose using their outstretched finger.

   Repeat these tests on the other side.

   What to look for:

   Look for intention tremor and past pointing as the patient touches the examiner's fingertip, which can indicate disease of the cerebellar hemispheres.

b. Finger-to-finger test – both shoulders are abducted to bring both the elbow extended, the patient is asked to bring both the hand toward the midline and approximate the index finger from opposing hand.

2. Adiadokokinesia or dysdiadokokinesia – the patient is asked to do rapidly alternating movements, e.g., forearm supination and pronation, hand tapping. Similarly, difficulty with rapid alternating movements (dysdiadochokinesia) or marked overshoot or undershoot when attempting to hit a target (intention tremor) suggests cerebellar problems on that side.

The patient needs to have one palm facing upwards.

They need to touch this palm with the palmar and then dorsal sides of the fingertips of the other hand as quickly as possible. Note that they must lift the second hand between each movement and touch the same point on the other palm without rolling the hand.

Test both sides. It is normal for the dominant hand to be a little faster at this test.

What to look for:

Look for dysdiadochokinesis. This is incoordination or slow movement when trying to perform this test.

3. Intention tremor – repetitive over and undershoot during voluntary movement may reflect as "intention tremor." Extreme slowness of movement can be produced by extrapyramidal disease (such as Parkinson's).

4. Rebound phenomena – the patient is with their elbow fixed, flex it against resistance. When the resistance is suddenly released the patient's forearm flies upward and may hit his face or shoulder.

1. What to look for:

Excessive rebound (or loss of checking) is suggestive of cerebellar injury on the side of the abnormality.

TESTING REFLEXES

I. Scientific basis of reflex testing

II. What are reflexes tested?

III. How are they done?

IV. How are the results to be interpreted?

I. Scientific basis of reflex testing.

Reflexes testing will tell us whether the paralysis or weakness of the muscle or group of muscles is due to a lesion and involvement of the upper motor neuronal pathway or the lower motor neuronal pathway.

The basic step of the reflex is that when a sudden stretch of the muscle is caused, a reflex is initiated, which results in the muscle contracting immediately. This is primarily to prevent undue stretching of the muscle and hence avoiding injury to the muscle fibres. This reflex contraction of the muscle that has been stretched is called the stretch reflex. The mechanism by which this stretch reflex occurs, involves two simple neuron arcs.

First, when the muscle is stretched, the afferent neuron transmits the sensation of stretch to the corresponding region of the spinal cord. From the spinal cord, the efferent neuron transmits the motor impulse to make the muscle contract. The components of this arc (Figure 4.4) are

1. End organs in the muscle and tendons

2. Afferent nerves

3. Spinal cord

4. Efferent nerves

5. Muscle fibres that contract

A. End organs of the muscle: These are two types of muscle fibres, the extrafusal fibres and the intrafusal fibres.
a. Extrafusal muscle fibres, which are the actual contracting fibres, make up the bulk of the muscle.
b. Intrafusal muscle fibres are muscle fibres within fusiform muscle spindles that are seen to lie parallel in between the extrafusal muscle fibres. The intrafusal fibres again are of two types – nuclear bag fibres and nuclear chain fibres, and about six to ten of these lie within the connective tissue sheath of the muscle spindle. The nuclear bag fibres are so called as they resemble a bag, and the nuclei are arranged in a cluster, while in the nuclear chain fibres, the nuclei are arranged one behind the other in the form of a chain. These fibres do not contract like the extrafusal fibres but respond to stretch of the neighbouring fibres. Together, the nuclear bag fibres and the nuclear chain fibres lie in a connective tissue cover in a structure known as the muscle spindle, so called, owing to the spindle shape.

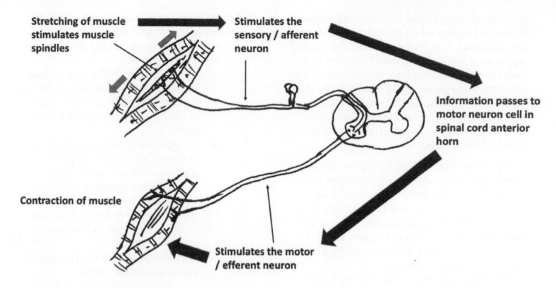

Figure 4.4 The stretch reflex components.

The muscle spindle (Figure 4.5) is a proprioceptor, a sense organ that receives information from muscle, that senses stretch and the speed of the stretch. When a muscle is suddenly stretched, and the endpoint of the stretch is reached, beyond which damage to the muscle may occur, a reflex occurs, by which, the spinal cord sends a message to muscle contract and shorten itself.

Impulses from these muscle spindles are carried by afferent nerves.

I. B. End organs in the tendons are known as the Golgi tendon organs (GTO). The GTO is attached between the extrafusal fibres and the tendon. Thus, the tendon organ is in series with the extrafusal fibres and will fire as the muscle contracts. The spindles,

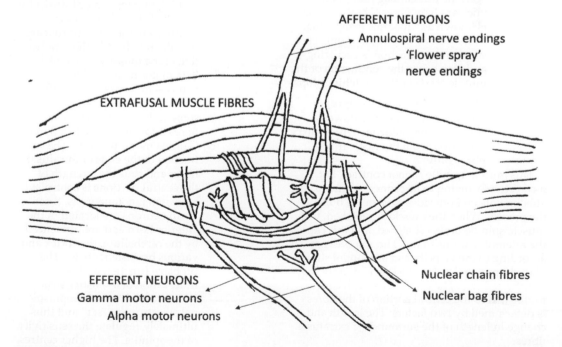

Figure 4.5 The muscle spindle and its parts.

in contrast, are parallel with the extrafusal fibres and so fire when the extrafusal fibres are stretched. The impulses from the tendon organ go through the dorsal horn and synapse on an inhibitory interneuron which in turn synapses on an alpha motoneuron that goes to the agonist. Therefore, the tendon organ ultimately causes relaxation of the agonist and, by way of interneurons, a facilitation of the antagonist.

Function: The GTO is a proprioceptor, a sense organ that receives information from the tendon, and it senses "tension." When a person lifts weights, the GTO senses how much tension the muscle is exerting, and if there is too much muscle tension, the GTO will inhibit the muscle from creating any further force via a reflex arc.

1. The afferent nerves: Nerves that innervate the spindle and have their cell body in a sensory ganglion are the afferent nerves in the stretch reflex. The afferent sensory terminals that innervate the spindle fibres are of two types: Primary and secondary.

    – The first type (primary) of afferent nerves are the annulospiral sensory neurons, which belong to Type Ia neurons which give information about "stretch" and "speed of stretch." These neurons arise from both the nuclear bag fibres and nuclear chain fibres. They do what is known as "dynamic firing," that is, they carry maximum impulses when the contraction is occurring and stop when the contraction of the muscle starts or the stretching stops.

    – The second type (secondary) of afferent nerves are the flower-spray sensory neurons which carry sensation from the nuclear bag fibres only.

This muscle spindle cannot contract, but it can stretch, owing to its connective tissue attachments on both sides, within the bulk of the muscle. When the muscle is stretched, the muscle spindle is also stretched, and this causes the afferent neurons to fire. The spindles fire according to the velocity and amount of stretch placed upon the central nuclear regions of the intrafusal fibres. The degree of stretch communicated to the central portion of the fibres is determined by two factors: The length and change in length of the surrounding extrafusal fibres.

These impulses are carried to the spinal cord.

2. Spinal cord: Impulses from the spindle receptors enter the dorsal horn, from where the information takes four routes:
    i. To the cortex.
    ii. To synapse directly on an alpha motoneuron, which causes immediate contraction of the muscle innervated by the spindle, the agonist.
    iii. To synapse on an inhibitory neuron which in turn synapses on an alpha motoneuron that goes to a muscle antagonistic to the one innervated by the spindle – thus there is concomitant relaxation of the antagonist as the agonist contracts.
    iv. To the cerebellum via the dorsal spinocerebellar tracts.

    The response from the spinal cord or the higher centres is through the efferent neurons.

3. The efferent neuron: There are two types of efferent neurons to the muscle. They are the alpha motor neuron and the gamma neuron.
    a. Alpha motor neurons: The alpha motor neuron causes the extrafusal muscle fibres to contract. These are alpha motoneurons in the anterior horn of the spinal cord which supply the muscle that is being tapped or transiently stretched. The alpha motor neurons are the neurons that are actually involved in the contraction of the muscle.
    b. Beta motor neurons: These neurons innervate the intrafusal fibres of muscle spindles with some collaterals to extrafusal fibres (type of slow twitch fibres).
    c. Gamma motor neurons: The contraction of the ends of intrafusal fibres and thus the strength of the central portions is controlled by gamma motoneurons. these small neurons are located in the anterior horn and are influenced by the cerebellum, the cortex and various brainstem nuclei. The probable function of this motor innervation of a sensory structure is to enable these supraspinal structures to "set" and thus ultimately regulate the sensitivity of the spindle. The higher centres, and in particular the cortex

thereby get sensory information from the muscle spindles and, in turn, through the gamma motoneuron, control the amount and quality of information received.

4. Muscle fibres that contract: In response to the impulses from the efferent motor neurons, the muscle fibres contract. The major response is by the extrafusal fibres. The agonist muscle relaxes, and the antagonist muscle contracts in response to the stimulus. This occurs in response to the alpha motor neurons.

The ends of the intrafusal fibres increase their tone in response to the impulses in the gamma motor neurons.

II. What are reflexes tested in the upper limb?
  a. "Deep tendon" (muscle stretch; myotatic) reflexes.

The commonly tested deep tendon reflexes include the biceps, triceps, brachioradialis (radial periosteal).
  b. Superficial and "pathologic" reflexes.

These are not very important or prominent in the upper limb. However, reflexes like the forced grasp or grope reflex and the palmomental reflex can be performed.

III. How are they done?

Before describing the methods of performing the different tests, there are certain principles that need to be understood about the testing.
  1. The muscle group to be tested must be in a neutral position (i.e., neither stretched nor contracted).

2. The tendon attached to the muscle(s) which is/are to be tested must be clearly identified. Place the extremity in a position that allows the tendon to be easily struck with the reflex hammer.
3. To easily locate the tendon, ask the patient to contract the muscle to which it is attached. When the muscle shortens, you should be able to both see and feel the cord like tendon, confirming its precise location.
4. Strike the tendon with a single, brisk, stroke. You should not elicit pain.
5. Note any asymmetric increase or depression.
6. The Jendrassik manoeuvre can be used to augment hypoactive reflexes. The patient can push the knees together against each other, or clench their teeth, while the upper limb tendon is tested.

Biceps Reflex (Testing C5,6 Myotome)

The forearm should be supported and resting either on the patient's thighs or resting on the forearm of the examiner. The arm is placed in 90° flexion at the elbow. The examiner places his thumb over the palpated biceps tendon and with his fingers curling around the elbow. With the reflex hammer, the examiner taps briskly over his own thumbnail which has been placed over the biceps tendon (Figure 4.6).

Normal response: The forearm will flex at the elbow.

Triceps Reflex (Testing C7 Myotome)

The patient's forearm is cradled over the forearm of the examiner. The arm of the patient is kept flexed to 90° at the shoulder, and the elbow flexed at 90°. The triceps tendon is palpated and

Biceps reflex   **Triceps reflex**   **Brachioradialis reflex**

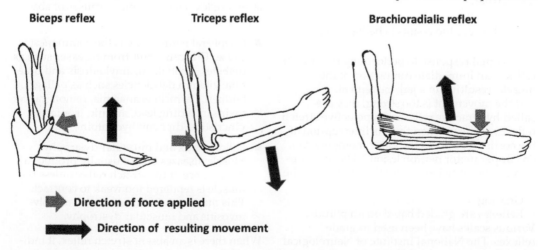

➡️ **Direction of force applied**

➡️ **Direction of resulting movement**

Figure 4.6 Demonstration of reflexes.

identified at its insertion on the olecranon, and the examiner taps just above the insertion.

Normal response: The elbow will extend.

Brachioradialis Reflex (Testing C5,6 Myotome)

The patient's arm should be supported. The brachioradialis tendon is identified at the wrist. It inserts at the base of the styloid process of the radius, usually about 1 cm lateral to the radial artery. If it is difficult to identify the tendon, the patient is asked to hold their forearm as in a sling and flex this semi-pronated forearm against resistance offered by the examiner. By this step, the brachioradialis muscle and tendon stand out. The examiner's hand supports the patient's forearm. The examiner then places the thumb of his hand on the biceps tendon while tapping the brachioradialis tendon with the other hand.

Normal response: There will be flexion and supination of the forearm due to contraction of the brachioradialis muscle. In some patients who may have a hyperactive biceps or finger jerk reflex, two other responses may also be seen along with the brachioradialis contraction.

a. Biceps reflex: Flexion of the forearm. You will feel the biceps tendon contract if the biceps reflex is stimulated by the tap on the brachioradialis tendon.

b. Finger jerk: Flexion of the fingers.

Finger Jerk (Testing C8 Myotome)

The patient is asked gently curl their fingers in opposition to the examiner's fingers. The examiner then taps briskly on his own fingers on the dorsal aspect so that the force will transmit to the patient's curled fingers.

Normal response: The patient's fingers will flex further.

V. How are the results to be interpreted?

The normal response to performing the stretch reflex is an immediate contraction of the muscle, resulting in a jerk movement.

If the movement is too strong, they are called hyperactive reflexes. Hyperactive stretch reflexes are seen when there is interruption of the cortical supply to the lower motor neuron, an "upper motor neuron lesion." The interruption can be anywhere above the segment of the reflex arc.

Grading

Reflexes are graded based on amplitude. Various scales have been used to grade reflexes. The National Institute of Neurological Disorders and Stroke (NINDS) Muscle Stretch Reflex Scale is frequently used and empirically supported:

NINDS scale:

Grade 0: Reflex absent: No evidence of contraction.

Grade 1: Reflex small, less than normal; includes a trace response or a response brought out only with reinforcement: Decreased, but still present (hypo-reflexic). Hyporeflexia is generally associated with a lower motor neuron deficit (at the alpha motor neurons from spinal cord to muscle) e.g., Guillain–Barré syndrome.

Grade 2: Reflex in the lower half of the normal range.

Grade 3: Reflex in the upper half of the normal range: Super-normal (hyper-reflexic). Hyperreflexia is often attributed to upper motor neuron lesions e.g., multiple sclerosis.

Grade 4: Reflex enhanced, more than normal; includes clonus if present, which optionally can be noted in an added verbal description of the reflex [7]. Clonus: Repetitive shortening of the muscle after a single stimulation.

Generally speaking:

■ Lower motor neurone lesions usually produce a diminished or absent response.

■ Upper motor neurone lesions usually produce hyperreflexia.

■ Isolated loss of a reflex can point to a radiculopathy affecting that segment – e.g., loss of biceps jerk if there is a C5–C6 disc prolapse.

If the movement does not occur, it indicates an absent reflex. There are many causes of absent reflexes.

■ Peripheral neuropathy is the commonest cause. This can result from diseases such as diabetes, alcoholism, amyloidosis and uraemia; vitamin deficiencies such as pellagra, beriberi, pernicious anaemia, remote cancer, toxins including lead, arsenic, isoniazid, vincristine, diphenylhydantoin.

■ Polymyositis and muscular dystrophy: Muscle diseases do not usually produce a disturbance of the stretch reflex unless the muscle is rendered too weak to contract. This may occur in diseases such as polymyositis and muscular dystrophy.

When there is an absent stretch reflex, it indicates a lesion in the reflex arc that has been described earlier. So, performing the stretch reflex helps us in two ways:

1. Finding the location of the lesion.

   Associated symptoms and signs usually make localization possible:
   a. Absent reflexes and sensory loss in the distribution of the nerve supplying the reflex indicates a lesion involving the afferent arc of the reflex. This could mean involvement of the afferent nerve or the dorsal horn.
   b. On the other hand, absent reflex with paralysis, muscle atrophy, and fasciculations would indicate involvement of the efferent arc, which could be the anterior horn cells or efferent nerve, or both.

2. Finding the level of the lesion.

   The stretch reflexes can provide excellent clues to the level of lesions along the neuraxis. Each muscle stretch reflex is related to a particular cord level. For example, the biceps and brachioradialis reflexes represent C5, 6 levels, the triceps reflex represents the C6, 7 levels and the finger jerk represents the C8–T 1 levels.

   A diagrammatic representation of the interpretation of an example is shown below.

   if the biceps and brachioradialis reflexes are normal, the triceps absent and all lower reflexes (finger jerk, knee jerk, ankle jerk) hyperactive, the lesion would be located at the C6–C7 level, the level of the triceps reflex. The reflex arcs above (biceps, brachioradialis, jaw jerk) are functioning normally, while the lower reflexes give evidence of absence of upper motor neuron innervation.

3. Finding the laterality of the lesion.

   If all the reflexes on the left side of the body are hyperactive and those on the right side are normal, then the lesion involves the corticospinal pathways to that side, somewhere above the level of the highest reflex that is hyperactive.

Pathological Reflexes

In addition to testing the normal physiological reflexes in the upper limb, we also need to look for the pathological reflexes that occur. The pathological reflexes of upper extremities

are less constant, more difficult to elicit and usually less significant diagnostically then lower extremity reflexes. They are mainly of two types:

1. Forced grasping or grasp reflex (GR) is known to be a primitive reflex not normally seen in adults and is caused by a pathological lesion located in the frontal lobe.

   A positive GR is defined as forced grasping of the examiner's hand by the patient in response to the examiner touching the patient's palm between the thumb and index finger. When a patient unintentionally grasps a visually presented object, it is called a groping reflex. Forced grasping and groping are usually performed by the hand contralateral to a destructive lesion in the frontal lobe, such as a lesion in the supplementary motor area (Brodmann area 6) or frontal-orbital area (Brodmann area 8).

2. The palmomental reflex (PMR) is a primitive reflex consisting of a twitch of the chin muscle elicited by stroking a specific part of the palm. It is present in infancy and disappears as the brain matures during childhood but may reappear due to processes that disrupt the normal cortical inhibitory pathways. Therefore, it is an example of a frontal release sign. This sign can be elicited by stroking the thenar eminence with a thin stick, from the wrist to the thumb base using moderate pressure. If there is a single visible twitch of the ipsilateral mentalis muscle, it is considered a positive response.

Other reflexes that may be seen in the upper limb:

a. The Hoffmann sign [1] is an involuntary flexion movement of the thumb and/or index finger when the examiner flicks the fingernail of the middle finger down. The reflex pathway causes the thumb to flex and adduct quickly. A positive Hoffmann sign can be indicative of an upper motor neuron lesion and corticospinal pathway dysfunction likely due to cervical cord compression. However, up to 3% of the population has been found to have a positive Hoffmann sign without cord compression or upper motor neurone disease.

   Method of testing: The wrist must be kept dorsiflexed, fingers partially flexed and holding the partially extended middle finger, a flick is given to the nail of middle finger. If there is flexion and adduction of the thumb with flexion of index finger sometimes, it is indicative of a positive Hoffmann sign.

b. The Trömner sign [2] is flexion of the thumb and index finger in response to tapping or flicking the volar surface of the distal phalanx of the middle finger held partially flexed between the examiner's finger and thumb. It is an established neurological sign for pyramidal response in the upper extremity and has been recognized as an alternative of Hoffmann's sign. Both the Trömner and Hoffmann signs are commonly used as clinical neurological examinations for upper motor neuron lesions above the fifth or sixth cervical segments of the spinal cord.

NEUROLOGICAL MOTOR EXAMINATION IN CHILDREN

Indications: A proper motor examination is indicated in children, if they have any of the following complaints:

- Headaches
- Blurry vision
- Change in behaviour
- Fatigue
- Change in balance or coordination
- Numbness or tingling in the arms or legs
- Decrease in movement of the arms or legs
- Injury to the head, neck or back
- Temperature of unknown source
- Seizures
- Slurred speech
- Weakness
- Tremor

In older children, it may be possible to carry out the motor examination as outlined above, but in infants, it may not be possible. For infants, testing the motor system may be done in the following ways.

Examination of Tone

Resting posture: For a term newborn the resting posture is flexion of the extremities with the extremities closely adducted to the trunk. After the first few days of life, the extremities are still predominantly in the flexed position, but they are not as tightly adducted as they are in the first 48 hours of life.

Upper extremity tone: We can begin assessing the motor function of the upper extremities by testing the passive range of motion. This can be done by rotating each extremity at the shoulder, elbow and wrist and feeling the resistance and the range of movement. Too little or too much resistance reflects hypotonia or hypertonia.

Arm traction: This is done with the baby in the supine position. The wrist is grasped, and the arm is pulled until the shoulder is slightly off the mat. Normally, there should be some flexion maintained at the elbow. If there is full extension at the elbow, it indicates hypotonia.

Arm recoil: This test relies on the action of the biceps muscle. The arms are held in flexion against the chest for a few seconds, then are quickly extended and released. Normally the arms should spring back to the flexed position. The hypotonic infant will have slow incomplete recoil. Asymmetry to this response with lack of recoil would be seen with Erb's or brachial plexus palsy.

Scarf sign: The tone of the shoulder girdle is assessed by taking the baby's hand and pulling the hand to the opposite shoulder like a scarf. The hand should not go past the shoulder and the elbow should not cross the midline of the chest.

Hand position: A newborn baby's hand is held in a fisted position with the fingers flexed over the thumb. The hand should open intermittently and should not always be held in a tight-fisted position. Rubbing the ulnar aspect of the hand or touching the dorsum of the hand will often cause extension of the fingers. Over the first one to two months of life, the baby's hand becomes more open. Persistence of a fisted hand is a sign of an upper motor neuron lesion in an infant.

Primitive Reflexes

To complete the examination (Table 4.4).

- Explain to the child and parents that the examination is now finished.
- Ensure the child is re-dressed after the examination.
- Thank the child and parents for their time.
- Explain your findings to the parents.
- Ask if the parents and child (if appropriate) have any questions.
- Dispose of PPE appropriately and wash your hands.
- Summarize your findings to the examiner.

Table 4.4: Method of Examining and Testing for Primitive Reflexes

Reflex	Normal Response
Blinking reflex	The infant will close his/her eyes in response to bright lights
Babinski reflex	As the infant's foot is stroked, his/her toes will extend upward
Crawling reflex	If the infant is placed on his/her belly, will make crawling motions
Moro's reflex	A quick change in the infant's position will cause the infant to throw his/her arms outward, open his/her hands, and throw back his/her head
Startle reflex	A loud noise will cause the infant to extend and flex his/her arms while his/her hands remain closed in a fist
Palmar and plantar grasp	His/her fingers or toes will curl around a finger placed in the area

REFERENCES

1. Floeter, MK. (2010). Structure and function of muscle fibres and motor units (PDF). In Karpati, G, Hilton-Jones, D, Bushby, K and Griggs, RC (eds), *Disorders of Voluntary Muscle* (8th edition). Cambridge University Press. Chapter 1, Motor Neurons, pp. 1–2

2. Ince, PG, Clark, B, Holton, J, Revesz, T and Wharton, SB (2008). "Chapter 13: Diseases of movement and system degenerations." In Greenfield JG, Love S, Louis DN and Ellison DW (eds), *Greenfield's Neuropathology*. 1 (8th edition). London: Hodder Arnold. p. 947.

3. Statland, JM, Barohn, RJ, McVey, AL, Katz, JS and Dimachkie, MM (2015). "Patterns of weakness, classification of motor neuron disease, and clinical diagnosis of sporadic amyotrophic lateral sclerosis." *Neurologic Clinics*. 33(4): 735–748.

4. Hoffmann P (1915). Über eine Methode, den Erfolg einer Nervennaht zu beurteilen. *Medizinische Klinik*, 11(13): 359–360.

5. Cooper MJ. (1933). Mechanical factors governing the Trömner Reflex. *Arch NeurPsych*, 30(1): 166–169.

5 Sensory Examination

J Terrence Jose Jerome

CONTENTS

SIMPLE SENSATIONS

There are four simple sensations: Pain, temperature, touch and vibration. These sensations are all called simple because their perception does not require a healthy contralateral cerebral cortex. The simple sensations have distinct sensory organs in the skin except for the vibration sense. Also, the pathways in the spinal cord are well defined except for the touch sensation. The sensation is a fascinating quality of every human where touch or pain can be perceived well but not light [1].

SENSORY RECEPTORS IN THE SKIN

Two sensory receptors convert the stimulus to encoded information in a stream of action potential transferring to the cerebral cortex for interpretation.

a. Pacinian corpuscles, which respond quickly to a stimulus and subsequently fade.

b. Merkel discs, which respond more slowly but continue to give a sustained response [2].

Superficial sensation (also termed exteroceptive sensation): Superficial sensation provides

DOI: 10.1201/9781003125938-5

information regarding external stimuli of the skin receptors (skin and mucous membranes). The superficial sensation is either fine and discriminative or gross. It has an essential role in informing and in discrimination of intensities of all qualities and particularly of local specifications. The superficial sensation has a protective function and brings about a regional response of defence termed withdrawal response [3].

Tactile or touch sensation (thigmesthesia):

- *Anesthesia:* Absence of touch appreciation

- *Hypoesthesia:* Decrease of touch appreciation

- *Hyperesthesia:* Exaggeration of touch sensation, which is often unpleasant

Pain sensation (algesia):

- *Analgesia:* Absence of pain appreciation

- *Hypoalgesia:* Decrease of pain appreciation

- *Hyperalgesia:* Exaggeration of pain appreciation, which is often unpleasant

Temperature sensation, both hot and cold (thermesthesia):

- *Thermanalgesia:* Absence of temperature appreciation

- *Thermhypesthesia:* Decrease of temperature appreciation

- *Thermhyperesthesia:* Exaggeration of temperature sensation, which is often unpleasant

Sensory perversions:

- *Paresthesia:* Abnormal sensations perceived without specific stimulation. They may be tactile, thermal or painful; episodic or constant.

- *Dysesthesia:* Painful sensations elicited by a nonpainful cutaneous stimulus such as a light touch or gentle stroking over the body's affected areas and sometimes referred to as hyperpathia or hyperalgesia. Often perceived as intense burning, dysesthesias may outlast the stimulus by several seconds.

Deep sensation (proprioceptive sensation):
The deep sensation of the hand provides information about the position of the skeleton and muscles with specific receptors located in muscles, tendons, ligaments and joints.

- *Joint position sense:* Absence is described as arthresthesia

- *Vibratory sense:* Absence is explained as pallesthesia

- *Kinesthesia:* Perception of muscular motion

Cortical sensory functions: Interpretative sensory functions that require analysis of individual sensory modalities by the parietal lobes to provide discrimination. Individual sensory modalities must be intact to measure cortical sensation.

- *Stereognosis:* Ability to recognize and identify objects by feeling them. The absence of this ability is termed *astereognosis.*

- *Graphesthesia:* Ability to recognize symbols written on the skin. The absence of this ability is termed *graphanesthesia.*

- *Two-point discrimination:* Ability to recognize simultaneous stimulation by two blunt points. It is measured by the distance between the points required for recognition.

- *Touch localization (topognosis):* Ability to localize stimuli to parts of the body. *Topagnosia* is the absence of this ability.

- *Double simultaneous stimulation:* Ability to perceive a sensory stimulus when corresponding areas on the opposite side of the body are stimulated simultaneously. Loss of this ability is termed *sensory extinction.*

THE TECHNIQUE OF SENSORY EXAMINATION

Sensory examination is a valuable neurological examination and should be performed carefully with optimal patient cooperation to achieve reliable results. The patient should be relaxed and comfortable. Accurate results are challenging to obtain in anxious or distracted patients. In cases of equivocal or exhausted patients, the examination should be repeated once the patient is relaxed.

The patient should be questioned as to whether abnormal sensations are experienced subjectively before starting the examination. Also, the examiner should ask the patient if any parts of the body feel numb or have different sensory perception such as pain, paresthesias or dysesthesias. The examination should be tailored to patients with positive replies and should focus on the specific anatomical areas. For peripheral nerve injuries, the goal of sensibility testing is to evaluate this recovery on a quantitative anatomical basis and a functional basis.

The testing sensation can be divided into three main categories: Threshold test, functional test and objective test (Table 5.1) [1–4].

QUICK SURVEY

A quick survey includes screening the patients with no sensory disturbances. This consists of a reliable survey by testing touch (with double

Table 5.1: Threshold Tests

Threshold Test	Methods Used for Test	Prerequisites	Test Results	Responses	Precaution
Pinprick	Safety pin	Patient should differentiate between sharp and dull pain	Nerve regenerating area will be hypersensitive to prick	1. Absence of awareness 2. Pressure sensation without distinguishing between sharp and dull 3. Hyperanalgesia with radiation 4. Sharp sensation with some radiation and gross localization 5. Sensation of sharpness with or without slight stinging or radiation and fair localization 6. Normal perception	Always test the normal side first
Temperature	Cold and hot water test tube	Patient should distinguish between hot and cold	Positive to test tube with hot and cold temperatures	Positive to test tube with hot and cold temperatures	Always test hot and cold at one level in the range
Light touch	Semmes-Weinstein monofilaments	Twenty filaments, graded in thickness, and numbers ranging from 1.65 to 6.65*	Except for the very largest, all filaments buckle as the examiner presses them against the skin	1. Normal 2. Diminished light touch 3. Diminished protective sensation 4. Loss of protective sensation	Avoid testing over the skin callus
Vibration	Tuning fork (128 or 256 Hz)	The tuning fork is struck against a surface and then one of the ends of the prong is held tangentially to the fingertip with eyes closed	Did the test feel different?	1. Felt "different" 2. "Didn't feel anything" 3. Felt "softer" 4. Felt "louder"	Always maintain the same striking force with each application of the tuning fork. Support the finger and compare the test with contralateral side

*The filament number represents the logarithm of 10 multiplied by the force in milligrams required to bow the filament.

120

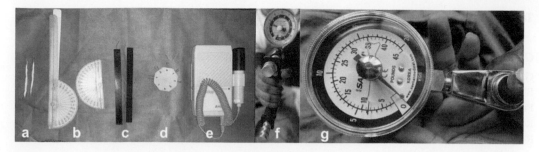

Figure 5.1 Instruments commonly necessary to complete a physical examination of the hand: (a) cotton wisps (b) finger and wrist goniometers used to measure joint range of motion. (c) Semmes-Weinstein monofilament (d) Two-point discriminator used to test sensation. (e) Doppler can be used to assess vascular flow to the hand or digits or both. (f) Dynamometer and (g) thumb-pinch meter used to measure strength.

simultaneous stimulation), pain or temperature, joint position and vibratory sensibilities in a few well-chosen locations. Also, check whether the patient has a protective sensation (ability to receive or perceive a sharp object, deep pressure), appreciates light touch or fine discrimination. This takes only 3 to 5 minutes (Figure 5.1).

DETAILED SURVEY

A thorough examination must be done in patients when disturbances are suspected after the history of uncovered screening examination. In such cases, the examiner should investigate the anatomic basis of the sensory findings.

SUPERFICIAL (EXTEROCEPTIVE) SENSATION

1. TACTILE SENSATION (TOUCH)

The upper limb, including the hand, should be touched lightly with a wisp of cotton, a small piece of paper or the gentlest possible touch of your finger pads. Care must be taken to touch lightly, as more potent stimuli may activate deep pressure receptors in addition to superficial tactile receptors. With eyes closed, the patient should be asked to reply "yes" each time a stimulus is applied. Tactile localization can be tested by having a patient point to the area stimulated or describe the area tested. Double simultaneous stimulation can be tested by touching each side of the body simultaneously.

On a screening examination, it is imperative to touch on three locations on the upper limb, and the proximal and distal responses should be compared. If an area of sensory loss is discovered, it is often helpful to have the patient outline the boundaries with their fingertips. Care should be taken not to apply the stimuli rhythmically to prevent the inattentive state

from being reached by the stimuli's rhythmic nature.

LIGHT TOUCH – DEEP PRESSURE

A Semmes-Weinstein pressure aesthesiometer contains nylon monofilaments (20) mounted in Lucite rods calibrated to exert specific pressures in eliciting the light touch (deep pressure) sensation. The examiner keeps varying numbers of monofilaments over the well supported patient's hand and exerts pressure until it bends. Here, the examiner should avoid force because first-order buckling is produced by the monofilaments' bending quality reaching a peak force. The monofilament bends the skin, and this mechanical information causes nerve ending firings. By repeatedly testing the patient with the same instrument and the same examiner, a Semmes-Weinstein monofilament monitors the sensory change or recovery. The advantage of this monofilament is that it provides a controlled, objective and reproducible force stimulus for testing peripheral nerve function.

Of the 20 available monofilaments in the testing kit, many authors have suggested that no more than five monofilament forces need to be used ordinarily for diagnosis and one or two for monitoring progress or recovery. Efforts are made so that the increasing size monofilaments are coloured and differentiated according to the numbers, force and use (Table 5.2). A mini kit contains five coloured elements for tests. Also, this monofilament can be utilized for two-point discrimination to assess the sensory grades (normal, diminished light touch, diminished protective sensation and loss of protective sensation).

Testing is begun with monofilament 2.83 (green colour), which is considered normal light-touch sensibility. Gradually the other coloured filaments are used to test the sensation. The results are noted in the areas of sensory loss and interpreted with the clinical

Table 5.2: Scale of Interpretation of Monofilaments

Colour	Sensation	Filament Markings	Calculated Force (gm)
Green	Normal	1.65–2.83	0.0045–0.068
Blue	Diminished light touch	3.22–3.61	0.166–0.408
Purple	Diminished protective sensation	3.84–4.31	0.697–2.06
Red	Loss of protective sensation	4.56–6.65	3.63–447
Red-lined	Untestable	>6.65	>447

findings. In cases of inconclusiveness, the examiner performs the test three times to get a reliable test. The examiner should apply the filaments holding them for about 1.5 seconds and uniformly removing them. Care must be taken not to touch the skin before pressing to bend the filament, bouncing the filament against the skin and removing the filaments too quickly, giving additional stimulus clues to the patient and misleading results. If a response is not obtained with the thickest filament (6.65 – red lined) in a particular hand area, the pinprick test is used as a final test of sensibility [1–8] (Figure 5.2).

2. PAIN SENSATION

The use of a sterile safety pin is the most common method to assess painful stimuli. Applying a safety pin randomly using the point and guard assesses reliability and attention. The patient should reply "sharp" or "dull" with their eyes closed. The examiner should evaluate the same areas tested in the screening examination for tactile sensation. Each side of the upper limb should be compared with the opposite, and distal and proximal portions of each upper limb should be tested. The examiner should stimulate from areas of diminished sensibility to the normal areas in areas of analgesia or hypoalgesia because the onset of the painful stimulus is better perceived than attenuation or cessation of the stimulus.

The drawback of this test is the transmission of communicable diseases by transferring small amounts of blood produced by the pinprick. Therefore, use a sterile safety pin, or the safety pin should be cleaned between patients.

3. TEMPERATURE SENSATION

Test tubes filled with warm and cold water is the traditional method of testing temperature sensation. Also, temperatures <5°C or >45°C elicit painful responses in addition to temperature and should be avoided. With their eyes closed, have the patient describe the stimulus; simple answers of hot or cold may mask subtle changes in temperature sensibility. In screening examinations, a tuning fork can be used to provide a cool object. Temperature testing is often a more sensitive measure of subtle dysfunction than pain testing.

PROPRIOCEPTIVE SENSATION

Famously called a "sixth sense," proprioception allows an individual to detect joint motion and limb position with their eyes closed. Proprioception has distinct sense organs and ascending pathways in the spinal cord.

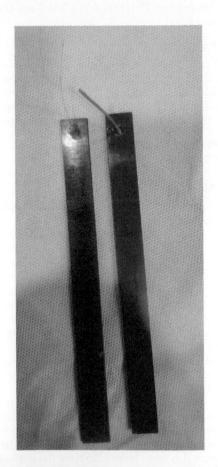

Figure 5.2 Purple- and red-coloured, and calibrated monofilaments, varying in pressure, are shown in the picture.

JOINT POSITION SENSE

The joint position sense is tested by the examiner with the patient closing their eyes. By moving the joints up and down, a patient with normal proprioception confirms the joint movements and position. The upper and lower limbs' most distal joints are tested first because most proprioception disturbances involve distal before proximal joints. If testing on the distal joint is abnormal, more proximal joints should be tested successively until a normal joint is reached. If the distal joint appears normal, there is rarely a need to try more proximal joints. Early proprioceptive dysfunction is seen in the third and fourth digits of both upper and lower limbs because they are more sparsely innervated than the first, second or fifth digits. The digit tested should be separated from the neighbour digits to prevent tactile clues of up and down movement mediated by the neighbour digits.

TECHNIQUE

The examiner lightly grasps the sides of the patient's finger or big toe and bends it slowly up and down. The patient is asked to indicate the sense of movement and direction of finger or toe movements. Examiners placing their hand over the patient's side of the finger or toe and parallel to the plane of motion prevent pressure stimuli on the digit's surface, which might provide clues to the patient. A normal individual can perceive movements of one or two degrees in the joints and even smaller excursions in more proximal joints (hip and shoulder joints). Up to 10% of normal individuals can indicate the wrong direction during the test.

For patients with decreased sensation or who are unable to understand the testing sequence, joint position sense can be roughly assessed in the upper extremity by placing the digits of one of the patient's hands in a particular position and asking them to imitate the position in the other with their eyes closed.

The Romberg test (test for joint position sense). The examiner stands firm behind the patient and instructs the patient to stand with their heels together and to close their eyes. The patient will sway severely or fall in a diminished position sense. Patients with cerebellar disease will swing with their eyes open or closed.

CLINICAL SIGNIFICANCE

Proprioceptive sensation loss is seen in peripheral neuropathy (e.g., diabetes mellitus), spinal cord disease (e.g., multiple sclerosis, vitamin B12 deficiency, tabes dorsalis) and severe hemispheric disease. In spinal cord unilateral disorder (e.g., Brown-Séquard syndrome), there is sensory loss on both sides of the body. Additionally, the pain and temperature sensation is lost on the side opposite to the lesion and tactile sensation is lost on the side of the lesion.

In patients with strokes, proprioceptive loss indicates extensive damage and correlates with a poorer functional recovery and higher mortality.

There is a disproportionate loss of vibration sensation and proprioception (compared with the pain and temperature sensation) that occurs in diseases of the dorsal columns of the spinal cord (e.g., tabes dorsalis, multiple sclerosis, vitamin B12 deficiency) and some peripheral neuropathies (e.g., diabetic polyneuropathy).

VIBRATORY SENSE

As humans are more sensitive to the vibration frequency of 200–300 Hz, it is preferred to test the vibration sensation using a tuning fork, usually 128 Hz and less often with 256 Hz. The examiner places the tuning fork on the patient's bony prominences. The patient starts feeling buzzing or like electricity. The examiner instructs the patient to indicate instantly when the sensation stops and notes the total elapsed time since the fork was struck.

Normal and healthy individuals of 40 years of age should perceive a 128 Hz tuning fork struck from a distance of 20 cm from the examiner for at least 15 seconds when held against the ulnar styloid. These values may decrease by 2 seconds for every decade of age. If vibration is not perceived on distal joints, testing should be continued proximally over joints or bony prominences until it is perceived and noted. Also, the clinician can demonstrate the test by tapping and holding the tuning fork on the abdominal wall. Traditional application against the bony wall is a mistaken belief because vibratory receptors are good in soft tissues.

CLINICAL SIGNIFICANCE

The vibratory sensation is preserved in diseases of the cerebral cortex and diminished in peripheral neuropathy and spinal cord disease.

CORTICAL SENSORY FUNCTION

Cortical sensations require high integration and processing. They also need a healthy contralateral cerebral cortex. Cortical sensory functions can be tested only when patients lack dementia and have normal exteroceptive and proprioceptive sensations.

STEREOGNOSIS (STEREOS IN GREEK MEANS "SOLID")

Tactile recognition is the ability to recognize everyday objects such as a pen, key, comb or paperclip when placed in the patient's hand. With eyes closed, the patient is asked to describe or identify the objects. Normal individuals can name >90% of such objects within 5 seconds. Touch and tactile sensations are quite different. Touch involves an appreciation of all the information at the level of the cortex. The contribution of elementary sensation is indispensable to the intellectual art of recognizing an object. Tactile sensation is an immediate symbolic perception that is not hindered by the detail and analytic perception. It supplements the information given by the symbolic perception.

GRAPHESTHESIA

Graphesthesia is the ability to identify letters or numbers written on the hand.

TWO-POINT DISCRIMINATION

Two-point discrimination, localization and the Moberg pick-up test are functional tests to assess sensation quality [9]. The function test helps find prevention, daily living activities recognizing and manipulating objects with vision occluded. Two-point discrimination is the ability to distinguish two points simultaneously applied to the skin and most helpful in the fingertips to quickly test normal versus abnormal sensation. The normal minimal distance is 3 cm for the hand or foot. With the patient's eyes closed, the examiner uses a pair of measured callipers or a bent paperclip to randomly touch the patient with either one or two points and indicate whether one or two points are perceived. Always compare the test with the opposite sides of the body. The following are the normal distances at which two points can be discriminated on various body parts:

Fingertip: 2 to 6 mm; dorsum of fingers: 4 to 6 mm; palm: 8 to 12 mm; Dorsum of hand: 20 to 30 mm.

STATIC (CONSTANT) TWO-POINT DISCRIMINATION

Ernst Heinrich Weber (1953) described the two-point discrimination test to measure the quality of the finger's sensation and ability to perform as a sensory organ [10]. The examiner uses Weber's calliper held against the skin at different distances apart. The static two-point discrimination test determines the minimum distance at which the patient can distinguish

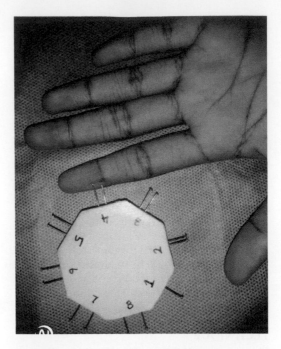

Figure 5.3 Examiner testing two-point discrimination using an instrument calibrated with defined measurements of separation between the points.

whether they are being touched with one or two points in contact with skin (Figure 5.3). The American Society for Surgery of the Hand clinical assessment recommendations and interpretations of scores:

Normal: Less than 6 mm

Fair: 6 to 10 mm

Poor: 11 to 15 mm

Protective: One point perceived

Anaesthetic: No point perceived

Usually, 5 mm is required for performing daily activities such as winding a watch or putting a nut on a screw, 6 to 8 mm for buttoning and sewing activities and 12 to 15 mm for small precision tools activities. Above 15 mm, gross tool handling is possible but with decreased speed and skill.

MOVING TWO-POINT DISCRIMINATION

Moving two-point discrimination depends on quickly adapting sensory fibres, which usually returns earlier than slow-adapting fibres responsible for constant touch (static two-point discrimination). It is 8 to 10 mm better than static two-point discrimination. The examiner starts the test using a Boley gauge set at an 8 mm distance between the two points moving proximal to distal direction on the fingertip parallel to the long axis of the finger. The examiner stops the test at 2 mm intervals because this is the normal value for moving two-point discrimination. The patient is required to respond to seven out of ten stimuli before the distance is narrowed. Moving two-point discrimination measures the hand's ability to feel objects when the hand is in motion. In contrast, static two-point discrimination indicates the hand capacity to be aware of static objects within the hand. Interestingly a patient with 8 to 10 mm of moving point discrimination can detect and identify objects with their eyes closed but unable to recognize the object lifted when the hands are held immobile or in a static position.

TOPOGNOSIS (LOCALIZATION)

Ask the patient to describe or point to various parts of the body tested with tactile stimulation. This can be done with tactile testing. With the patient's eyes closed, the examiner touches their skin using a monofilament. If the patient receives the stimulation, they open their eyes and localize the touchpoint. The examiner marks a dot in the corresponding zone on a worksheet. If the patient fails to recognize it then an arrow is marked on the worksheet. Thus, the mapping of responses gives the patient's level of localization. Bilateral tactile stimulation is the ability to recognize the touch of both sides of the body simultaneously. Tactile extinction is the patient's failure to appreciate the touch on one side of the body.

TACTILE GNOSIS

Tactile gnosis is the delicate sensation of the finger pulp, which recognizes touch with the eyes closed. Touch and palpation together give us knowledge ("gnosis") of an object. The "tactile gnosis" provides the third dimension and educates the eye to appreciate the object's contours.

MOBERG PICK-UP TEST

The patient must pick up nine objects of different shape and size one at a time as quickly as possible and place them in a container. The test is done both with eyes open and closed. The examiner records the time using a stopwatch and observes the manner of prehension while picking up objects. The Moberg pick-up test assesses general sensation, tactile gnosis, hand in active motion, active manipulation and recognition of an object, e.g., the patient uses

thumb, ring and little finger instead of thumb and index finger in the median nerve palsy. The patients usually avoid using those fingers with poor sensation [9].

APPRECIATION OF WEIGHTS

It is the ability to perceive differences in weight between two objects placed sequentially in the patient's hand.

NINHYDRIN TEST

Aschan and Moberg developed the ninhydrin sweat test to detect sudomotor activity in the fingers. Sweating in an area supplied by a peripheral nerve is generally indicative of peripheral nerve regeneration and the absence of sweating is a sign of peripheral nerve lesion. The patient's hand is cleaned and wiped with alcohol and kept dry for 5 minutes (some prefer 20–30 minutes). Now the fingers are pressed against a good quality bond paper and the fingertips are traced with a pencil held in place for 15 seconds. The paper is sprayed with ninhydrin spray reagent and allowed to dry for 24 hours. The amino acids and lower peptide components of the sweat stains purple by the ninhydrin.

WRINKLE TEST

A normal hand placed in warm water (40°C) for 30 minutes wrinkles and a denervated hand does not. This phenomenon is associated with an absence of sensory function in denervation and return of wrinkling in reinnervation. The reliability of the test is limited and not used nowadays. It might be useful in children who are unable to respond to other tests.

DERMATOMES

A dermatome is defined as the area of skin innervated by a single nerve root or spinal segment. It determines the limb's sensory loss corresponding to that single spinal segment confirming the lesion to a particular nerve route (radiculopathy) or assigning a neurological level for a spinal cord lesion (Figure 5.4).

Sensitive skin territories corresponding to a dermatome have ill-defined boundaries, and adjacent dermatomes may overlap extensively. Thus, radial nerve injury or palsy produces little or no sensory loss on the dorsum of the hand. This explains that the autonomous zone for a particular nerve is much smaller than its potential sensory territory. The autonomous zone (signatory zone) is this small area in which sensory loss is specific to one nerve or nerve root [11, 12] (Table 5.3).

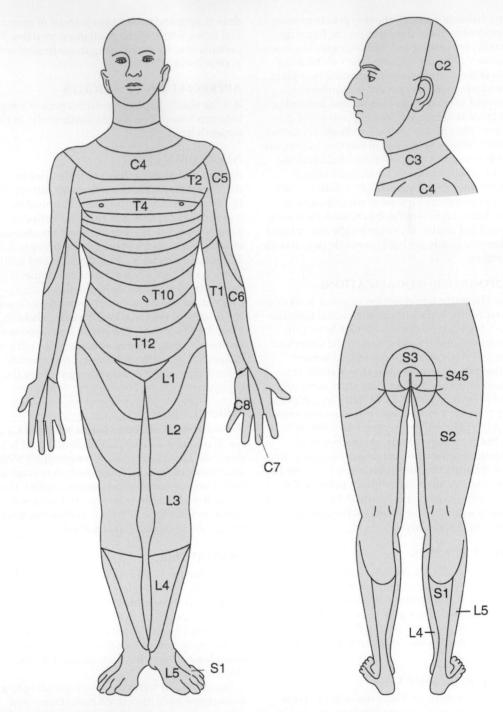

Figure 5.4 Dermatomes. This is the dermatome map recommended by the American Spinal Injury Association. A printable copy is available at http://www.asia-spinalinjury.org/learning/.

Tactile dermatomes are larger than pain dermatomes. So, testing for pain sensation is more sensitive than abnormal touch.

Significance of Sensation Levels and Loss is shown in Table 5.4.

SENSORY EXAMINATION IN PERIPHERAL NERVE LESIONS

The British Medical Research Council scale assesses sensibility similar to motor grading in peripheral nerve lesions (Table 5.5). A visual

Table 5.3: Autonomous Zone in the Upper Limb

C3	Supraclavicular fossa
C4	Top of the acromioclavicular joint
C5	Lateral side of the antecubital fossa
C6	Thumb
C7	Middle finger
C8	Little finger

Note: When the sensory and motor levels disagree, the motor level is a more reliable indicator of level of injury and future disability. In some patients with spinal cord disease, the most accurate indicator of the spinal segment affected is the site of the patient's vertebral pain and tenderness or the level of the patient's radicular pain.

analogue score (VAS) helps in measuring the intensity of pain (0 = no pain, 10 = intolerable pain).

SYMPATHETIC FUNCTION ASSESSMENT IN PERIPHERAL NERVE LESIONS

Trophic disorders depend on both sensory and sympathetic fibres. Lesions of the sympathetic nerve fibres have a direct action on sweating and circulation. Thus, we always appreciate dry skin with elasticity loss and thinner epithelium in a peripheral nerve injury. The skin is often stretched and shiny with features of causalgia such as cyanosis because of reduced blood flow. The nails become brittle and striated with retarded growth. Skin temperature is lower in the nerve-injured zone and remains cold-sensitive even after reinnervation. Also, the consistency of the subcutaneous tissue, fat pad and palm pulp get atrophied. In a median nerve injury, the index finger subcutaneous tissue and pulp shows these changes.

TROPHIC ASSESSMENT

Trophic ulcers are caused by skin atrophy, changes in blood flow, loss of sensation and impairment of protective reflexes, which are prone to injury and poor healing. The examiner should observe the atrophy and nail changes, blisters, burns, cuts or bruises, which indicate an insensitive hand. Dry, scaly, moist, mottled, pale and shiny are the trophic changes noted in the skin.

SKIN SWEATING

Sweating is not seen in peripheral nerve-injured skin areas, and they are dry in appearance. The appearance of sweating in an area supplied by the peripheral nerve is an indicator of nerve regeneration.

SENSORY TEST IN PERIPHERAL NERVE COMPRESSION

Carpal tunnel syndrome is the most common peripheral nerve compression seen in clinical practice. Most patients who present with carpal

Table 5.4: Sensory Loss Significance

Sensory loss both sides	Polyneuropathy Spinal cord disease
Sensory loss one side	Contralateral disease of the brainstem, thalamus or cerebral cortex
Sensory loss both sides Pain and temperature loss (opposite side) touch, vibratory, tactile sensation loss (same side of lesion)	Brown-Séquard syndrome Syringomyelia, spinal stroke
Sensory level Loss at and below the level, normal sensation above the level	Spinal cord disease
Sensory loss on the same side of face	Disease of the thalamus or cerebral hemisphere
Sensory loss on the opposite side of face	Brainstem disease (e.g., lateral medullary syndrome)

Table 5.5: Sensory Recovery

S0	Absence of sensibility in the autonomous area
S1	Recovery of deep cutaneous pain sensibility within autonomous area of nerve
S2	Return of some degree of superficial cutaneous pain and tactile sensibility within the autonomous area of the nerve
S3	Return of superficial cutaneous pain and tactile sensibility throughout the autonomous area, with disappearance of any previous over-response
S3+	Return of sensibility as in S3, with some recovery of two-point discrimination within the autonomous area
S4	Complete recovery

tunnel syndrome have normal sensation or no conduction studies because they avoid wrist positions (repetitive movements, sleeping with the wrist flexed) which triggers the symptoms. The sensory test can be evaluated by doing electrodiagnostic evaluation and sensory evaluation in normal resting wrist position and stressed position. Sensibility is tested with the Semmes-Weinstein monofilaments and followed by nerve conduction testing [3, 13]:

1. Test at rest or neutral position

2. Test in end-range dorsal and volar flexion

3. Retest in end-range position following 5–8 minutes of therapy (putty squeezing)

4. Compare testing of responses in the respective situations before and after dynamic activity and against resting baseline responses

REFERENCES

1. McGee S. *Evidence-Based Physical Diagnosis*, 4th edition. Examination of the Sensory System. Elsevier, Philadelphia, PA 2017, 569e–581.

2. Bell-Krotoski JA, Weinstein S and Weinstein C. Testing sensibility, including touch-pressure, two-point discrimination, point localization and vibration. *J Hand Therapy* 1993; 6:114–123.

3. Tubiana R, Thomine JM and Mackin E. *Examination of the Hand and Wrist*. CRC Press, Boca Raton, FL 1996, 328e–354.

4. Callahan AD. Sensibility testing: Clinical methods. In: Hunter JM, Schneider LH, Mackin, EJ, et al., (eds), *Rehabilitation of the Hand: Surgery and Therapy*, 3rd edition. St Louis, MO: CV Mosby, 1990, 432–442.

5. McCloskey DI. Kinesthetic sensibility. *Physiol Rev.* 1978; 58(4):763–820.

6. Rayan G, Akelman E. *The Hand: Anatomy, Examination and Diagnosis*. Philadelphia, PA: Lippincott Williams & Wilkins, 2011, 1e–160.

7. Elfar JC, Petrungaro JM, Braun RM, Cheng CJ, et al. Nerve. In: Hammert WC, Calfee RP, Bozentka DJ, Boyer MI, (eds), *ASSH Manual of Hand Surgery*. Philadelphia, PA: Lippincott Williams & Wilkins, 2010, 294e–342.

8. Virk MS and Rodner CM. History and physical examination. In: Weiss APC, Goldfarb CA, Hentz VR, Raven III RB, Slutsky DJ, Steinman SP, (eds), *The American Society for Surgery of the Hand: Textbook of Hand & Upper Extremity Surgery*. Chicago, IL: American Society for Surgery of the Hand, 2013, 33e–48.

9. Moberg E. Criticism and study of methods for examining sensibility in the hand. *Neurology* 1962; 12:8.

10. Weber EH. Uber den Tastinn. *Arch Anat Physiol Wissensch Med.* 1835; 152–160.

11. Kirshblum SC, Waring W, Biering-Sorensen F, et al. Reference for the 2011 revision of the International Standards for Neurological Classification of Spinal Cord Injury. *J Spinal Cord Med.* 2011; 34:547–554.

12. Lee MW, McPhee RW and Stringer MD. An evidence-based approach to human dermatomes. *Clin Anat.* 2008; 21:363–373.

13. Gelberman RH, Szabo RM, Williamson RV and Dimick MP. Sensibility testing in peripheral-nerve compression syndromes: An experimental study in humans. *J Bone Joint Surg Am.* 1983; 65(5):632e–638.

6 Dupuytren's Contracture

Clinical Examination and Classifications

Patrick Houvet

CONTENTS

INTRODUCTION

Dupuytren's contracture results in the thickening of the palmar fascia (middle palmar aponeurosis), a structure which is located under the skin of the palms and fingers. This thickening is accompanied by tissue retraction which limits the extension of the fingers and can infiltrate the skin.

A Swiss physician from Basel first described the condition in 1614. Platter postulated that the contracture of the ring and little fingers was due to flexor tendon shortening. Henry Cline, a student of John Hunter who is considered the father of English surgery, first described the disease in 1787 from a cadaveric study and proposed that it could be corrected with a surgical procedure. The surgery was first performed by Sir Astley Cooper in 1822 and consisted of a short vertical incision between the distal palmar crease and the base of the middle finger. In 1826, in France, Baron Boyer who was the master of Guillaume Dupuytren, described the affliction in a case report as "the tendon crispation of the fingers" (crispatura tendinum). Subsequently, the disease was fully described, and the procedure was performed by Baron Guillaume Dupuytren, a surgeon at the Hotel-Dieu Hospital in Paris in 1831. The patient was his cab driver who displayed the typical deformity [8–10].

ETIOLOGY

The prevalence of this affliction is 0.6 to 31.6%, increases with age and is more common in men than in women. In the Caucasian population, it affects between 10 and 20% of men over the age of 60, compared to 5% of women.

The difference in prevalence observed between men and women decreases with age, the ratio being only 1.3 beyond the age of 80 [3, 11, 20, 26].

The etiology of Dupuytren's contracture (DC) is still unknown to this day, but many factors have been implicated [13].

The only certainty is the existence of a genetic predisposition to the disease. The study of the patient's families shows the importance of heritability where the transmission is autosomal dominant with variable penetrance. Some studies have shown a positive association with specific classes of the human leukocyte antigen (HLA) system, namely: HLA-B12, 17 HLA-A1 and DR4, 18 HLA-DR3,19 HLA-DRB1, 15 (HLA-DR2) 20 and HLA-DRB1, 01 (HLA-DR1) [2].

Also, when a family history is present, the disease is more likely to progress faster than usual [19].

Several favouring mutations have been identified, most of them encoding Wingless Integration (WgINT)-like proteins. Rare in Asian and African populations, the disease most frequently occurs in white Caucasians, mainly Northern European individuals with light eyes, e.g., blue. Invasions by the Vikings and Celts remain the predominant factor in the distribution of the disease in Europe. Very often, another member of the family has also presented with the disease, but this is very often unknown to the patient and should be investigated during the first consultation [13, 33].

Diabetes mellitus appears to be a risk factor as well. The risk is higher for type 1 diabetes, which justifies the fact that the pathology is more common in insulin-dependent patients, compared to those taking oral antibiotics [4].

Smoking and alcohol both have a dose-response association with the malady. The

DOI: 10.1201/9781003125938-6

interaction between the two factors is not yet corroborated in the literature [5, 18].

The development of Dupuytren's disease has been linked to certain manual labour tasks, such as the use of vibratory tools. From these observations, it can be postulated that trauma can trigger Dupuytren's disease in a patient with risk factors. No relationship has been established, however, except in a few specific situations summarized by McFarlane [6, 12, 25, 29, 30, 32].

The relationship between epilepsy and antiepileptic drugs and the development of this disorder is not clearly defined [4].

In 1963, Hueston proposed the concept of Dupuytren's diathesis in relation to patients who develop the pathology at a younger age, have bilateral disease, a positive familiar history and a higher rate of recurrence [22–24].

PATHOPHYSIOLOGY

The pathogenesis of this disorder has been compared to wound healing, which correlates with the theory of micro-traumatisms where the body generates an inflammatory response which produces free radicals of superoxide and hydrogen peroxide which in turn stimulates a restorative response [7].

Dupuytren's contracture is a fibromatosis of the middle palmar fascia caused by the overgrowth of myofibroblasts that produce excess neocollagen. These cells are not of the muscular type but rather a derivative of the fibroblasts provided in their cytoplasm with microfilaments capable of contractions. The existence of "fibronectin" on the surface of these cells creates a link between them that produces the capability for retraction to occur.

Histological study of the palmar fascia shows the existence of type III collagen as compared with type I in the tendon collagen. Several forms of thickening can be described, and cell density is correlated with disease activity. Luck correlated this criterion and proposed a classification in three stages [14, 16, 17, 27, 37, 38]:

- Stage 1: This stage is characterized by a fibroblast proliferation. There is a nodular thickening of cells with high density where many fibroblasts and fibrocytes populations are enclosed in a rich network of collagen fibres and local hypervascularization, generally located in the metacarpophalangeal and proximal interphalangeal (PIP) joints.

- Stage 2: This stage of the evolution appears with the progressive organization of collagen. When collagen production increases, myofibroblasts become the predominant cell type and nodule-cord units are developing.

- Stage 3: The terminal or residual stage is characterized by low fibroblastic activity but with the presence of collagen cords. There is low cell density but there is lamellar fascia thickening with dense collagen in parallel fibres and sparse fibrocytes between the collagen fibres.

Most pathological studies confirm that the condition follows the anatomical pathways of the fascia, both in the palm and in the digits. Joint retractions mainly affect the MCP and PIP joints but rarely the distal interphalangeal joint (DIP).

In a pathological hand extremity, a pretendinous cord develops from the pretendinous band and is responsible for the flexion contractures of the MCP joints.

The most common cord is the central cord. The lateral cord, which originates from the lateral leaflet, causes contracture of the PIP joint and has the potential to deflect the neurovascular pedicle if the cord is coiled (Figure 6.1).

The septa of Legueu and Juvara (fibrous node of connective tissue), when affected, gives rise to a vertical cord. The abductor digiti minimi muscle-tendon can also be a source of an isolated cord [28, 34].

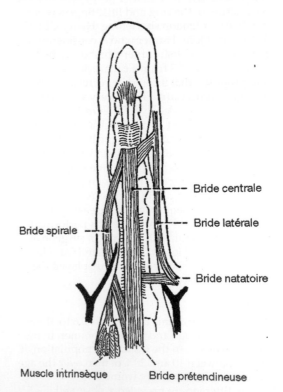

Bride centrale

Bride latérale

Bride spirale

Bride natatoire

Muscle intrinsèque

Bride prétendineuse

Figure 6.1 Different types of cord.

PHYSICAL EXAMINATION AND CLASSIFICATIONS OF DUPUYTREN'S CONTRACTURE

The diagnosis of Dupuytren's contracture is clinical. The physical examination makes it possible to evaluate functional impairment, evaluate the deformities and classify the lesions and finally, inform the patient of a therapeutic strategy.

The disease is characterized by symptoms related to the retraction of the integuments.

The lesions are painless, without other associated symptoms [28, 34, 36].

One can find in the examination:

- Nodules which are mainly palmar, more rarely digital (Figure 6A)

- Cords which for the most part, are palmar and/or digital (Figure 6B)

- Skin umbilications commonly called pitting

- Mainly located between the proximal and distal palmar crease and the distal insertion of the longitudinal fibres

In early stages, retraction and pitting may be absent.

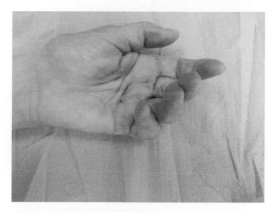

Figure 6A Dupuytren's classic deformities.

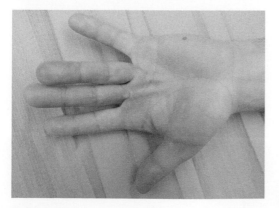

Figure 6B Dupuytren's cords.

The ailment begins with the fifth and fourth fingers in 75% of cases, but all fingers may be affected with bilateral lesions in 50% of cases. In particular, the location at the fifth finger is known to be difficult and recurrent.

The examination reveals the appearance in the palm of one or more nodules located at the base of the fourth or fifth finger. These nodules are firm, adherent to the skin and deeper structures. Nodules are the most notable characteristic of the disease and where the retraction occurs. If nodules are absent and there is only a thickening of the fascia, the diagnosis of Dupuytren's contracture should be questioned and a re-evaluation should be performed. This situation is frequently observed with a wrist fracture. In this case, the aponeurotic thickening is most often reversible and is not indicative of a future retraction of the fingers.

Fibrosis transforms the palmar and digital fascia and results in the formation of fibrous bands. Palmar cords cause flexion of the MCP joints: Digital cords where pure digital involvement is a rare cause of flexion of the proximal and sometimes distal interphalangeal joints. Fibrosis worsens gradually and discontinuously with successive outbreaks. The extension of the fingers gradually becomes more and more limited. Eventually extension is not possible, and the fingers become totally flexed and permanently remain in this position, causing functional impairment [38].

The extent of the impairment is assessed using the classification described in 1961 by Tubiana and Michon who established a five-stage rating scale which has been widely distributed and adopted in Europe [21, 39].

Referencing the middle fingers, each stage corresponds to the progression of retraction of 45° by adding the three joints MCP + PIP + DIP with a total of six stages (Figure 6.2):

Stage 0: No lesion

Stage N: Palmar or digital nodule without retraction

Stage I: Total retraction of the three joints between 0 and 45°

Stage II: Total retraction of the three joints between 45 and 90°

Stage III: Total retraction of the three joints between 90 and 135°

Stage IV: Total retraction of the three joints greater than 135°, with the additional letter H when the DIP is fixed in hyperextension

Referencing the thumb column, Tubiana offers a double assessment at the first intermetacarpal space, in five stages corresponding to losses of 15° (Figures 6.3 and 6.4):

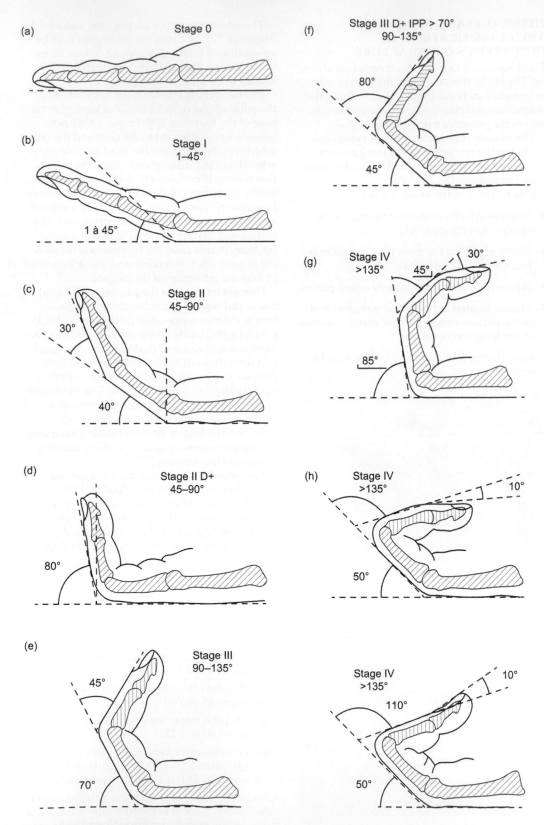

Figure 6.2 Middle fingers classification.

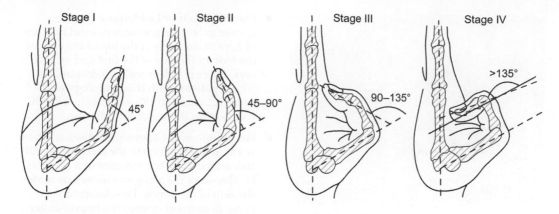

Figure 6.3 Tubiana's thumb classification.

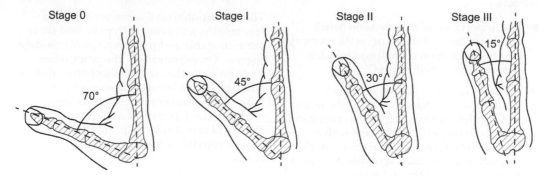

Figure 6.4 Tubiana's thumb classification.

Stage 0: No lesion

Stage N: Nodule without retraction

Stage I: Separation angle between 45 and 30°

Stage II: Separation angle between 30 and 15 °

Stage III: Lower separation angle <15°

Tubiana proposes the following observations in relation to his method by specifying the following points [21, 39, 40]:

- The palmar lesions are indicated by the letter P and the digital lesions are indicated by the letter D, the letter D followed by the + sign indicates that the PIP retraction is equal to greater than 70° and therefore of random correction.

- If the lesions are both palmar and digital, the number designating the stage is followed by the letters PD.

The letter H (for hyperextension) designates advanced cases in which the distal phalanx is fixed in hyperextension. It is necessary to differentiate between fixed cases and cases where active and/or passive IPD flexion exist.

During the physical examination, it is necessary to distinguish the following conditions:

- Pure nodular palmar forms which should be monitored and there is no indication of disease if the patient can put their hand in a flat position on a table.

- The digito-palmar form with extension deficit relating only to CMP joint (group I) for which complete recovery after fasciectomy is highly likely.

Although the two previously mentioned forms do not present serious problems, they are unlike the following two difficult cases:

- The digital forms with extension deficit predominant on the PIP (group II), which is much more difficult to treat because it is impossible to foresee pre-operatively a complete recovery of the extension, particularly on the fifth ray.

- The digito-palmar forms with MCP and PIP extension deficit (group III).

Summarizing, the difficult forms of the disease [1, 35, 41]:

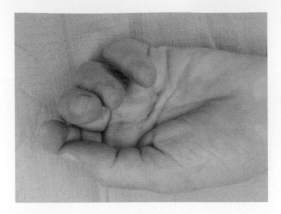

Figure 6C Difficult form with huge retraction.

- The importance of the extension deficit which can be moderated, or on the contrary lead to a retraction of the finger which is stuck in the palm (Figure 6C).

- The importance of fibrosis with the less severe problem characterized by the long band under the skin, and on the other hand with the more difficult problem with a more diffuse form with skin invasion. Skin invasion must be taken seriously because it constitutes one of the problems encountered with the surgical treatment of Dupuytren's contracture.

- As a rule, the extension of the fibrosis makes it possible to define localized forms in the fourth and fifth fingers and extensive forms reaching the other fingers, the thumb and the first intermetacarpal space.

Other lesions can be associated with the following characteristics:

- The disease can be localized on the dorsal face of the fingers opposite the PIP joints in the form of Garrod dorsal pads or "Knuckle pads" (Figure 6D).

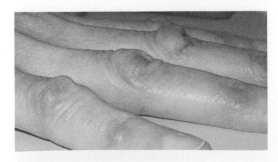

Figure 6D Knuckle pads.

- Plantar lesions or Ledderhose disease appear as large, sometimes painful nodules of 2 cm in diameter at the top of the arch of the foot, in the axis of the first and second rays. There is a clear male predominance: 50% of patients with this pathology also have DC. And 2 to 15% of patients with DC will express this associated disease.

- Penile lesions or Lapeyronie's disease: There is a bent deformation of the erect penis and characterized by the presence of a non-elastic fibrosis of the albuginea (envelope under the skin of the penis). This deformity can cause discomfort or even the impossibility of penetration. The frequency is 1 to 3% of the population in Europe.

This condition usually appears within a few months and often with pain, and then remains stable and may even spontaneously regress. On examination, the practitioner finds on palpation, a plate most often dorsal and sometimes lateral. Ultrasound associated with Doppler makes it possible to specify the anatomical relationships and the vascularization. MRI can also be helpful. The association with Dupuytren's disease is common (30% of cases).

DIFFERENTIAL DIAGNOSIS

A certain number of diagnoses can be determined by a retraction in the flexion of the MCP and PIP of the fingers that is not accompanied by pain, except sometimes localized in the palmar nodules.

Clinical examination and questioning can easily determine the following:

- Stiffness in flexion, a sequel of a complex regional syndrome most often involving PIPs and DPIs.

- Diffuse retraction with joint locations in certain diabetes especially in young subjects.

- Fibroblastic rheumatism.

- A tumour of an undetermined nature on the palmar side of the hand: Cyst of the flexor sheath (cyst of the pulley A1), giant cell tumour. In the latter case, ultrasound can be an easy diagnostic aid.

ISOLATED FIFTH RAY INVOLVEMENT IN DUPUYTREN'S DISEASE

In its location at the fifth ray, the type of cord is variable, but isolated digital involvement without palmar involvement is not uncommon, unlike other fingers. Indeed, some bands do not present any continuity with the middle palmar fascia [5, 31].

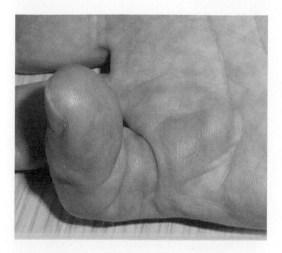

Figure 6E Isolated form of the fifth finger.

Four varieties of cord can be found at the fifth ray: The central, spiral, lateral and retro-vascular cords. However, some formations are specific to this location (Figure 6E).

The ulnar cord attached to the abductor digiti minimi is specific and almost constant. This cord is always superficial in relation to the vasculo-nervous bundle at the finger base.

However, it can remain lateral at the base of the finger and be associated with a spiral strap. It retracts the MCP joint and medially deviates the axis of the fifth finger.

Hyperextension of the DIP can be found, but it is rare. It is secondary to a retraction of the retinacular ligament, making a buttonhole by progressive distension of the central band and dislocation of the collateral bands.

The radial digital cord can be isolated and terminate on the pulleys or on the periosteum of the middle phalanx.

Finally, the association of different cords is frequent, producing significant retractions with often poor quality of the skin.

REGARDING DIFFICULT FORMS

One can use the term "difficult forms" with consequences for therapy and can result in [1, 35, 41]:

- Stage III or IV forms with a predominantly extension deficit on the PIP joint, whether or not associated with hyperextension of the DIP, whether it is reducible or not.

- The forms of the fifth ray that have been treated.

- The radial forms reaching the thumb and the first intermetacarpal fold.

- The extensive forms of the young, occurring in a subject of 20 to 30 years old, are often bilateral.

- Recurrent forms with:

- The stiffness at the PIP presents a complex problem because it is often impossible to know if the only excision of the aponeu-rotic lesions will allow the extension of the PIP.

- Fixed DIP hyperflexion: Distal interphalangeal flexion can be seen but is rare and more common in DIP hyperextension.

- Vascular and trophic disorders: It is important to be vigilant about the indication for surgery in recurrent forms, especially at the fifth ray with significant extension deficit because there may be preoperative trophic lesions with interruption of a vascular axis where the Allen test and a Doppler study can be very helpful. Surgery can create additional trauma which can unfortunately result in necrosis and even amputation.

Therefore, it is prudent to warn the patient of the possible difficulties in treating the problem and it is prudent to limit oneself to correcting the MCP extension and perhaps performing the intervention in two steps reserving the PIP problem for the second step.

CONCLUSION

Dupuytren's contracture produces a retractile fibrosis of the superficial palmar fascia and should not be confused with another diagnosis. Its essential problem is etiological, pathogenic and the extra-palmar manifestations clearly show that it is not simply a local disease but a general affliction, especially in certain extensive forms in young patients.

The genesis of the disease is not yet fully understood despite numerous molecular studies on collagen and fibroblast.

Questioning the patient is not always helpful but can contribute to a better understanding of the patient's situation, namely, family medical history, work and leisure activities. This is part of the Hueston diathesis.

A clinical examination is the cornerstone of determining a diagnosis. It must be detailed and meticulous by reporting each joint-by-joint extension evaluation/deficit. This not only makes it possible to determine the stage of the disease in each finger, but also to establish a preoperative prognosis and above all, an element of comparison with the postoperative result. Finally, the importance of pictures should be emphasized.

REFERENCES

1. Alnot JY. *Maladie de Dupuytren: formes difficiles. Cahier d'enseignement de la SFCM.* Expansion Scientifique Publications, 1998.

2. Bobinski R, Olczyk K, Wisowski G and Janusz W. Genetic aspect of Dupuytren's disease. *Wiad Lek* 2004; 57: 59–62.

3. Bergenudd H, Lindgarde F and Nilsson BE. Prevalence of Dupuytren's contracture and its correlation with degenerative changes of the hands and feet and with criteria of general health. *J Hand Surg [Br]* 1993; 18B(2): 254–257.

4. Broekstra DC, Groen H, Molenkamp S and Werker P. A systematic review and meta-analysis on the strength and consistency of the association between Dupuytren disease and diabetes mellitus, liver disease and epilepsy. *Plast Reconstr Surg* 2018; 141(3): 367–379.

5. Burge P, Hoy G, Regan P and Milne R. Smoking, alcohol and the risk of Dupuytren's contracture. *J Bone Joint Surg [Br]* 1997; 79B(2): 206–210.

6. De La Caffinière JY, Wagner R, Etscheid J and Metzger F. Manual labor and Dupuytren disease. The results of a computerized survey in the field of iron metallurgy. *Ann Chir Main* 1983; 2(1): 66–72.

7. Chiu HF and McFarlane RM. Pathogenesis of Dupuytren's contracture: A correlative clinical-pathological study. *J Hand Surg [Am]* 1978; 3:1–10.

8. Cline H Jr. *Notes of John Windsor (student) from a lecture by Henry Cline* Jr. Manuscript collection, John Pylands University Library of Manchester, Manchester, 1808, pp. 485–489.

9. Dupuyren G. De la rétraction des doigts par suite d'une affection de l'aponévrose palmaire. Description de la maladie. Opération chirurgicale qui convient dans ce cas. Compte rendu de la Clinique Chirurgicale de l'Hôtel Dieu par Messieurs les Docteurs Alexandre PAILLARD et MARX. *Journal Universel et Hebdomadaire de Médecine et de Chirurgie Pratique et des Institutions Médicales* 1831; 5: 349–365.

10. Elliot D. The early history of contracture of the palmar fascia. In: Mc Farlane RM, Mc Grouther DA and Flint MH, (eds), *Dupuytren's Disease.* Churchill Livingstone, Edinburgh, 1990, 1–9 and 413–419.

11. Finsen V, Dalen H and Nesheim J. The prevalence of Dupuytren's disease among two different ethnic groups in northern Norway. *J Hand Surg [Am]* 2002; 27A(1): 115–117.

12. Fisk G. The relationship of manual labour and specific injury to Dupuytren's disease. In: Hueston J, (ed.), *Dupuytren's Disease.* Churchill Livingstone, Edinburgh, 1985, pp. 104–105.

13. Geoghegan JM, Forbes J, Clark DI, Smith G and Hubbard R. Dupuytren's disease risk factors. *J Hand Surg [Br]* 2004; 29B(5): 423–426.

14. Gosset J. Maladie de Dupuytren et anatomie des aponévroses palmo-digitales. *Annales de Chirurgie* 1967; 21: 554–565.

15. Goubier JN, Le Bellec Y and Cottioas P. L'atteinte isolée du ve rayon dans la maladie de Dupuytren. *Chir main* 2001; 20(3): 212–217.

16. Goyrand G. Nouvelles recherches sur la rétraction permanente des doigts. *Mémoires de l'Académie Royale de Médecine* 1834; 3: 489–496.

17. Grazina R, Texeira S, Ramos R, Sousa H, Ferreira A and Lemos R. Dupuytren's disease: Where do we stand? *EFORT Open Rev* 2019; 4(2): 63–69.

18. Gronbaek M. A prospective study linked both alcohol and tobacco to Dupuytren's disease. *J Clin Epidemiol.* 2004; 57(8): 858–863.

19. Gudmundsson KG, Arngrimsson R and Jonsson T. Eighteen years follow-up study of the clinical manifestations and progression of Dupuytren's disease. *Scand Rheumatol* 2001; 30: 31–34.

20. Hindocha S, McGrouther DA and Bayat A. Epidemiological evaluation of Dupuytren's disease incidence and prevalence rates in relation to etiology. *Hand (NY)* 2009; 4: 256–269.

21. Hindocha S, Stanley JK and Watson JS. Revised Tubiana's staging system for assessment of disease severity in Dupuytren's disease-preliminary clinical findings. *Hand (NY)* 2008; 32: 80–86.

22. Hueston JT. Dupuytren diathesis. In: Mc Farlane RM, Mc Grouther DA and Flint MH, (eds), *Dupuytren's Disease*. Churchill Livingstone, Edinburgh, 1990, pp. 191–200.

23. Hueston JT. The management of recurrent Dupuytren's disease. *Eur Med Bibliog* 1991; 1(4): 7–16.

24. Hueston JT. Dupuytren's contracture and occupation. *J Hand Surg [Am]* 1987; 12A: 657–658.

25. Liss GM and Stock SR. Can Dupuytren's contracture be work-related? Review of the évidence. *Am J Ind Med* 1996; 29(5): 521–532.

26. Lanting R, Broekstra DC, Werker PM and van den Heuvel ER. A systematic review and meta-analysis on the prevalence of Dupuytren disease in the general population of Western countries. *Plast Reconstr Surg* 2014; 133: 593–603.

27. Ledderhose G. Zur Pathologie der Aponeuvrose des Fuses und der Hand. *Av Ch Klin Chir* 1897; 55: 694.

28. Luck JV. Dupuytren's contracture. *J Bone Joint Surg* 1959; 41: 635–664.

29. Mcfarlane RM. On the origin and spread of Dupuytren's disease. *J Hand Surg [Am]* 2002; 27A(3): 385–390.

30. Mcfarlane RM, Botz JS and Cheung H. Epidemiology of surgical patients. In: Flint MH, McFarlane RM and McCrouther DA, (eds), *Dupuytren's Disease*. Churchill Livingstone, Edinburgh, 1990, pp. 201–238.

31. Medhi KS, King JD and Keshtvarz S. Isolated small finger DIP Dupuytren's contracture. *Case Report Orthop* 2019; 4. doi: 10.1155/2019/7183739.

32. Mikkelsen OA. Dupuytren's disease: The influence of occupation and previous hand injuries. *Hand* 1978; 19: 1.

33. Mikkelsen OA. Epidemiology of a Norwegian population. In: Flint MH, McFarlane RM and McGrouther DA, (eds), *Dupuytren's Disease*. Churchill Livingstone, Edinburgh, 1990, pp. 191–200.

34. Rayan GM. Dupuytren disease: Anatomy, pathology, presentation, and treatment. *J Bone Joint Surg Am* 2007; 89(1): 189–198.

35. Rombouts JJ, Noel H, Legrain Y and Munting E. Prediction of recurrence in the treatment of Dupuytren's disease: Evaluation of a histologic classification. *J Hand Surg [Am]* 1989; 14: 644–652.

36. Shaw RB, Chong AK and Zhang A. Dupuytren's disease: History, diagnosis and treatment. *Plast Reconstr Surg* 2007; 120(3): 44–54.

37. Thomasek JJ, Sehultz RJ, Episalla CW and Newman SA. The cytoskeleton and extracellular matrix of the Dupuytren's disease «myobroblast: An inmmuno fluorescence study of a non-muscle cell types. *J Hand Surg* 1986; 11A: 365–371.

38. Thomine JM. Conjonctif d'enveloppe des doigts et squelette fibreux des commissures interdigitales. *Ann Chir Plast* 1965; 3: 194–203.

39. Tubiana R and Michon J. Evaluation chiffrée précise de la déformation dans la maladie de Dupuytren. *Mém Acad Chir* 1961; 87: 886–888.

40. Tubiana R, De Frenne H. Les localisations de la maladie de Dupuytren à la partie radiale de la main Chirurgie 1976; 102: 989–993.

41. Tubiana R and Leclercq C. Les récidives dans la maladie de Dupuytren. In: Tubiana R. and Hueston JT, (eds), *La Maladie de Dupuytren*, Expansion Scientifique Française, Paris, 1986, 3rd ed., pp. 203–207.

7 Digital Deformities in Rheumatoid Arthritis

Physical Assessment and Clinical Classifications

Patrick Houvet

CONTENTS

INTRODUCTION

Rheumatoid arthritis (RA) typically affects the hand and/or the wrist in 90% of cases. It can affect these anatomical structures to varying degrees of severity. In the absence of treatment, joints and tendons can become compromised and result in deformities causing a loss of function which in turn can lead to disability/handicap [4, 7, 10, 12, 13, 15, 19, 23, 34].

Recent therapeutic advances in RA treatment have resulted in vast improvements for severe cases and deformities are now practically non-existent.

ETIOLOGIES

RA is the most common form of chronic inflammatory rheumatism. RA is a systemic immune-mediated inflammatory disorder that alters the synovium around the joints and tendons through a proliferation of synovial lining cells, angiogenesis and increased lymphocytes in the perivascular area. It usually manifests itself between the ages of 40 and 50, but it can occur at any age, as early as the age of 16 as well as late onset after 65 years of age.

RA is three times more common in women before the age of 60 but this sex ratio imbalance gradually diminishes with time. Its prevalence in the adult population is 0.3 to 0.8%.

Its prevalence in first-degree relatives of a patient with RA is on the order of 2 to 4%, which means despite the increased risk of a genetic predisposition due to the existence of a family history, more than 95% of first-degree relatives of a patient with RA will be free from the disease [15, 29, 53].

The genetic link appears to be established with HLA-DR4.4, HLA-DRB1.4, the PTPN22 gene and the C5-TRAF1 gene. Overall, these factors represent 30% of the risk of developing RA [55].

Environmental factors are thought to contribute to the onset of the disease:

- European studies have shown that the incidence of RA is generally higher in Northern Europe than in Southern Europe.

- Hormonal factors play a role in this disease because it occurs more frequently in women during menopause. Additionally, remission

DOI: 10.1201/9781003125938-7

has been observed during pregnancy, often with a relapse after childbirth. Finally, it has been observed that oral contraceptives may decrease the severity of RA.

■ Psychological stress factors can also increase the likelihood of developing RA: In 20 to 30% of cases it is noted that RA occurs after a significant stress-inducing event such as bereavement or divorce.

■ Smokers have a slightly higher risk of RA than non-smokers.

ASSESSMENT AND CLASSIFICATION OF DEFORMITIES

In 70 to 80% of cases, the clinical diagnosis is an acromelic arthritis which is bilateral and generally symmetrical, without extra-articular or systemic manifestations ("naked" polyarthritis), evolving in a chronic mode (>6 weeks), characterized by inflammatory joint pain (waking up at the end of the night and accompanied with morning stiffness >30 minutes), most often localized to the wrist, metacarpophalangeal joint (MCP) and proximal interphalangeal joints (PIP), but can also affect the ankles and metatarsophalangeal joints.

Digital deformities in rheumatoid arthritis are common and functionally well tolerated.

They are always multi digital and different depending on the rays concerned [4, 7, 10, 13, 19, 23, 33, 39, 46, 53].

An extensive and thorough physical examination is required:

■ The wrist should be positioned in alignment to assess its impact on the ulnar deviation of the digital chains. Before performing a direct gesture of realignment at the MCP level, it is imperative to first correct the radial deviation of the carpus which only aggravates the dislocation of the extensor muscle-tendons [5, 18, 28, 29, 36, 41, 51, 57].

■ The localization of the different synovitis is evaluated, joint by joint. The spontaneously painful joints are most often on the lateral side (squeeze test).

■ Instability and joint dislocation.

■ The function of the extensor apparatus; the sub-dislocation or the dislocation of the extensor tendons in the intermetacarpal grove must be systematically corrected because they contribute to the deficit of extension of the digit chain, in the "ulnar side" and promote the palmar subluxation of the first phalanx.

■ The function of the wrist and finger flexors.

■ The intrinsic muscles: The interosseous retraction is assessed by the Finochietto test.

When the MP is in extension and passive flexion of the PIP is impossible or severely limited and while the MCP is in flexion, the test is considered positive [17, 21, 30].

■ Buttonhole or swan-neck deformities must be taken into account in the surgical procedure as well.

WRIST AND METACARPOPHALANGEAL JOINTS

There are many factors that contribute to palmar dislocation and ulnar translation of the first phalanx as well as its ulnar deviation of the fingers and this requires an accurate analysis of wrist and MCP deformities [6, 8, 45, 47–49, 54, 56, 57] Figures 7A and 7B).

Pathophysiology

As rheumatoid disease progresses, the wrists are affected in more than 80% of cases and bilaterally in 95% of cases. The pathophysiology of wrist deformities has been well studied. The degradation of the radio-ulnar fibrocartilage associated with the volar dislocation of the extensor carpi ulnaris muscle-tendon induces a dorsal subluxation of the ulnar head. Palmar dislocation of the internal carpal column places the hand into supinate with respect to the forearm. As the extensor carpi radialis longus muscle becomes predominant, the carpal bones accentuate their radial inclination.

At this stage, by the compensation phenomenon according to Landsmeer theory, the digital chains can initiate their ulnar deviation although this mechanism is not the unique etiology [25].

The scapholunate ligament rupture, the horizontalization of the scaphoid, the accordion-like dislocation of the carpal rows will cause a collapse, weakening the flexor and extensor system and strengthening the intrinsic system which give rise to such finger deformities as swan-neck. This cascade of deformations partly

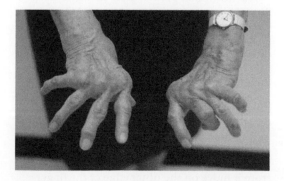

Figure 7A Wrist and hand deformities.

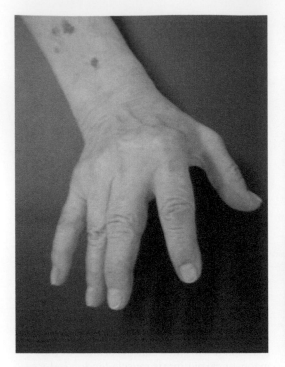

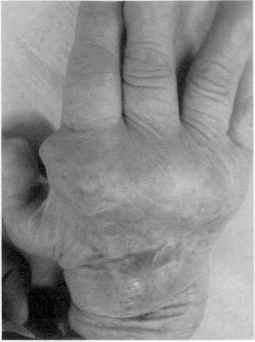

Figure 7B Wrist and hand deformities.

Figure 7C MCP deformity.

explains the mechanisms of the deformity of the digital chains and need to be corrected before any digital therapeutic is attempted.

The MCP joints, under the action of the synovitis proliferation, first present a palmar subdislocation of the first phalanx with respect to the metacarpal head and then possibly develop an ulnar deviation with translation of the first phalanx. During the development of the synovitis on the dorsal surface of the metacarpal head, in the cul-de-sac of the palmar plate, around the collateral ligaments and at the level of their metacarpal insertion, the joint capsule will distend and then rupture Figure 7C.

Joint instability will be aggravated by the elongation and then the rupture of the collateral ligaments.

The infiltrated palmar plate detaches from its metacarpal attachments and contributes, through the flexor sheath, to aggravate the palmar dislocation of the first phalanx. Radial elongation of the extensor hood will result in ulnar dislocation of the extensor tendon in the intermetacarpal grove.

The ulnar interossei and more specifically the abductor digiti minimi of the fifth finger, contribute not only to the MCP flexion but also to its ulnar deviation. At the level of the long and middle fingers, the palmar plate and the neighbouring structures which are detached from it move on the ulnar edge of the finger under the action of the flexors whose path

is oblique with respect to the axis of the A1 pulley. Radial tilt of the wrist, collapsed wrist and flexion of the fourth and fifth metacarpals contribute to the aggravation of the ulnar deviation.

MIDDLE FINGER DEFORMITY
Buttonhole deformity
(bouttonnière deformity)

The elongation of the median band of the extensor apparatus progressively leads to an extrusion of the PIP between the two lateral bands which move apart under the pressure of the convex edges of the first phalangeal head like a buttonhole forced open by a button. It was Milch who in 1931, gave it the name of "buttonhole deformity" (Figure 7D).

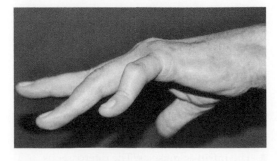

Figure 7D Buttonhole deformity.

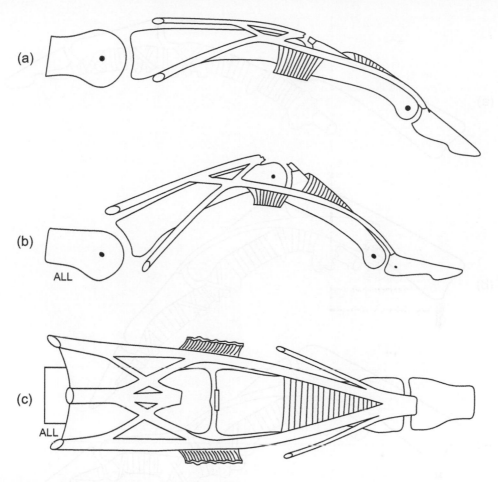

(a)

(b)

ALL

(c)

ALL

Figure 7.1 Buttonhole (boutonnière) deformity.

This deformity is characterized by a flexion of the PIP and hyper-extension of the distal interphalangeal joint (DIP) [1, 16, 22, 31, 32, 52] (Figure 7.1).

Pathophysiology

In RA, the pathological process always begins with intra-articular proliferation of the synovium (synovitis). This will distend the capsulo-ligamentous apparatus which, progressively, will interfere with the weakest points of the extensor apparatus, between the lateral bands and the median band. This proliferation lifts the medial band, distending it until it breaks. The strong lateral ligaments will resist the pressure and the hypertrophic synovial tissue will tend to grow below at the level of the accessory collateral ligaments.

This explains (unlike metacarpophalangeal synovitis) that it is rare to observe at the level of PPIs an instability secondary to the destruction of the lateral ligaments.

There is hyperextension of DIP. This is not only due to excessive traction of the extensor apparatus, but also to a voluntary compensatory extension of the patient, to put the end of the affected finger at the same level as the others.

The lateral bands ultimately migrate below the axis of motion of the PIP joint, where they become PIP flexors rather than extensors, promoting dorsal protrusion of the PIP.

At this point, Stack's triangle with the triangular ligament located at the dorsal base of P2 keeps widening, which can only worsen the hyperextension of the DIP joint and the flexion of the PIP.

Classification

Nalebuff and Millender proposed a classification of buttonhole deformation [34, 36]:

- Stage 1: The deformation is reducible or partially reducible with moderate deficit of extension of –10 to –15° of the PIP, with a loss of extension of the DIP.

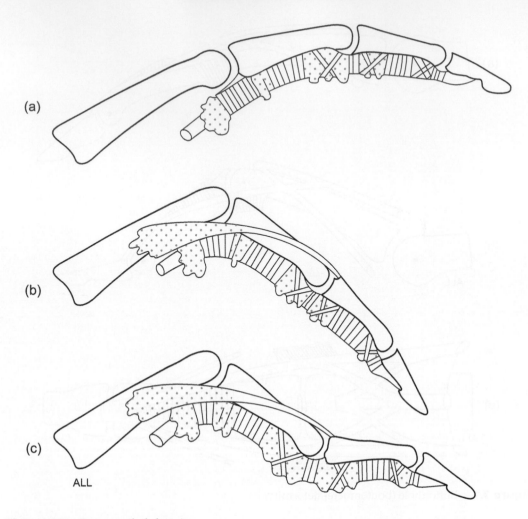

(a)

(b)

(c)

ALL

Figure 7.2 Swan-neck deformity.

The passive extension of the PIP should be tested by applying the extension force to the middle phalanx, while leaving the DIP free:

- If the hyper-extension of the DIP is corrected by passively extending the PIP, the transverse retinacular ligaments are not yet retracted and allow the dorsal displacement of the lateral bands.

- When extending the PIP, the DIP remains in hyper-extension, then the lateral strips are already fixed in the palmar position.

- Stage 2: The PIP is flexed at 40° and the deformity is not passively reducible. The hyperextension of the DIP is installed, and the degree of flexion is limited. At this stage, the transverse retinacular structures are retracted and fibrotic.

- Stage 3: Joint destruction and stiffness are established in the PIP in flexion and the DIP in hyperextension.

The MCP develops, by compensation, and hyperextension particularly at the fourth and fifth rays, as a deformation which is better tolerated here than at the index.

Swan-neck deformity

In the early stages of the disease, the diagnosis is uncomplicated since it is manifested by hyperextension of the PIP joint and flexion of the DIP joint. It becomes a more disabling lesion at the functional level which alerts the patient more quickly to the disease than a buttonhole deformity [22, 26, 37, 50] (Figure 7.2).

Pathophysiology

Several mechanisms can induce swan-neck deformity during rheumatoid arthritis. Deformities resulting from carpal collapse, metacarpophalangeal dislocations, specific lesions of the PIP and DIP should be distinguished (Figure 7E).

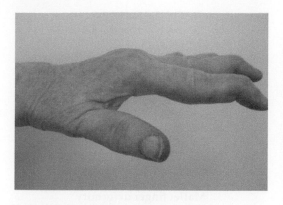

Figure 7E   Swan-neck deformity.

• The carpal rows collapse:

Shapiro observed that carpal collapse can induce swan-neck deformity through the distension of the extrinsic flexor and extensor apparatus, which puts tension on the intrinsic system and therefore, as a result, causes hyperextension of the PIP. This disruption of the balance between the intrinsic system is very common in the MP joints, but much less so as a result of carpal collapse.

Shapiro observes that when it reduces carpal collapse, the swan-neck corrects itself.

- Metacarpophalangeal dislocations and retraction of the intrinsic muscles:

Palmar dislocation of the first phalanx can gradually migrate under the metacarpal head and relax the extensor apparatus and put tension on the intrinsic muscles, which helps to dorsalize the lateral bands and increase traction on the median band.

The dislocation of the extensor apparatus on the ulnar side of MCP displays the same pattern.

At the palmar level of MCP joint, the detachment of the synovitis at the palmar plate and the flexor apparatus will flex the joint, placing the hand in an "intrinsic plus" position which can only develop the swan-neck. When the MCP dislocation is reducible, the swan-neck is also reducible in its early stages. It is understood that the correction of the swan-neck also requires the treatment of its etiology.

The very relative retraction of the intrinsic muscle-tendons is easily evaluated by the Finochietto test.

• Synovitis PIP and tenosynovitis of the flexors muscle-tendons:

PIP joint synovitis has been implicated by the elongation of the palmar plate and the retinacular ligaments, which would induce dorsalization of the lateral bands. All of these lesions are effectively sufficient to create hyperextension of the PIP and its corollary, flexion of the DIP. In fact, this pathophysiological mechanism remains exceptional because the first lesion created by the PIP synovitis is the elongation or even the rupture of the median band, which causes the appearance of a buttonhole deformation.

In reality, it is most often the tenosynovitis of the flexor muscle-tendons of the fingers in their digital sheath that is involved. This tenosynovitis can be seen in the palm of the hand at the emergence of the A1 pulley. The pressure of the examiner's middle finger or thumb at the distal palmar crease arouses the pain, and the attempt to flex the fingers by the patient makes a crackle appear under the examiner's finger. It is more difficult to physically perceive this synovitis volume in the digital sheath, which explains why this lesion is very frequently underestimated or even unrecognized. When the patient wants to actively flex the PIPs the amplitudes are limited, while passively, they are almost normal. This blocking of the flexors will lead to compensation by flexion of the MCPs using the intrinsic muscles. Their overuse will induce the extension and hyperextension of the PIP by elongation of the palmar plate which has been weakened by the synovitis of the flexor sheaths.

The progressive appearance of an intrinsic hand (+) with a positive Finochietto test, shows that the action of the intrinsic muscles is secondary to the tenosynovitis of the flexors which can lead to a rupture of the superficial flexor aggravating the hyperextension of the PIP [17].

- Elongation and rupture of the terminal insertion of the extensor tendon:

DIP joint synovitis is rarely significant in rheumatoid arthritis. However, it can induce elongation or even a rupture of the extensor tendon, creating a mallet finger which, secondarily, will induce PIP hyperextension.

Classifications

As there are multiple etiologies, there are multiple classifications resulting from these pathophysiological interpretations:

■ Nalebuff and Millender classified the deformities according to the range of motion of the PIP assessed from the position of the MCP and according to the degenerative lesions which are observed [34, 36]:

■ Type I: The flexion of the PIP is normal. There is a hyperextension of the PIP with full active mobility and flexion of the DIP.

These are patients who have probably presented with tenosynovitis of the flexor tendons, with distension of the palmar plate of the PIP having progressed towards recovery spontaneously or after treatment.

■ Type II: The flexion of the PIP is limited in certain positions.

■ The patient may actively flex the fingers, but the precise physical examination shows a retraction of the intrinsic musculature. When the MCPs are extended, active and passive flexion of the PIP is limited. When there is an ulnar deviation, the intrinsic musculature on its ulnar side is more shortened. The flexion of the PIP is then more difficult when the MCP is in extension in the axis than in extension with an ulnar inclination, it is then added to the anatomical lesions of Type I, the retraction of the intrinsic musculature.

■ Type III: The flexion of the PIP is limited in all positions.

■ The patient cannot passively flex the PIPs, even when the MCPs are flexed to relax the intrinsic musculature. The duration of the evolution progression causes a retraction of the dorsal joint capsule and the fibres uniting the median band to the lateral bands (transverse ligament), preventing them from moving laterally to allow the joint to flex. In addition to the anatomical lesions of the anterior groups, there is then a retraction of the capsule and the extensor apparatus at the dorsum of the PIP.

■ Type IV: The stiffness of PIPs is complete with alteration of the articular surfaces. In this case, the PIPs are stiff not only for extra-articular reasons, but especially from the destruction of the articular surfaces (ankylosis). Sometimes joints present a lateral instability, secondary to ligament and/or subchondral bone destruction.

The osteo-articular destruction of PIP is in addition to the anatomical lesions of the preceding groups.

■ Zancolli in 1979, classifies swan-neck deformities, according to the mechanisms of deformations (extrinsic, intrinsic, articular) [56, 57].

■ Tonkin, using Nalebuff's classification, takes into account, in five stages, the flexion of the PIP in relation to the position of the MCP and according to the articular degeneration [50].

● Type 1a: The bending of the PIP is complete.

● Type 2a: The flexion of the PIP decreases with the extension of the MCP (intrinsic cause).

● Type 3a: Flexion of the PIP decreases with flexion of the MCP (extrinsic cause).

● Type 4a: Flexion of the PIP decreases in all positions of the MCP (intrinsic and extrinsic cause).

● Type 5a: Flexion of the IPP is impossible.

Degenerative changes are noted below.

Mallet finger deformity

In 1880, the French physician, Segond, was the first to describe the digital deformation secondary to the rupture of the extensor tendon at the base of the distal phalanx. In 1948, Bunnell called this flexion deformation of the DIP "drop finger." Later, Boyes popularized it by giving it the name "mallet finger" [43] (Figure 7F).

Pathophysiology

DIP joints have anatomy comparable to PIP joints in terms of the skeleton and capsulo-ligament structures and only their dimensions and the synovial cul-de-sacs are smaller. Their mobility is also slightly less since it varies between 70 and 90° of flexion. Synovitis is less common with DIP than with PIP. It causes distension of the distal extensor tendon with progressive loss of joint extension. The deformation can be very important and can secondarily induce hyperextension of the PIP according to Landsmeer's joint chain balance theory. A secondary swan-neck deformity can also appear [25].

THUMB DEFORMITY IN RA

The thumb represents one of the predominant locations for RA to occur and is reported in:

■ 57% of cases for Swanson et al. [49]

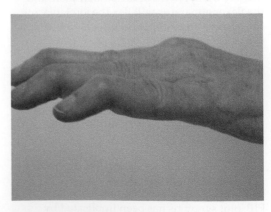

Figure 7F Mallet finger deformity.

- 60% of cases for Nalebuff [35]
- 62% of cases for Alnot [2, 3]

The deformities of the thumb are almost always significant and associated with deformities of the wrist and middle finger. Paradoxically, these anatomical lesions are functionally well tolerated in the early stages of the disease. In the following section, the different anatomical lesions are described and classified in order to outline important surgical therapeutic procedures. Surgical management is never isolated and is always a part of comprehensive strategy for the wrist and middle fingers [2, 3, 11, 27, 35, 38, 42, 44].

Pathophysiology

There are several different deformities of the thumb in RA, and they are specific entities: The first two are differentiated according to the position of the first metacarpal bone (M1):

- If the M1 is displaced in abduction, the terminology of a Z-thumb is used, which can

be considered for the thumb as an equivalent of the buttonhole middle finger.

- When the M1 is positioned in adduction, the terminology of adductus thumb, equivalent to the deformity of the swan-neck for the middle finger.

- The third type of deformity is called "unstable thumb" and is the result of tendon ruptures, either from the flexor pollicis longus or from the extensor pollicis longus.

Classifications

It has been attempted to establish classifications of the deformities of the thumb pillar encountered in rheumatoid arthritis. These different classifications have the merit of giving an accurate view of the condition of the thumb pillar at any given time. In addition to the Ratliff classification, these classifications do not include states of tendon rupture, flexor or extensor.

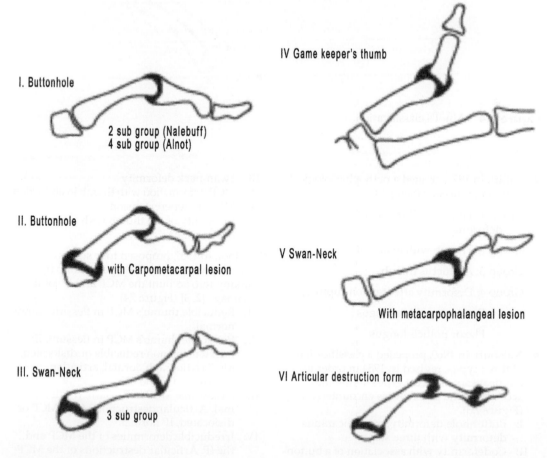

I. Buttonhole
2 sub group (Nalebuff)
4 sub group (Alnot)

II. Buttonhole
with Carpometacarpal lesion

III. Swan-Neck
3 sub group

IV Game keeper's thumb

V Swan-Neck
With metacarpophalangeal lesion

VI Articular destruction form

Figure 7.3 Nalebuff's classification.

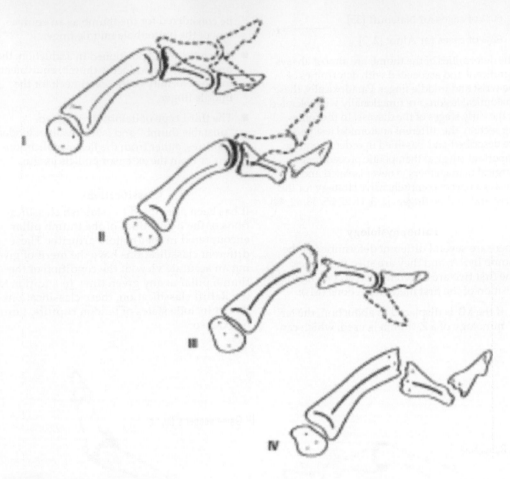

Figure 7.4 Alnot's classification.

■ Ratliff, in 1971, created a pathophysiological four-stage classification [38]:

Group 1: Thumb in Z shape or buttonhole deformity

Group 2: Thumb with instability

Group 3: Adductus thumb

Group 4: Deformity after tendon ruptures

Extensor pollicis longus

Flexor pollicis longus

■ Nalebuff, in 1969, proposed a classification of three types, revised in 1984 in order to delineate six different types taking into account all the possibilities encountered [35] (Figure 7.3).

I: Buttonhole deformity; extrinsic minus deformity with three stages

II: Codeformity with association of a buttonhole and swan-neck

III: Swan-neck deformity

IV: MCP deformation with thumb in abduction

V: MCP in hyperextension

VI: Instability of the thumb with articular destructions

■ Alnot, in 1987, proposed four stages of development of the Z-shaped thumb by taking into account the MCP and IP joint damage [2, 3] (Figure 7.4).

I: Reducible thumb's MCP in flessum. X-ray normal.

II: Reducible thumb's MCP in flessum, IP in extension non reducible or dislocated. MCP radiograph normal, articular destruction of the IP.

III: Irreducible MCP in flessum, IP subnormal. Articular destruction of the MCP or dislocated, IP normal.

IV: Irreducible deformities of the MCP and the IP. Articular destructions of the MCP and IP.

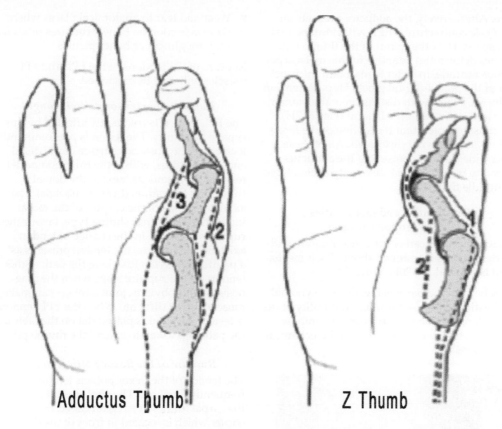

Figure 7.5 Thumb deformities in rheumatoid arthritis, from Tubiana et al. **Right:** Thumb in "Z" shape or buttonhole deformity. (1) Extensor pollicis brevis muscle. (2) Extensor pollicis longus muscle, dislocated on the ulnar side of the thumb. **Left:** Adductus thumb or swan-neck deformity. (1) Extensor pollicis brevis muscle. (2) Extensor pollicis longus muscle. (3) Flexor pollicis longus.

Thumb in "Z"

This is the most frequently encountered deformity of the thumb, accounting for nearly 80% of cases. The productive synovitis on the dorsal side of the MCP joint will gradually distend the tendon of the extensor digitorum brevis muscle (without any rupture) causing this joint to flexion. Concomitantly, the extensor pollicis longus tendon of the thumb is dislocated on the ulnar side of the thumb, the fibrous expansions of the adductor muscle of the thumb that attach to this tendon will cause hyperextension of the IP joint. This deformity is often associated with the "buttonhole" encountered with middle fingers, although the tendon of the extensor brevis does not disengage towards the radial side of the thumb but distends and becomes ineffective (Figure 7.5).

Along with these tendon abnormalities, joint damage occurs in both joints, leading to a radial inclination of the distal phalanx (during the pollici-digital pinch movements).

The functional discomfort is tolerated well enough by the patient for a long time, although the pollici-finger grip function is first impaired and aggravated by the ulnar deviation of the MCP joints of the middle fingers, causing "leakage" in relation to the thumb (Figure 7G).

Adductus thumb

Much less common than a thumb in "Z" (7 to 20%), this deformation is explained by an initial deterioration of the trapezo-metacarpal joint and all the surrounding elements (Figure 7.5). The productive synovitis of the trapezo-metacarpal joint will distend the joint capsule and cause instability. The combined forces of traction of the abductor pollicis longus (APL) and the pressures exerted during the pollici-digital grip will gradually succeed the first metacarpal base to subdislocation in the dorsal and radial position. This results in an articular destruction (trapezo-metacarpal joint) and the permanent adduction of the first metacarpal

147

bone. Alternatively, the adductor presents an analgesic contracture which will close the first web space. The other joints of the thumb will present deformities adaptive to this metacarpal vicious attitude, in order to maintain the function of the pollici-digital pinch: Hyperextension of the MCP joint with distension of the palmar plate and stiffness of the IP joint (Figure 7H).

It must be noted that the tendon of the flexor pollicis longus is not dislocated. All of these deformities lead to comparing the adductus thumb to the swan-neck deformity encountered for middle fingers [24].

Deformities and instabilities due to tendon ruptures

Tendon ruptures can occur concomitantly with the deformities mentioned above. Their mechanism is twofold [14, 20] (Figure 7I):

- Ischemia: The pannus invades the synovial sheaths and causes segmental fragility of the tendon, leading to its rupture or compressions (change in anatomical and mechanical relationship).

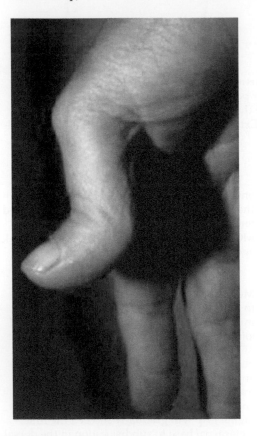

Figure 7G "Z" thumb deformity.

- Wear and tear in anatomical places where there is friction on bone structures provided with roughness or bone spicules.

Rupture of the tendons of the EPL and FPL muscles will now be discussed.

Rupture of extensor pollicis longus

The EPL tendon is frequently affected by this type of deformity. The lesion is predominantly located on the posterior surface of the distal end of the radius, within the third compartment of the extensors, next to the dorsal tubercle of the radius (Lister's tubercle). The axial deviations of the carpus, of the radial inclination and ulnar sliding type, favour these ruptures (increase in the change of tendon axis). Before rupture, the tendon presents as a painful tenosynovitis along the path of this tendon. At the rupture stage when the diagnosis is most obvious, joint damage can make muscle testing difficult. When the EPL tendon is tested, the hand is placed flat on the table and the patient is asked to extend the thumb pillar.

Rupture of the flexor pollicis longus

The tendon of the flexor pollicis longus is also frequently involved. The ruptures take place in the carpal tunnel in a region called the critical corner which is located in front of the distal pole of the scaphoid bone. Here, the tendon changes direction on the radial side. Intracarpal instability, which results in a misalignment of the carpus and a horizontalization of the scaphoid bone (appearance of bone spicules on its distal pole), directly affects this tendon. The diagnosis is usually not difficult with the sudden inability to IP flexion of the thumb. However, stiffness in the joints of the thumb pillar can lead to a delay in diagnosis. Another diagnostic marker is the discovery of an associated rupture of the deep flexor tendon of the index finger.

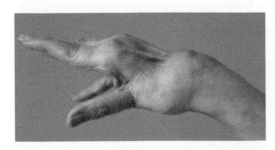

Figure 7H Adductus thumb.

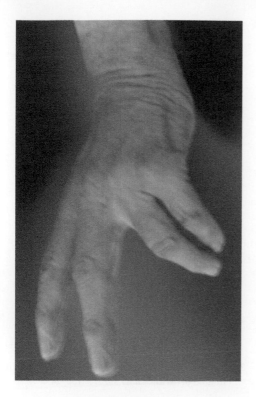

Figure 7I Tendon rupture.

CONCLUSIONS

Deformities of the hand and wrist linked to the inflammatory process in RA were caricatures before the rapid and effective management of new therapies.

Careful clinical examination and the use of an appropriate classification are even more relevant today.

An overall assessment of the upper limb will not be able to take into account only the pain phenomenon and the radiological lesions but will have to be part of a more global study, evaluating the pathological context and the reaction to rheumatological treatment.

REFERENCES

1. Aiache A, Barsky AJ and Weiner DL. Prevention of « boutonniere » deformity. *Plast Reconstr Surg* 1979; 46: 164–167.

2. Alnot JY. Le pouce rhumatoide. *Ann Chir Main* 1987; 6: 67–68.167.

3. Alnot JY and Masmejean E. Le pouce rhumatoïde. In: Allieu Y, *La main et le poignet rhumatoïde – traitement chirurgical, traitement médical, rééducation et réadaptation fonctionnelle.* Monographie de la Société Française de Chirurgie de la Main n° 23, Paris: Expansion Scientifique Française, 1998, pp. 154–163.

4. Apfelberg DB, Maser MR and Lash H. Rheumatoid hand deformities: Pathophysiology and treatment. *West J Med* 1978; 129(4): 267–272.

5. Bachdahl M. The carpit ulnare syndrome in rheumatoid arthritis. *Acta Rheumatol Scand* 1963; 5: 1–75.

6. Backhouse KM. Mechanical factors influencing normal and rheumatoid metacarpophalangeal joints. *Ann Rheum Dis* 1969; 28(5): suppl: 15–19.

7. Brewerton DA. Hand deformities in rheumatoid disease. *Ann Rheum Dis* 1957; 16: 183–197.

8. Burke FD. The rheumatoid metacarpophalangeal joint. *Hand Clin* 2011; 27(1): 79–86.

9. De la Caffiniere JY, Mazas F and Achach PC. The stage of articular destruction in the rheumatoid hand. *Rev Chir Orthop Reparatrice Appar Mot* 1975; 61(1): 61–74.

10. Dorwart BB and Schumacher HR. Hand deformities resembling rheumatoid arthritis. *Semin Arthritis Rheum* 1974; 4(1): 53–71.

11. Dyer GSM and Simmons BP. Rheumatoid thumb. *Hand Clin* 2011; 27(1): 73–77.

12. Eberhardt K, Johnson PM and Rydgren L. The occurrence and significance of hand deformities in early rheumatoid arthritis. *Br J Rheumatol* 1991; 30(3): 21–23.

13. Eiken O. Aspects of rheumatoid hand surgery. *Acta Orhtop Bely* 1912; 38: 53–59.

14. Ertel RG, Millender RH and Nalebuff EA. Flexor tendons ruptures in patients with rheumatoid arthritis. *J Hand Surg Am* 1988; 13: 860–866.

15. Feldon P. Rheumatoid arthritis. In: Manske PR, (ed.), *Hand Surgery Up Date*. American Society for Surgery of the Hand, 1996, pp. 173–181.

16. Ferlic DC. Boutonniere deformities in rheumatoid arthritis. *Hand Clin* 1989; 5(2): 215–222.

17. Finochietto R. Retraccion de Volkmann de los musculos intrinsecos de la mano. De la Sociedad de Cirugia de Buenos-Aires, Tomo IV, 1920.

18. Flatt AE. Some pathomechanics of ulnar drift. *Plast Reconstr Surg* 1966; 37: 295–303.

19. Fowler SB. The hand in rheumatoid arthritis. *Am Surg* 1963; 29: 403–404.

20. Harris R. Spontaneous rupture of the tendon of extensor pollicis longus as a complication of rheumatoid arthritis. *Ann Rheum Dis* 1951; 10: 298–306.

21. Harris C Jr and Riordan DC. Intrinsic contracture of the hand and its surgical treatment. *J Bone Joint Surg* 1954; 36A: 10–20.

22. Harrison SH. Rheumatoid deformities of the PIP joints of the hand. *Ann Rheum Dis* 1969; 28(5): suppl: 20–22.

23. Henry J, Roulot E and Gaujoux-Viala. The rheumatoid hand. *C Presse Med* 2013; 42(12): 1607–1615.

24. Kessler I. Aetiology and management of adduction contracture of the thumb in rheumatoid arthritis. *The Hand* 1973; 2: 170–174.

25. Landsmeer JM. The coordination of finger-joint motion. *J Bone Joint Am* 1963; 45: 1654–1662.

26. Leach RE and Baumgard SH. Correction of swan-neck deformity in rheumatoid arthritis. *Surg Clin North Am* 1968; 48: 661–666.

27. LeViet D. *Traitement chirurgical du pouce rhumatoïde. Cahier d'enseignement de la Société française de Chirurgie de la main.* Paris: Elsevier, 2000, pp. 9–23.

28. Lindscheid RL and Dobyns JH. Rheumatoid arthritis of the wrist. *Orthop Chir North Ann* 1971; 2: 649–665.

29. Littler JW. The hand and wrist. In: Howorth MB, (ed.), *A Textbook of Orthopaedics.* Philadelphia: W.B. Sawnders Company, 1952, p. 284.

30. Littler JW. Intrinsic contracture in the hand and its surgical treatment. In: Harris C and Riordan DC. *J Bone Joint Surg* 1954; 36A: 10–20.

31. Littler JW and Eaton RG. Redistribution of forces in the correction of the boutonniere deformity. *J Bone Joint Surg* 1967; 49A: 1267–1274.

32. Littler JW. The finger extensor mechanism. *Surg Clin North Am* 1967; 47: 428.

33. Lluch A. Les deformations des chaines digitales et leur traitement dans la polyarthrite rhumatoïde. In: Allieu Y. La main et le poignet rhumatoïdes. Paris: Expansion Scientifique Francaise, 1996, pp. 85–104.

34. Millender LH and Nalebuff EA. Evaluation and treatment of early rheumatoid hand involvement. *Orthop Clin North Am* 1975; 6: 697–708.

35. Nalebuff EA. Diagnosis, classification and management of rheumatoid thumb deformities. *Bull Hosp Joint Dis* 1968; 29(2):119–137.

36. Nalebuff EA, Feldon PG and Millender LH. The rheumatoid arthritis in the hand and wrist. In: Green DP, (ed.), *Operative Hand Surgery,* 2nd edition. Edinburgh: Churchill Livingstone, 1988, pp. 1655–1766.

37. Nalebuff EA. The rheumatoid swan-neck deformity. *Hand Clin* 1989; 5: 203–214.

38. Ratliff AHC. Deformities of the thumb in rheumatoid arthritis. *Hand* 1971; 3: 138–143.

39. Rizio L and Belsky MR. Finger deformities in rheumatoid arthritis. *Hand Clin* 1996; 12(3): 531–540.

40. Shapiro JS. Wrist involvement in rheumatoid Swan-neck deformity. *Hand Surg* 1982; 7: 484–491.

41. Shapiro JS. The wrist in rheumatoid arthritis. *Hand Clin* 1996; 12(3): 477–498.

42. Stanley JK and Trail IA. Thumb dysfunction in systemic arthritis. In: Peimer CA, (ed.), *Surgery of the Hand and Upper Extremity.* New-York: Mac Graw-Hill, 1996, pp. 1691–1703.

43. Stark HH, Boyes JH and Wilson JN. Mallet finger. *J Bone Joint Am* 1962; 44-A: 1061–1068.

44. Stein AB and Terrono AL. The rheumatoid thumb. *Hand Clin* 1996; 72: 541–550.

45. Stirrat CR. Metacarpophalangeal joints in rheumatoid arthritis on the hand. *Hand Clin* 1996; 12: 515–529.

46. Straub LR. The rheumatoid hand. *Clin Orthop* 1959; 75: 127–139.

47. Straub LR. The etiology of finger deformity in the hand affected by rheumatoid arthritis. *Bull Hosp Joint Dis* 1960; 27: 322–329.

48. Smith RJ and Kaplan EB. Rheumatoid deformities at the metacarpophalangeal joints of the fingers. *J Bone Joint Surg Am* 1967; 49(1): 31–47.

49. Swanson AB and Swanson GG. Pathogenesis and pathomechanics of rheumatoid deformities in the hand and wrist. *Orthop Clin North Am* 1973; 4(4): 1039–1056.

50. Tonkin MA, Hughes J and Smith KL. Lateral band translocation for Swan-Neck deformity. *J Hand Surg Am* 1992; 17(2): 260–267.

51. Tubiana R, Kuhlmann N, Fahrer M and Lisfranc R. Etude du poignet normal et ses déformations au cours de la polyarthrite rhumatoide. *Chirurgie* 1980; 106: 257–264.

52. Valentin P. Mechanism of finger deformities in the rheumatoid hand. *Rev Chir Orthop Appar Mot* 1972; 58(5):445–451.

53. Wilson RL. Rheumatoid arthritis of the hand. *Orthop Chir N Ann* 1986; 77: 313–343.

54. Wilson RL and Carlblom ER. The rheumatoid metacarpophalangeal joint. *Hand Clin* 1989; 5: 223–237.

55. Yoshida M, Belt EA and Kaarela K. Prevalence of mutilans-like hand deformities in patient with seropositive rheumatoid arthritis. A prospective 20-year study. *Scand J Rheumatol* 1999; 28(1): 38–40.

56. Zancolli EA. *The Structural and Dynamic Bases of the Hand Surgery*, 2nd edition. Philadelphia, JB Lippincott, 1979, pp. 64–78.

57. Zancolli EA, Zancolli ER, Kohut GN and Cagnone JC. The wrist and metacarpal arch in rheumatoid arthritis. The supination collapse of the hand. *Hand Surg* 1996; 2: 219–237.

8A Peripheral Nerve Examination

Radial Nerve Palsy

*Mohammed Tahir Ansari, Santanu Kar, Devansh Goyal,
Dyuti Deepta Rano and Rajesh Malhotra*

CONTENTS

INTRODUCTION

The radial nerve is the largest branch of brachial plexus innervating the posterior compartment of the arm and forearm. The nerve is most frequently paralyzed from penetrating trauma to the upper limb with or without associated fractures. There may be wide variation in clinical presentation according to the site of affection of the nerve. The treatment modality can be altered significantly according to the etiology and anatomical integrity of the nerve. Hence, a meticulous history and clinical examination supplemented with appropriate investigations is of paramount importance for a proper diagnosis and management of such injuries. This chapter hopefully can guide the clinician to manage radial nerve injury in a comprehensive manner in an emergency trauma setting as well as in outpatient clinics.

Another purpose of writing this chapter is to develop set of skills among the candidates to pass examinations as radial nerve palsy is a common clinical case in most of the examinations (Video 8A.1). It is essential to know what an examiner expects from the students. The examiner wants to pass a well-behaved, safe surgeon who has the decision-making capability to deal with common clinical conditions.

The objectives of this chapter are: 1) To know about applied anatomy of the radial nerve. 2) Clinical examination of the patient with radial nerve. 3) To develop skills for decision making in patients with radial nerve palsy. 4) To know about the investigations related to such cases. 5) The surgical part will be discussed in short

DOI: 10.1201/9781003125938-8

Video 8A.1   This is the usual case scenario given in the examinations. The history may vary depending upon individual case scenarios. It can be noticed that the patient is not able to extend the wrist and the fingers. Slight extension due to tenodesis effect of EPL and extensor of the index finger is visible. During examination the wrist should be supported so that the manifestation of the finger and thumb drop may become prominent.

www.routledge.com/9780367647162.

as the examination is also a key for decision-making in a particular type of surgery.

CONCEPT OF VERY HIGH, HIGH AND LOW RADIAL NERVE PALSY

The innervations of the triceps muscle vary significantly. The branches to the long head, medial head and lateral head about 7.1, 9.5 and 10.1 cm respectively, below the tip of acromion. Another branch to the medial head arises about 11.2 cm below the tip of the acromion [1]. These branches to the triceps usually remain between the heads of the triceps muscle and the main stem remains very close to the bone (shaft of humerus) leading to stretching of the nerve by the shaft of the humerus fracture but minimal stretching of the triceps innervating collaterals [2]. Hence the triceps are usually spared in the shaft of humerus fractures but they can be compressed in axilla against the latissimus dorsi and teres major muscles or in the triangular interval where the nerve is against the humeral shaft and two muscles (long head of triceps and teres major) [2]. Hence, compression in the axilla leading to total paralysis including triceps comprising of **"very high" radial nerve palsy** and compression/stretching around/below the spiral groove but above the elbow leads to sparing of the triceps (hence elbow extension is normal) leading to **"high radial" nerve palsy**. The nerve to the brachioradialis (BR) and extensor carpi radialis longus (ECRL) is almost always supplied by branches above or at the level of the lateral epicondyle [2]. Hence wrist extension is spared in lesions below the elbow designating **"low" radial nerve palsy**.

CLINICAL EXAMINATION CAN OFTEN DETERMINE PATHOLOGY OF NERVE INJURY

It is paramount to determine the conduction block (neuropraxia) and axonotmesis or neurotmesis by clinical examination. This can be confirmed, as well as followed up, with subsequent electrodiagnostic studies.

1. Low-energy trauma, incomplete motor palsy, partial loss of sensation (usually dull pinprick sensation preserved), preserved sympathetic function below the injury level and absent Tinel's sign are suggestive of CONDUCTION BLOCK.

2. On the other hand, high-energy trauma, complete motor and sensory loss, loss of sympathetic tone below the injury level (the area becomes warm as well as there being no sweating at the area due to loss of sweat gland innervations) and presence of Tinel's sign are suggestive of AXOTMESIS or NEUROTMESIS.

APPLIED ANATOMY AND SURFACE ANATOMY

The radial nerve is the largest branch of the brachial plexus and originates as a terminal branch of posterior cord carrying fibres from ventral rami of C5–T1 with the largest contribution from C7. The nerve descends into the arm after passing anterior to the latissimus dorsi insertion lying posterior to the axillary artery. Then it leaves the axilla and enters the arm through lower triangular interval bounded superiorly by the teres major, medially by medial head of triceps and laterally by the shaft of the humerus to lie on the posterior surface of the humerus (Figure 8A.1). It gives off the posterior cutaneous nerve of the arm in the axilla. The nerve lies on the upper part of medial head of the triceps separated from spiral groove by a 3.4 mm thick cuff of muscle [3]. The nerve is in direct contact with the humerus only in the distal part where it pierces the lateral intermuscular septum. The nerve travels along the posterior aspect of the humerus from 20.7 ± 1.2 cm proximal to the medial epicondyle (74% of the length of humerus) to 14.2 ± 0.6 cm proximal to the lateral epicondyle (51% of the length of the humerus) and pierces the lateral intermuscular septum about 10.2 ± 0.4 cm proximal to the lateral epicondyle and enters the anterior arm between the brachialis and brachioradialis [4]. The radial nerve in the spiral groove is the least mobile throughout its course. It is commonly compressed by spiral fractures at the junction of the middle and distal one third of the shaft of the humerus (Holstein–Lewis fracture) [5]. This part of the nerve must be explored

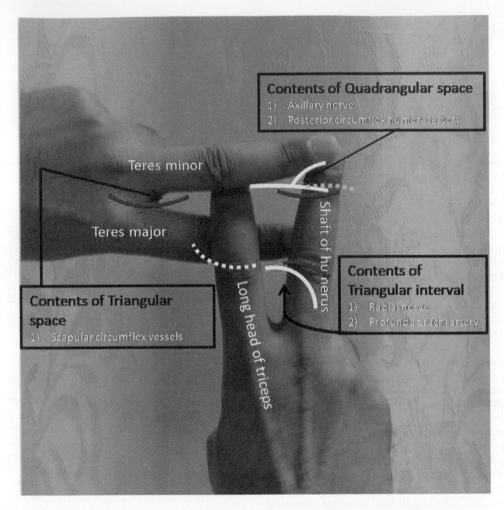

Contents of Quadrangular space
1) Axillary nerve
2) Posterior circumflex humeral artery

Teres minor

Teres major

Shaft of humerus

Contents of Triangular interval
1) Radial nerve
2) Profunda brachi artery

Contents of Triangular space
1) Scapular circumflex vessels

Long head of triceps

Figure 8A.1 The spaces around the axilla are a commonly asked question in the examination. This can be easily remembered by crossing your fingers as depicted. The spaces formed are usually the triangular space, quadruangular space and triangular structure as depicted.

routinely for open reduction and fixation of humeral shaft fractures with plating through the posterior approach. In the spiral groove, the radial nerve sends off a branch to the medial head of the triceps. This branch is considered as an expendable donor and used to gain shoulder abduction by transferring the fibres to the axillary nerve [6]. Motor branches to the brachioradialis, the ECRL and one branch to brachialis are given off in this area above the elbow (Figure 8A.2). Then it passes between the brachialis and brachioradialis and divides into its terminal branches (superficial radial nerve and posterior interosseous nerve) anterior to the lateral epicondyle of the humerus. This division occurs proximal to the radiocapitellar joint in most cases [7]. There is controversy regarding nerve supply of the extensor carpi radialis brevis (ECRB). The most recent literature suggests

that nerves to the ECRB may originate from the radial nerve proper before its terminal division, from the posterior interosseous nerve (PIN) [8, 9] however, it can also be supplied from superficial branch of the radial nerve [10, 11]. In some series it has been found that the ECRB is supplied by the PIN in 45% of cases, radial nerve proper in 30% of cases and from the superficial branch of the radial nerve (SBRN) in 25% of cases [12] but there may be variations in the innervation [13]. When the nerve to the ECRB is a branch from the SBRN, then the ECRB will not be affected in posterior interosseous nerve syndrome (compressive neuropathy of the PIN). Injury to the SBRN around the elbow will lead to isolated paralysis of the ECRB (partial weakness in wrist extension) and sensory loss in the first web space. These variations of nerve supply must be taken into consideration during

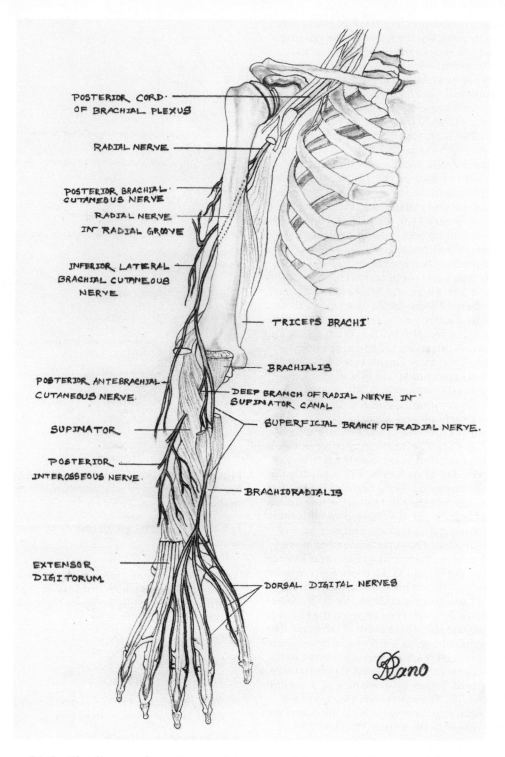

Figure 8A.2 The diagram shows the complete course of the nerve in the arm and forearm.

clinical examination [14]. The PIN reaches the posterior aspect of the forearm after passing around the neck of the radius between the superficial and deep heads of the supinator to supply the extensor compartment of forearm. The course of the PIN from radiocapitellar joint to supinator muscle is imagined as a tunnel – RADIAL TUNNEL [15] which is bounded by the brachialis muscle and biceps tendon medially, and brachioradialis and ECRB and longus muscles laterally, the floor is formed by the elbow joint capsule proximally and distally by the supinator (it passes between the two heads of supinator and comes out in the posterior aspect of forearm) [16]. At the distal border of extensor pollicis brevis (EPB), it passes deep to extensor pollicis longus (EPL) and descends on the interosseous membrane to the dorsum of the corpus and supply carpal ligaments and articulations. Three and four fingers must be remembered for the surface marking of these nerves as it forms an important guide during surgery. The radial nerve is approximately four fingers breadth above the lateral epicondyle and the PIN is three fingers breadth below the lateral epicondyle. The PIN successively innervates the supinator, ECRB, extensor digitorum communis, extensor digiti minimi, extensor carpi ulnaris, abductor pollicis, extensor pollicis brevis (EPL) and extensor indicis proprius (EIP). The innervating order of PIN is to be kept in mind to evaluate the recovery of the nerve. The branch to the EIP is usually the last motor branch and the branch to the EPL is supplied before the EIP. Hence, for assessment of recovery, the EIP is evaluated and if is found functioning it denotes near complete gain of nerve function. The superficial radial nerve passes deep to the brachioradialis and emerges between the BR and ECRL about 8.64 cm (with average 7.8–9.0 cm) proximal to the radial styloid [17] and becomes subcutaneous. It crosses the anatomical snuff box between the EPL and EPB and supplies the dorsum of the hand. The dorsal digital nerves, the terminal branches of the superficial branch, supply sensation to the dorsal skin of the first, second and radial side of the third fingers up to the base of the middle phalanx [18]. The autonomous region of the superficial radial nerve (SRN) is the dorsal web space closest to the thumb [19] (Figure 8A.3).

HISTORY TAKING

The patient should be allowed to narrate the history of the ailments in his/her own words from the beginning to the present condition. The salient points are to be picked up and the patient is allowed to elaborate each point with specific leading questions. In a patient with

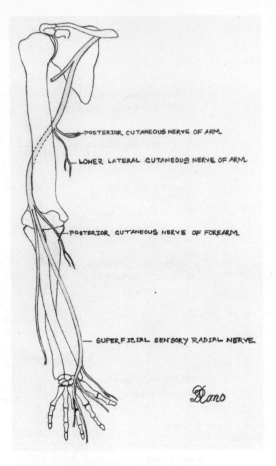

POSTERIOR CUTANEOUS NERVE OF ARM.

LOWER LATERAL CUTANEOUS NERVE OF ARM.

POSTERIOR CUTANEOUS NERVE OF FOREARM.

SUPERFICIAL SENSORY RADIAL NERVE.

Dano

Figure 8A.3 The figure depicts the large branches of the nerve which are usually raised in the examination.

radial nerve injury, careful history of trauma must be elicited.

History of trauma

1. Circumstances and mechanism of the injury must be elicited which includes injury to other organ systems (suggests high or low velocity trauma)

2. Closed vs open injury

3. Gunshot injury

4. Thermal and crush injury

5. Injury by sharp objects – superficial radial nerve is most prone to injury

6. History of head injury

Interpretation

This gives insight as to whether the nerve is damaged by physiological interruption of conduction (neuropraxia) or anatomical discontinuity of nerve fibres. Injury by sharp objects leads to clean-cut nerve injury that may warrant immediate exploration and repair. On the contrary, open wounds, crush injuries and gunshot wounds may lacerate the nerve and need wound exploration and secondary repair. The clinician must determine the extent of nerve tissue as well as limb destruction which is the single most important prognostic factor to determine the timing of intervention, as well as recovery of function. Classification of the wound according to contamination of the wound is desirable at the first visit to the emergency and photographic documentation is a must for future references.

1. Tidy wound – This is a clean-cut injury. There is no or little contamination. Usually caused by sharp objects (knife, glass or iatrogenic by surgeon's scalpel).

2. Untidy wound – This is a contaminated wound. The damage to soft tissue is usually extensive and deep. The possibility of underlying infection is usually very high, precluding acute repair of the nerve. The most common causes of such injuries are projectile injury (gunshot wound), open fractures.

3. Closed traction injury – The most destructive injury to the nerves and vessels. This is due to retraction of the nerve trunk after injury. There is variable loss of axons according to the severity of injury.

B. History of fracture

Ask for the site of the fracture (if any) and whether the palsy was immediately after trauma, after manipulative reduction or after surgical treatment.

Interpretation

Most commonly the radial nerve is injured in association with humeral fractures and typically these fractures are at the junction of middle and distal one third (Holstein–Lewis type) [5]. The radial head, neck, shaft of radius or ulna can be a cause of posterior interosseous nerve palsy [20, 21] Rarely, the radial nerve can be paralyzed when being entrapped by a healing callus [22].

C. History of surgery

The nerve can be damaged by hardware [23, 24] or from poor positioning on the operating table [25–29]. The longer screws must be looked at carefully in radiographs as nerves can be explored directly in such cases (Figure 8A.4). Blood pressure cuffs may damage the

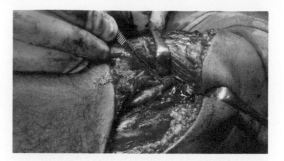

Figure 8A.4 The surgical photograph shows a longer screw, which has caused the radial nerve palsy in postoperative period.

vascularity of the radial nerve, leading to radial palsy [30]. Surgical fixation of the radial head, radial neck, total elbow arthroplasty and elbow arthroscopy (anterolateral portal is near the PIN) can lead to PIN palsy [31].

K wire fixation of distal radius fractures [32, 33] as well as shoulder arthroscopy [34] may lead to superficial radial nerve injury. The K wire fixation for supracondylar fracture can also give rise to radial nerve palsy if the medial wire perforates the lateral cortex and K wire is kept too long.

D. History of intramuscular injections

Intramuscular injections can lead to radial nerve palsy and the triceps muscle can also be involved [35, 36]. Symptoms usually appear immediately after the injection [5]. The natural history after injection palsy may be different for oil-based preparation than for water-based preparation. Hence it also becomes important to know the name of the preparation.

Interpretation

The oil-based preparation causes irreversible damage to the nerve tissue and prognosis is usually guarded in such cases, while neurolysis may be considered in patients of post injection radial nerve palsy after water-based injection.

E. Past history

The history related to the arm must be asked. Sometimes, a prior history of tumour removal or any apparent swelling which the patient ignored for long time may come out.

F. Personal history

Smoking/occupation/hand dominance should be asked.

Interpretation

Smoking carries important significance in the prognosis of nerve recovery and fracture healing. The prognosis is usually poor in smokers who must be informed about it and counselled to stop smoking until complete recovery. The occupation of the patient carries significance as the internal splinting (pronator teres transfer to ECRB) may be considered in a patient who wants to return to their job early as the loss of wrist extension significantly alters the grip. Hand dominance also pays an important role as the choice and timing of surgery can be preponed or postponed for a short duration.

1. G. Medical history

The available medical records may be requested from the patient.

Interpretation

The history of diabetes mellitus is important, as the wound healing, postoperative complication and the nerve recovery may be prolonged. Similarly, the use of steroids for various diseases is common and steroids also impair the nerve healing. Autoimmune diseases and inflammatory conditions are not rare and these should be ruled out. The use of anticoagulant or anti-platelet agents should be asked as a part of preoperative planning.

1. H. Patient expectations

It is important to know the patient's expectations as the decision for the surgery is a mutual decision and patient may decide as per his or her own circumstances.

EXAMINATION

Prerequisites of the Examination

The prerequisites of the examination are usually the same as of other orthopaedic examination related to a particular site. It is important to revise these here, as no examination should proceed without fulfilling the prerequisites. The candidate appearing for examination may be asked about these; moreover, the examiner will expect demonstration.

1. Greet the patient, approach the patient after introducing yourself.

2. Take verbal consent.

3. Clean hands with sanitizers.

4. Position the patient appropriately and expose neck to fingers.

5. Simultaneously both upper limbs to be examined.

6. Be sincere and professional to the patient and do not cause any pain.

7. There should be adequate light.

8. Do not forget to ask for female staff or a relative of the patient to be present all the time during examination of female patients if it is the hospital policy of the country.

Sequence of Examination

The examination should be followed in a sequence, and it should be repeated every time in same sequence in the clinic too so that none of the steps are forgotten and the examinee can do it smoothly during the examination. The examination should be: A) Inspection. B) Palpation. C) Movements. D) Neurological examination. E) Special tests.

A. Inspection

The examination findings should be compared with the opposite side.

1. Attitude of the limb in resting position will suggest wrist drop, finger drop and thumb drop of the affected side.

2. Look for any muscle wasting in the arm and forearm area. In patients with radial nerve palsy the girth of proximal forearm will look wasted.

3. Look for any swelling of elbow, wrist or small joint of hand.

4. May suggest chronic inflammatory arthritis like rheumatoid arthritis, synovitis or space-occupying lesions.

5. Must look for signs of trauma as deformity of arm.

6. Scar mark (healing with primary intention, signs of compound fracture/burn/blast injury, etc.). The surgical mark also gives an indication about the surgical approach which was used during surgery. Most of the cases that are a surgical candidate for secondary exploration of the nerve are those cases where an antero-lateral approach has been used.

7. Dilated veins, redness, swelling around the arm or axilla which is suggestive of any tumour.

8. Whether patient is with any splint.

B. Palpation

Palpation of the arm and forearm should be carried out to look for the local site of trauma, compression, tumour, etc.

The local temperature and tenderness should be checked. The tenderness along the shaft may be because of trauma, callous, periosteal elevation. The bone thickening and irregularity of the ridges may be a sign of previous trauma and callous formation.

If non-union is suspected in the old trauma, then the examination regarding the signs of non-union must be carried out. The key findings include abnormal mobility of the arm in both planes, loss of transmitted movement and pain-free movement at the fracture site.

The surgical mark should be palpated for its adequate healing and sometimes the signs of infection may be noticed if there is history of compound fracture or postoperative wound infection.

C. Movements

Each joint is examined for a passive range of motion and determination of any fixed joint contracture must be taken in account. It is important as 1) tendon transfer can be carried out in the presence of supple joints and 2) the need for splinting in functional positions can be carried out.

D. Neurological Examination

TINEL'S SIGN AND ITS INTERPRETATION [36]

Paraesthesia (fornication) is experienced by the patient along the nerve distribution by gentle percussion over the nerve from distal to proximal location (Video 8A.2). The Tinel's sign helps in three aspects as: 1) Localization of site of injury. 2) Complete or partial nerve injury. 3) Assessment of regeneration of the nerve. The interpretations still hold valid as mentioned in the landmark work done by Tinel [36].

Interpretation

1. A non-progressive area of tingling over a substantial period of time (for weeks or months) along the nerve trunk pathway is suggestive of neuroma formation. The tingling area is often quite small (around 2–3 cm). The nerve fibres, despite their regeneration, are unable to bridge the gap between the proximal and distal nerve segment – that implies complete transaction of the nerve.

2. A regenerating nerve is signified by gradually increasing the area of tingling that is perceived distal to the site of injury and gradually extending towards the periphery over months along the path of the injured nerve. The feature should be noted during the course of the treatment (after operative or conservative management).

3. In rare circumstances, one traumatic insult can injure the same nerve in two different sites. In these cases, there will be two separate areas of tingling on that nerve. The interpretation remains the same and serial examination can delineate the regeneration of the nerve at different injury sites.

4. In some cases, it is seen that partial damage of the nerve fibres leads to neuritis. The tingling experienced by the patient with neuritis is very painful or there might be a painful swelling present. The clinician must be cautious to differentiate between neuritic pain and a tingling sensation due to nerve fibre regeneration. On serial examination over months, the neuritic pain is usually diminished in intensity and replaced with tingling sensation on percussion on the nerve trunk. Another important differentiating feature is the neuritic pain is often disabling in comparison to the tingling sensation of nerve regeneration.

5. Tingling caused by pressure on the nerve usually starts after four to six weeks from injury.

6. The tingling is sensed by the patient due to hyperexcitable axons in the initial period of regeneration. Hence it is a usual finding that when the axons are completely matured the tingling sensation is resolved. It may take about eight or ten months for the tingling to be resolved (complete nerve regeneration). It is important for a clinician to determine

 Video 8A.2 The demonstration of Tinel's sign has been done. The correct way to do it is from proximal to distal.

www.routledge.com/9780367647162.

Video 8A.3 Tenodesis effect: The extension of the wrist leads to flexion of the fingers and flexion of the fingers leads to extension of the wrist.

www.routledge.com/9780367647162.

whether the nerve is regenerating or not but the time to be elapsed for a complete nerve recovery depends on many variables like the velocity of injury, extent of nerve damage, soft tissue conditioning, nutritional status of the patient and are extremely difficult to determine accurately.

7. Tingling is not a universal phenomenon. It may not be perceived by a few patients although it is rare. This may suggest two extremely opposite clinical scenarios. Tingling may not be experienced if there is subtle nerve injury that caused minimal nerve fibre destruction. On the other hand, with severe malnutrition, old age and patients with chronic diseases there might be no nerve regeneration leading to no evidence of Tinel's sign (no tingling experienced by the patient).

8. A rapidly advancing Tinel's sign is suggestive of axonotmesis (around 2 mm/day) which is faster than nerve grafting or nerve repair. It is also faster in proximal aspect of the limb (in axilla the nerve regeneration may be as fast as 3 mm/day) than a distal one.

Tinel's sign should be examined repeatedly in the course of the treatment and single examination does not have any clinical implication.

MOTOR EXAMINATION

It is essential to know the tenodesis effect in the hand and wrist as sometimes the patient uses this effect to compensate his loss of functions. These sometimes manifest as trick movements. The extension of the wrist leads to flexion of the fingers and flexion of the fingers leads to extension of the wrist (Video 8A.3).

Examination of Muscles Innervated by the Radial Nerve

Do not forget to compare the muscle strength with the normal side.

1. Triceps – Forward flex the shoulder and elbow at 90° (this manoeuvre eliminates the action of gravity) and extend the elbow.

Video 8A.4 The finger extension should be tested by holding the wrist of the patient in a neutral degree as wrist flexion will produce extension of the fingers due to the tenodesis effect.

www.routledge.com/9780367647162.

The fibres of triceps are palpated to note contraction.

2. Brachioradialis (BR) – Semi pronate the forearm and flex the elbow against resistance. The fibres of BR are palpated. Keep the elbow supported against the patient's trunk. This is a common fallacy that the patient moves the elbow away from the body. The distance between the radial nerve injury (fracture site or plate/screw causing the nerve compression) and the nerve supply to the BR may be calculated and the time period of regeneration of the BR is calculated as (1 mm/day plus one month). Regeneration of the BR helps the surgeon in decision-making for secondary exploration of the nerve.

3. Supinator – Extend the elbow completely (to negate the function of biceps brachii) and supinate the forearm from the mid prone position. Palpation of the muscle fibres can be done, although it may be difficult to interpret.

4. ECRL and ECRB – These are palpated when the wrist is extended and abducted against resistance when the forearm is pronated. Beware of the trick movements that few patients can produce false extension of the wrist up to a neutral degree due to finger flexion, as the tenodesis effect of extensor tendons may lead to this false extension. The patient is requested to do wrist extension while maintaining the fingers extended, the patient will not be able do extension due to trick movements.

5. ECU – It is palpated when wrist is extended and adducted against resistance when the forearm is pronated at the lateral groove that overlies the posterior subcutaneous border of the ulna.

6. Extensor digitorum communis – Tendons are usually seen better and felt when the fingers are extended against resistance and the forearm is pronated. The finger extension should be tested by holding the wrist of the patient in a neutral degree as wrist flexion will produce extension of the fingers due to the tenodesis effect (Video 8A.4).

7. Extensor digiti minimi – Extend the little finger while maintaining flexion of the metacarpophalangeal joint of the other three fingers.

8. Extensor indicis – Extend the index finger while maintaining flexion of the metacarpophalangeal joint of other fingers.

9. Abductor pollicis longus (APL) – Thumb abduction is done at the carpometacarpal joint and the tendon is seen and felt at the radial aspect of the anatomical snuffbox.

10. Extensor pollicis longus – When the thumb is extended at the interphalangeal joint against resistance, the tendon is palpated at the ulnar border of the anatomical snuff box. The wrist should be supported at a neutral degree.

11. Extensor pollicis brevis (EPB) – When the metacarpophalangeal joint of the thumb is extended against resistance, the EPB tendon is felt at the radial border of the anatomical snuff box, lying medial to the tendon of the APL. The wrist should be supported at neutral degree.

Examination of Donor Tendons

The donor tendons are tested by activating the muscle and resisted force is given to undo the movement. Simultaneously, the muscle belly is palpated to reconfirm its activation. Most commonly, the donor tendons for tendon transfer for radial nerve palsy are:

1. Pronator teres (PT) – The patient is asked to fully extend the forearm and pronate it. The examiner tries to supinate the forearm, which the patient resists, and pronator teres is palpated at proximal forearm (Video 8A.5).

2. Flexor carpi ulnaris (FCU) – The patient is asked to clench the fist and asked to do palmar flexion and ulnar deviation of the wrist.

Video 8A.5 The examiner tries to supinate the forearm, which the patient resists, and pronator teres is palpated at proximal forearm.

www.routledge.com/9780367647162.

The muscle belly of FCU is palpated (Video 8A.6).

3. Flexor carpi radialis – The patient is asked to clench the fist and asked to do palmar flexion and radial deviation of the wrist. The tendon of the flexor carpi radialis (FCR) is palpated (Video 8A.6).

4. Palmaris longus (PL) – The patient is asked to touch their little finger and thumb and to do palmar flexion of the wrist against resistance (Video 8A.7). If the wrist is painful then the wrist is supported, and resisted finger flexion is done (Video 8A.8). Both the manoeuvres lead to tenting of the PL in the forearm. The tendon of the PT is absent in 30% of population.

5. Flexor digitorum superficialis (FDS) – This tendon integrity is tested by examination of active flexion of the proximal interphalangeal joint. The patient's hand and forearm are kept flat on the table with the forearm supinated. The examiner stabilizes the other fingers (except the finger to be tested) and the patient is asked to flex the proximal interphalangeal (PIP) joint against resistance and the tendon of the FDS is palpated (Video 8A.9).

SENSORY EXAMINATION

The sensory branches of radial nerve are as follows (Figure 8A.5):

1. Posterior cutaneous nerve of arm.

First sensory branch of the radial nerve, which arises from axilla.

2. Lower lateral cutaneous nerve to the arm.

Originates from the radial nerve in the spiral groove and supplies the lateral arm area below the deltoid.

Video 8A.6 The patient is asked to clench the fist and asked to do palmar flexion and ulnar deviation of the wrist for FCU testing, and to do palmar flexion and radial deviation of the wrist for FCR testing. The respective muscles are palpated during the examination.

www.routledge.com/9780367647162.

Video 8A.7 The patient is asked to touch their little finger and thumb and to do palmar flexion of the wrist against resistance. The manoeuvre leads to tenting of the palmaris longus in the forearm.

www.routledge.com/9780367647162.

Video 8A.8 If the wrist is painful, then the wrist is supported and resisted finger flexion is performed. The manoeuvre leads to tenting of the palmaris longus in the forearm.

www.routledge.com/9780367647162.

Video 8A.9 The examiner stabilizes the other fingers (except the finger to be tested) and the patient is asked to flex the PIP joint against resistance and the tendon of the FDS is palpated.

www.routledge.com/9780367647162.

3. *Posterior cutaneous nerve to forearm.*

Originates at the brachioaxillary angle, proximal to the origin of the lower lateral cutneous nerve of the arm and pierces the brachial fascia posterior to the lateral epicondyle and lateral to the olecranon. It supplies the dorsolateral aspect of the forearm.

4. *Superficial sensory radial nerve.*

Provides sensation to the dorsal skin of the first, second and radial side of the third digits up to the base of the second phalanx [37].

Pinprick and light touch to be tested along the posterior arm, posterior forearm and posterior lateral hand and thumb.

Changes in vibration and pressure thresholds are seen in early nerve compression but are unreliable in evaluating nerve lacerations.

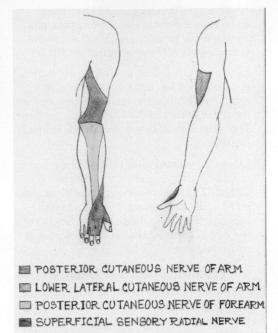

POSTERIOR CUTANEOUS NERVE OF ARM
LOWER LATERAL CUTANEOUS NERVE OF ARM
POSTERIOR CUTANEOUS NERVE OF FOREARM
SUPERFICIAL SENSORY RADIAL NERVE

Figure 8A.5 The sensory distribution of the sensory branches of the radial nerve is shown. Knowledge about it also helps in diagnosing the site of injury. The dorsum of the first web space is considered the autonomous zone of the radial nerve.

Changes in sensory receptor innervations density (2 PD) are seen in chronic nerve compression but are reliable for evaluating nerve laceration (Table 8A.1).

EXAMINATION OF OTHER NERVES

No examination should complete without complete examination of other peripheral nerves

Table 8A.1: Table Depicting the Clinical Tests, Perception, Main Receptors and Important Comments Related to the Tests

Test	Perception	Main Receptor	Comments
Static two-point discrimination (2 PD)	Tactile	Merkel cell	Evaluates sensory receptor innervations density (normal distance 6 mm)
Moving two-point discrimination (2 PD)	Tactile	Meissner corpuscle	Normal distance 3 mm
Tuning fork (250 Hz)	Vibration	Pacinian corpuscle	
Tuning fork (30 Hz)	Vibration	Meissner corpuscle	
Semmens–Weinstein monofilament test	Pressure	Merkel cell	
Ten test (moving light touch)	Pressure	Merkel cell	Reliability comparable to monofilament test
Cold–heat test	Temperature	Free nerve endings	

which specifically include the median and ulnar nerves. Sometimes, partially recovered brachial injury patients have similar presentations as those with radial nerve palsy. The motor only involvement as asymmetric muscle involvement should give rise to suspicion of motor neurone disease.

EXAMINATION OF ADJACENT AREA

The examination of the neck and shoulder is part of examination to diagnose associated conditions, or some conditions that can mimic the radial nerve palsy. The examination of the neck and shoulder is not a mandate of this chapter.

E. Special Tests

Special tests are sometimes used to diagnose compressive neuropathies of the radial nerve.
The tests are:

1. Motor examination

2. Tenderness over radial tunnel

3. Pain at origin of ECRB after resisted middle finger extension

4. Pain with resisted elbow supination

5. Pressure over supinator is very painful

6. Scratch collapse test

The opposite side must be examined meticulously by the examiner and repeated examination at the same site of possible entrapment as well as non-entrapment sites should be examined to rule out other pain generators to arrive at a precise diagnosis.

To exclude any concomitant radial nerve affection, deep palpation between the brachioradialis and brachialis just above the elbow should be performed and no pain should be generated on this palpation.

EXAMINATION RELATED TO NERVE TRANSFER

Wrist and finger extension are essential functions that has to be gained in low radial palsy to provide a power grip to the patient. Tendon transfers have been performed since to accomplish the loss of functions, but tendon transfers may impair pronation (due to pronator teres to ECRB transfer). Hence, intact expendable nerves are directed to muscles that perform specific functions. Currently, re-innervation to ECRB (for wrist extension) is done from the nerve supplying the FDS muscle (median nerve). The wrist

and thumb extension is a function of the PIN for which nerves supplying the PL and FCR are coaptated to the PIN.

Meticulous examination of donor nerves (median nerve) is performed to plan for a nerve transfer. Examination and intactness of the PL and FCR as well as FDS nerve supply to be performed and documented in the case sheet.

EVALUATION OF SENSORY ONLY SYMPTOMS

1. Sensory branch of radial nerve involvement (Wartenberg's syndrome).
   a. Suspicion if –

1. Paraesthesia, pain or numbness over dorso-radial aspect of forearm including first web space. The pain usually aggravates with forearm pronation and ulnar wrist flexion.

2. On examination, sensation over dorso-radial aspect is decreased, Tinel's sign is seen over the compression site of the nerve.
   b. Causation –

1. Tight bands around wrist may lead to compression.

2. Work that repeatedly needs pronation and supination, approximates the tendons of ECRL and BR during pronation and ulnar sided wrist flexion, can compress the nerve and produce symptoms.
   c. Differential diagnosis –

1. Cervical disc disease (C7 neuropathy) – examination of cervical spine and MRI can be ruled out.

2. Lateral antebrachial cutaneous nerve involvement – differential nerve blockade can rule out this.

3. de Quervain's disease – the affected first dorsal compartment tendons of the wrist may cause neuritis or scarring of the distal sensory component of the superficial radial nerve that may cause coexistence of both the conditions. Finkelstein's test can also be positive in SRN neuropathy,. But the differentiating factors between the two separate clinical entities are an absence of sensory symptoms and no Tinel's sign in de Quervain's disease.

HOW TO INVESTIGATE

1. *Radiographs:* This is usually the primary investigation in an emergency after trauma to delineate the fracture site (if any), bony

spur, excessive callus or it may indicate any soft tissue mass.

2. *Computed tomography (CT) scan* It can be used to determine bony architecture in detail. It helps to better understand fracture morphology and in surgical planning; it can also determine fracture union if it is doubtful, with radiography in the presence of hardware.

3. *Electrodiagnostic testing (EDT):*

The most commonly used electrodiagnostic testing methods are:
Usefulness of EDT

1. Electromyography (EMG)

2. Nerve conduction study (NCS)

   a. Documentation of injury

   b. Localization of injury

   c. Severity of injury

   d. Serial testing at six weeks to three months interval helps in monitoring the nerve recovery. A proper time of intervention or observation may be chosen as per the recovery of the nerve [10, 11].

4. *High frequency ultrasound (HFU):*

High frequency ultrasound is a powerful modality for evaluation of peripheral nerve pathologies. This suggests anatomic continuity as well as morphology of the nerve. Evaluation of surrounding soft tissues also helps the clinician in decision-making before embarking on surgical intervention when electrophysiological testing is not conclusive. HFU is particularly valuable in previously operated cases with implants in situ making the magnetic resonance neurography less useful to visualize the nerve structure.

HFU is a dynamic examination that can help eliciting Tinel's sign on pressing the ultrasound probe [38]. It is extremely important to sonoghraphically visualize at least a long segment of radial nerve as well as surrounding soft tissue – muscles, bones and tendons.

APPLICATIONS
HFU is especially helpful in trauma scenarios and compressive neuropathy syndromes. The nerve fascicles can be visualized, and interpretations can be made as 1) Complete transection/incomplete injury. 2) End neuroma/neuroma in continuity/fascicle disruptions

due to fibrosis. 3) Intraneural hematoma/traction injury. 4) External compression by fracture end, bone fragment, screw or another hard. 5) Compressive neuropathy due to any aberrant compressive lesion, etc. [38–40].

5. *Magnetic resonance neurography (MRN)*

A pathologic nerve is hyperintense in comparison to adjacent vessels, focal or diffuse nerve enlargement is often present due to differential oedema along the faciculi, epineurial or perineurial heterogenous thickening and fascicular disruption with intraneural and/or perineural fibrosis [41–44].

1. Differentiation of pseudo-neuroma and true neuroma with MRI.

2. Compression neuropathy.

3. Undetermined pathology – when there is discrepancy between the electrodiagnostic finding and clinical examination then MRI may be decisive to determine the pathology.

4. MRI is of particular significance in evaluation of the post-surgical nerve compression.

HOW TO INTERPRET FROM A BATTERY OF TESTS

1. Take a meticulous history with special emphasis on handedness and occupation.

2. Do a comprehensive clinical examination (muscles paralyzed, sensory loss).

3. Determine the site of injury from history and clinical examination and apprehend the depth of the nerve injury (only conduction block or axonotmesis or neurotmesis).

4. Determine the nerve status whether anatomically intact or not (HFU and MRN).

5. If the nerve injury is old, evaluate for recovering/partially recovering or non-recovering (from serial Tinel's sign and EDT.

6. Assess for the joint contracture (of elbow or wrist or MCP joint).

7. Evaluate for intactness of donor tendons (for possible tendon transfer), median nerve intactness (for possible median to radial nerve transfer).

Amalgamate all the information along with photographic documentation of wound (if any) in the patient file for future reference.

DIFFERENTIAL DIAGNOSIS IN PATIENTS OF RADIAL NERVE INJURY

1. **Very high radial nerve palsy:**
   a. Crutch palsy/Saturday night palsy
   b. Aneurysm of axillary vessels

2. **High radial nerve palsy:**
   a. Fracture shaft of humerus
   b. Prolonged application of tourniquet
   c. Injection palsy
   d. Excessive callus formation from fracture
   e. Iatrogenic

3. **Low radial nerve palsy:**
   a. Dislocation of elbow
   b. Fracture neck of radius
   c. Enlarged bursae around the elbow
   d. Rheumatoid synovitis of elbow
   e. Iatrogenic (injury due to surgery of radial head or neck)

CONCLUSION

Radial nerve examination needs a systematic approach which needs to be supplemented with a battery of tests. The examination is directed not only on the diagnosis of the disease but it should help in making a decision about further management. A recovering radial nerve can be identified by diligent examination. The nerve exploration or tendon transfer is a tricky decision. The type of tendon transfer can be determined by the availability of the tendons. The palmaris longus must be examined as its absence can lead to a change in plan about the type of tendon transfer. Investigations further help as a supplement for the diagnosis and management plan. Radiographs, CT scans, EDT, HFU and MRN are usual investigations, which should be chosen on a case-by-case basis.

REFERENCES

1. Linell EA. The distribution of nerves in the upper limb, with reference to variabilities and their clinical significance. *J Anat* 1921; 55(Pt 2–3):79.

2. Sunderland S. Metrical and non-metrical features of the muscular branches of the radial nerve. *J Comp Neurol* 1946; 85:93–111. doi: 10.1002/cne.900850108.

3. Whitson RO. Relation of the radial nerve to the shaft of the humerus. *JBJS*. 1954; 36(1):85–88.

4. Gerwin M, Hotchkiss RN and Weiland AJ. Alternative operative exposures of the posterior aspect of the humeral diaphysis with reference to the radial nerve. *J Bone Joint Surg Am* 1996;78-A:1690–1695

5. Bumbasirevic M, Palibrk T, Lesic A and Atkinson HD. Radial nerve palsy. *EFORT Open Rev* 2016; 1(8):286–294.

6. Wells ME, Gonzalez GA, Childs BR, Williams MR, Nesti LJ and Dunn JC. Radial to axillary nerve transfer outcomes in shoulder abduction: A systematic review. *Plast Reconstr Surg - Global Open* 2020; 8(9):e3096.

7. Tornetta III P, Hochwald Neal, Bono C and Grossman M. Anatomy of the posterior interosseous nerve in relation to fixation of the radial head. *Clin Orthop Relat Res* 1997; 345: 215–218.

8. Last RJ. *Anatomy: Regional and Applied*, 7th edition. Edinburgh: Churchill Livingstone, 1984, p. 89.

9. Lister G. *The Hand: Diagnosis and Indications*, 2nd edition. Edinburgh: Churchill Livingstone, 1984, p. 218.

10. Albrecht S, Cordis R and Kleihues H. Functional neuroanatomy of the radial nerve in the region of the long wrist and finger joint extensors and the supinator groove. Sportverletz Sportschaden 1998; 12:1–7.

11. Al-Qattan MM. The nerve supply to extensor carpi radialis brevis. *J Anat* 1996; 188:249–250.

12. Abrams RA, Ziets RJ, Lieber RL and Botte MJ. Anatomy of the radial nerve motor branches in the forearm. *J Hand Surg Am* 1997; 22(2):232–237. doi: 10.1016/S0363-5023(97)80157-8. PMID: 9195420.

13. Nayak SR, Ramanathan L, Krishnamurthy A, Prabhu LV, Madhyastha S, Potu BK and Ranade AV. Extensor carpi radialis brevis origin, nerve supply and its role in lateral epicondylitis. *Surg Radiol Anat* 2010; 32(3):207–211. doi: 10.1007/s00276-009-0526-7. Epub 2009 Jun 25. PMID: 19554250.

14. Binhammer P, Manktelow RT and Haswell T. Applications of the extensor carpi radialis brevis for facial reanimation. *J Reconst Microsurg* 1994; 10: 109.

15. Tsai P and Steinberg DR. Median and radial nerve compression about the elbow. *JBJS* 2008; 90(2):420–428.

16. Ferdinand BD, Rosenberg ZS, Schweitzer ME, Stuchin SA, Jazrawi LM, Lenzo SR, Meislin RJ and Kiprovski K. MR imaging features of radial tunnel syndrome: Initial experience. *Radiology* 2006; 240(1):161–168.

17. Folberg CR, Ulson H and Scheidt RB. The superficial branch of the radial nerve: A morphologic study. *RevistaBrasileira de Ortopedia (English Edition)* 2009; 44(1):69–74. ISSN 2255-4971. doi:10.1016/S2255-4971(15)30052-5.

18. Hu SY, Choi JG and Son BC. Cheiralgia paresthetica: An isolated neuropathy of the superficial branch of the radial nerve. eISSN2465-891X *The Nerve* 2015; 1(1):1–4. doi: 10.21129/nerve.2015.1.1.1.

19. Pećina MM, Krmpotić-Nemanić J and Markiewitz AD. *Tunnel Syndromes: Peripheral Nerve Compression Syndromes*, 3rd edition. BocaRaton: CRC Press, 2001, pp. 141–145.

20. Li H, Cai QX, Shen PQ, et al. Posterior interosseous nerve entrapment after Monteggia fracture-dislocation in children. *Chin J Traumatol* 2013; 16:131–135.

21. Serrano KD, Rebella GS, Sansone JM and Kim MK. A rare case of posterior interosseous nerve palsy associated with radial head fracture. *J Emerg Med* 2012; 43(2):e115–117.

22. Holstein A and Lewis GM. Fractures of the humerus with radial-nerve paralysis. *J Bone Joint Surg Am* 1963; 45(7):1382–1388.

23. Noger M, Berli MC, Fasel JH and Hoffmeyer PJ. The risk of injury to neurovascular structures from distal locking screws of the Unreamed Humeral Nail (UHN): A cadaveric study. *Injury* 2007; 38(8):954–957.

24. Blyth MJ, Macleod CM, Asante DK and Kinninmonth AW. Iatrogenic nerve injury with the Russell–Taylor humeral nail. *Injury* 2003; 34(3):227–228.

25. Hassan DM and Johnston GH. Safety of the limited open technique of bone-transfixing threaded-pin placement for external fixation of distal radial fractures: A cadaver study. *Can J Surg* 1999; 42:363–365.

26. Steinberg BD, Plancher KD and Idler RS. Percutaneous Kirschner wire fixation through the snuff box: An anatomic study. *J Hand Surg Am* 1995; 20:57–62.

27. Carlan D, Pratt J, Patterson JM, et al. The radial nerve in the brachium: An anatomic study in human cadavers. *J Hand Surg Am* 2007; 32:1177–1182.

28. Zhang J, Moore AE and Stringer MD. Iatrogenic upper limb nerve injuries: A systematic review. *ANZ J Surg* 2011; 81:227–236.

29. Lim R, Tay SC and Yam A. Radial nerve injury during double plating of a displaced intercondylar fracture. *J Hand Surg Am* 2012; 37:669–672.

30. Lin CC, Jawan B, de Villa MV, Chen FC and Liu PP. Blood pressure cuff compression injury of the radial nerve. *J Clin Anesth* 2001; 13(4):306–308.

31. Gupta A and Sunil TM. Complete division of the posterior interosseous nerve after elbow arthroscopy: A case report. *J Shoulder Elbow Surg* 2004; 13(5):566–567.

32. Singh S, Trikha P and Twyman R. Superficial radial nerve damage due to Kirschner wiring of the radius. *Injury* 2005; 36(2):330–332.

33. Ali AM, El-Alfy B and Attia H. Is there a safe zone to avoid superficial radial nerve injury with Kirschner wire fixation in the treatment of distal radius? A cadaveric study. *J Clin Orthop Trauma* 2014; 5(4):240–244.

34. Singh VK, Singh PK and Azam A. Intraoperative positioning related injury of superficial radial nerve after shoulder arthroscopy–a rare iatrogenic injury: A case report. *Cases J* 2008; 1(1):47.

35. Pandian JD, Bose S, Daniel V, Singh Y and Abraham AP. Nerve injuries following intramuscular injections: A clinical and neurophysiological study from Northwest India. *J Peripher Nerv Syst* 2006; 11(2):165–171.

36. Tinel J. "Tingling" signs with peripheral nerve injuries. *J Hand Surg* 2005; 30(1):87–89.

37. Ndiaye A, Diop M, Dia A, Seye SI and Sow ML. La branche sensitive du nerf radial au tiers inférieur de l'avant-bras et au poignet. Applications cliniques [The sensitive branch of the radial nerve at the inferior third of the

forearm and at the wrist. Clinical applications]. *Bull Assoc Anat (Nancy)* 1996; 80(249):27–30. French. PMID: 9102055.

38. Kele H. Ultrasonography of the peripheral nervous system. *Persp Med* 2012; 1(1–12): 417–421. ISSN 2211-968X. doi:10.1016/j.permed.2012.02.047.

39. Kopf H, Loizides A, Mostbeck GH and Gruber H. Diagnostic sonography of peripheral nerves: Indications, examination technique and pathological findings. *Ultraschall Med* 2011; 32:242–263.

40. Tas S, Staub F, Dombert T, Marquardt G, Senft C, Seifert V and Duetzmann S. Sonographic short-term follow-up after surgical decompression of the median nerve at the carpal tunnel: A single-center prospective observational study. *Neurosurg Focus* 2015; 39(3):E6.

41. Filler AG, Maravilla KR and Tsuruda JS. MR neurography and muscle MR imaging for image diagnosis of disorders affecting the peripheral nerves and musculature. *Neurol Clin* 2004; 22:643–682.

42. Lee PP, Chalian M, Bizzell C, Williams EH, Rosson GD, Belzberg AJ, et al. Magnetic resonance neurography of common peroneal (fibular) neuropathy. *J Comput Assist Tomogr* 2012;36:455–461.

43. Petchprapa CN, Rosenberg ZS, Sconfienza LM, Cavalcanti CF, Vieira RL and Zember JS. MR imaging of entrapment neuropathies of the lower extremity. Part 1. The pelvis and hip. *Radiographics* 2010; 30:983–1000.

44. Keen NN, Chin CT, Engstrom JW, Saloner D and Steinbach LS. Diagnosing ulnar neuropathy at the elbow using magnetic resonance neurography. *Skeletal Radiol* 2012; 41:401–407.

8B Peripheral Nerve Examination

Median Nerve Palsy

J Terrence Jose Jerome and Dafang Zhang

CONTENTS

MEDIAN NERVE ANATOMY

The median nerve arises from contributions from the medial cord and the lateral cord of the brachial plexus, with contributions from the nerve roots of C5 to T1 [1–3]. In the upper brachium, the median nerve descends lateral to the brachial artery and deep to the biceps brachii, until it crosses medial to the brachial artery at approximately the level of the mid-brachium. Its course continues medial to the brachial artery as it crosses the antecubital fossa, making it the most medial structure beneath the flexor-pronator musculature [3]. The median nerve splits the humeral and ulnar heads of the pronator teres as it crosses the elbow and continues in the forearm superficial to the flexor digitorum profundus and deep to the flexor digitorum superficialis. At the distal forearm, the median nerve emerges from beneath the flexor digitorum superficialis to travel radial to the palmaris longus tendon and ulnar to the flexor carpi radialis tendon. The palmar cutaneous branch emerges approximately 5 cm proximal to the wrist flexion crease and travels ulnar to the flexor carpi radialis tendon to supply sensation to the palm and thenar eminence. The median nerve traverses the carpal tunnel along with the nine extrinsic digital flexors before dividing into its terminal branches [3, 4].

The median nerve gives off motor innervation to the humeral head of the pronator teres proximal to the elbow. Distal to the elbow, the median nerve gives off branches to the ulnar head of the pronator teres, palmaris longus, flexor carpi radialis and flexor digitorum superficialis, as well as the anterior interosseous nerve branch. The anterior interosseous nerve and one branch to the pronator teres are generally the only branches that arise laterally from the median nerve proper, and all other branches arise medially at this level. The anterior interosseous nerve travels deep to the flexor-pronator musculature along with the anterior interosseous artery on the volar aspect of the interosseous membrane; as it descends, the anterior interosseous nerve innervates the flexor pollicis longus, the flexor digitorum profundus to the index finger and middle finger, and the pronator quadratus before supplying sensory innervation to the volar wrist capsule [3].

The carpal tunnel is bound by the transverse carpal ligament superficially, the carpal bones deeply, the trapezium radially, and the hook of the hamate ulnarly. The median nerve traverses the carpal tunnel with the flexor carpi radialis tendon, the four flexor digitorum superficialis tendons and the four flexor digitorum profundus tendons. The recurrent motor branch of the median nerve, which supplies the thenar muscles of the hand, most commonly arises distal to the carpal tunnel; however, in a notable minority of cases, the recurrent motor branch arises within the carpal tunnel or pierces the transverse carpal ligament [5, 6]. The terminal sensory branches of the median nerve are the common digital nerves to the first, second and third web spaces. The first and second lumbricals are supplied by the digital branches of the median nerve.

Internervous Communications

Anatomic variations exist in the internervous communications between the median nerve and the ulnar nerve at the levels of the forearm and the hand. It is important to be aware of the existence of these communications, as their presence can confound the diagnosis of a median nerve palsy.

The most common median nerve communication at the level of the forearm is the Martin–Gruber anastomosis. The Martin–Gruber anastomosis is a communication between the median nerve and ulnar nerve, in which axons

DOI: 10.1201/9781003125938-9

from the median nerve cross to join the ulnar nerve at the forearm level. This communication is estimated to be present in as high as 30 to 40% of the population [2]. Clinically, a median nerve lesion proximal to a Martin–Gruber anastomosis may affect the thenar muscles, whereas a median nerve lesion distal to the communication may not. A less common communication is the Marinacci communication, in which axons from the ulnar nerve cross to join the median nerve at the forearm level.

Communications between the recurrent motor branch of the median nerve and the deep motor branch of the ulnar nerve at the level of the hand are called Riche–Cannieu anastomoses. The incidence of this neural communication is estimated to be as high as 80%. The Berretini anastomosis refers to communications between common digital nerves arising from the median and ulnar nerves at the level of the hand. Berretini anatomoses are so commonplace that they are thought to be a part of normal anatomy [2].

HIGH MEDIAN NERVE PALSY

High median nerve palsy arises from a lesion of the median nerve proximal to the branching of the anterior interosseous nerve. These injuries may occur from a variety of mechanisms. Sharp laceration of the median nerve may occur from penetrating trauma or iatrogenic injury. Alternatively, compressive neuropathy may occur from pronator syndrome [1].

The sensory examination of a high median nerve injury typically consists of hypoesthesia or paraesthesia in the volar aspect of the thumb, index finger and middle finger, and the radial half of the ring finger. In that the median lesion is proximal to the take-off of the palmar cutaneous branch, patients may report numbness in the palm and thenar eminence as well, although this is not uniformly the case [7].

The motor examination of a high median nerve injury should focus on deficits in the median nerve innervated muscle groups, and the examiner should assess forearm pronation, wrist flexion, finger flexion, thumb flexion and thumb opposition. The motor examination of an isolated high median nerve injury can be complicated by redundant innervation patterns from an intact ulnar nerve [1]. Deficits in the flexor carpi radialis and palmaris longus are well compensated for by a functioning flexor carpi ulnaris. Deficits in flexor digitorum superficialis to the ring finger and small finger are compensated for by a functioning flexor digitorum profundus.

Patients with high median nerve palsies have diminished pinch and grasp strength, due to deficits in the median nerve-innervated thenar muscles. High median nerve palsies uniformly result in a lack of distal interphalangeal joint flexion in the thumb and index finger. While the middle finger flexor digitorum profundus is thought to be innervated by the anterior interosseous nerve. Bertelli et al., have shown that deficits in middle finger flexion are not functionally observed in isolated high median nerve palsies, likely due to redundant innervation from the ulnar nerve. Moreover, while the strength and excursion of forearm pronation can be limited, pronation function is largely preserved in these injuries, despite paralysis of the pronator teres and pronator quadratus. The drivers of this pronation are unclear but may result from a concerted effort from the brachioradialis, ulnar nerve-innervated flexor digitorum profundus, extensor carpi ulnaris and extensor digiti minimi [7].

Pronator Syndrome

Pronator syndrome refers to proximal compression of the median nerve at the level of the elbow. Compression of the median nerve at this level can be caused by the ligament of Struthers (a fibrous band connecting a supracondylar process of the distal humerus to the medial epicondyle), the bicipital aponeurosis (lacertus fibrosis), the two heads of the pronator teres, an accessory head of flexor pollicis longus (Gantzer's muscle) and the proximal edge of flexor digitorum superficialis. The treatment of pronator syndrome typically involves a trial of nonoperative treatment with rest, stretching of the flexor-pronator musculature and/or anti-inflammatory medications, but refractory cases may benefit from surgical decompression [8].

The examination for pronator syndrome consists of a sensory examination, a motor examination and provocative manoeuvres. In addition to numbness or paraesthesia in the radial digits, patients may report sensory symptoms in the palm or thenar eminence due to entrapment proximal to the take-off of the palmar cutaneous branch. Weakness in the median nerve-innervated thenar muscles and weakness in the proximal volar forearm may be elicited. A number of provocative manoeuvres are helpful for the diagnosis of pronator syndrome. Patients often exhibit a positive Tinel's sign over the proximal volar forearm over the compressed median nerve. The pronator compressive test is performed by applying manual compression over the median nerve proximal and lateral to the proximal edge of the pronator teres. Reproduction of painful paraesthesia is considered a positive test (Figure 8B.1). Reproduction of painful paraesthesia

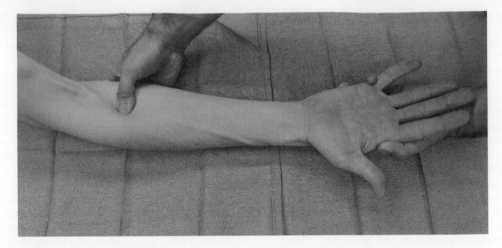

Figure 8B.1 The pronator compression test is performed by manual compression over the median nerve, proximal and lateral to the proximal aspect of the pronator teres.

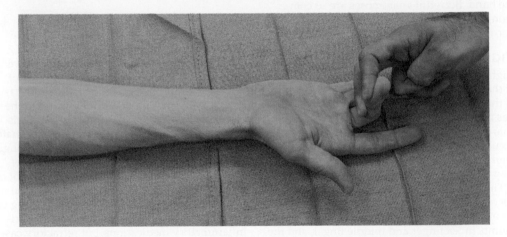

Figure 8B.2 Reproduction of painful paraesthesia with resisted middle finger flexor digitorum superficialis is a provocative manoeuvre for proximal median nerve compressive neuropathy.

with resisted pronation or resisted supination may signify compression of the median nerve by the pronator teres or bicipital aponeurosis, respectively. Finally, reproduction of painful paraesthesia with resisted middle finger flexor digitorum superficialis may signify compression of the median nerve by the proximal edge of flexor digitorum superficialis (Figure 8B.2).

Anterior Interosseous Nerve Syndrome

Anterior interosseous nerve syndrome is an isolated lesion to the anterior interosseous nerve fibres, which innervates the flexor pollicis longus, the flexor digitorum profundus to the index finger and middle finger, and the pronator quadratus. The cause of anterior interosseous syndrome is varied and unclear. While direct compression of the anterior interosseous nerve has been reported, a pseudo-anterior

interosseous nerve syndrome can arise from a brachial neuritis or Parsonage–Turner syndrome. The etiology of Parsonage–Turner syndrome may be autoimmune, post-viral or post-traumatic, and may involve an interplay of genetic and environmental factors. In the absence of direct compression, the mainstay of treatment of anterior interosseous nerve syndrome is observation before performing surgical decompression, as spontaneous recovery has been reported even after one year of symptoms [8].

The sensory examination in anterior interosseous nerve syndrome is unremarkable, since the anterior interosseous nerve does not supply skin sensation. The hallmark of the physical examination is weakness of the flexor pollicis longus and flexor digitorum profundus to the index finger. Weakness in forearm pronation is typically not seen due to the functional prona- tor teres, and weakness in flexor digitorum pro- fundus to the middle finger is frequently not observed due to redundant innervation from the ulnar nerve. The Kiloh–Nevin sign refers to the physical examination finding of the inability to make an "OK" sign with the thumb and index finger due to weakness of the flexor pollicis longus and flexor digitorum profundus to the index finger (Figure 8B.3).

LOW MEDIAN NERVE PALSY

Low median nerve palsy manifests as sensory deficits in the radial digits and motor weakness in the median nerve-innervated thenar mus- cles. Similar to high median nerve palsies, low median nerve palsies can result from a number of mechanisms, ranging from sharp laceration penetrating trauma to compressive neuropathy from carpal tunnel syndrome [4].

The sensory examination of a low median nerve injury typically consists of hypoesthesia or paraesthesia in the volar aspect of the thumb,

index finger and middle finger, and the radial half of the ring finger. Patients may complain of numbness in the palm and thenar eminence when the palmar cutaneous branch is affected.

The thenar muscles are comprised of the abductor pollicis brevis, the flexor pollicis bre- vis and the opponens pollicis, which together contribute more than 30% of grip strength and 60% of pinch strength in a normal hand [3]. The thenar muscles allow for opposition of the thumb, which is the placement of the thumb in a plane opposite the lesser digits [9]. Opposition is a composite motion that combines flex- ion, pronation and palmar abduction at the thumb trapeziometacarpal joint and flexion at the thumb metacarpophalangeal joint [9, 10]. The abductor pollicis brevis has the greatest contribution to thumb opposition due to its superficial position and resultant mechanical advantage. The flexor pollicis brevis frequently has redundant innervation from the ulnar nerve, particularly its deep head which has supply from the ulnar nerve in nearly 80% of patients [9].

In low median nerve palsies, atrophy of the the- nar muscles can be noted on inspection. Thenar atrophy is most apparent when viewed in profile from the radial side [9, 11]. The thumb metacarpal lies in unopposed supination and external rota- tion in patients with low median nerve palsies, and over time, a first web space contracture may be observed [9]. Weakness in palmar abduction is noted in low median nerve palsies. To assess for palmar abduction weakness, the thumb is positioned perpendicular to the plane of the palm, and a force is applied to the thumb meta- carpophalangeal joint, attempting to collapse the

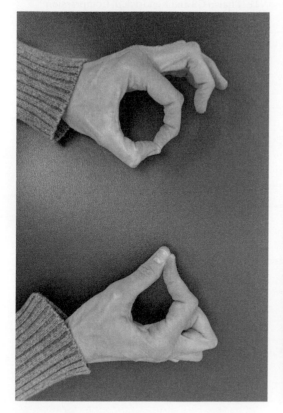

Figure 8B.3 Patients with anterior interos- seous nerve syndrome exhibit an inability to make an "OK" sign with the thumb and index finger due to weakness of the flexor pollicis longus and flexor digitorum profundus to the index finger.

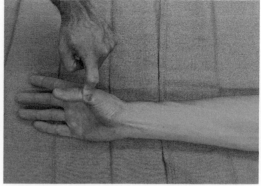

Figure 8B.4 Palmar abduction strength is tested by positioning the thumb perpendicular to the plane of the palm and applying a force to the thumb metacarpophalangeal joint, attempt- ing to collapse the thumb towards the index finger.

thumb towards the index finger. Weakness is noted as the inability to keep the thumb out of the plane of the palm [4] (Figure 8B.4)

REFERENCES

1. Isaacs J and Ugwu-Oju O. High median nerve injuries. *Hand Clin.* 2016; 32(3):339–348.

2. Unver Dogan N, Uysal II and Seker M. The communications between the ulnar and median nerves in upper limb. *Neuroanatomy.* 2009; 8(1):15–19.

3. Mazurek MT and Shin AY. Upper extremity peripheral nerve anatomy: Current concepts and applications. *Clin Orthop Relat Res.* 2001; (383):7–20.

4. Doughty CT and Bowley MP. Entrapment neuropathies of the upper extremity. *Med Clin North Am.* 2019; 103(2):357–370.

5. Kozin SH. The anatomy of the recurrent branch of the median nerve. *J Hand Surg Am.* 1998; 23(5):852–858.

6. Papathanassiou BT. A variant of the motor branch of the median nerve in the hand. *J Bone Joint Surg Br.* 1968; 50(1):156–157.

7. Bertelli JA, Soldado F, Lehn VL and Ghizoni MF. Reappraisal of clinical deficits following high median nerve injuries. *J Hand Surg Am.* 2016; 41(1):13–19.

8. Rodner CM, Tinsley BA and O'Malley MP. Pronator syndrome and anterior interosseous nerve syndrome. *J Am Acad Orthop Surg.* 2013; 21(5):268–275.

9. Chadderdon RC and Gaston RG. Low median nerve transfers (Opponensplasty). *Hand Clin.* 2016; 32(3):349–359.

10. Seiler JG 3rd, Desai MJ and Payne SH. Tendon transfers for radial, median, and ulnar nerve palsy. *J Am Acad Orthop Surg.* 2013; 21(11):675–684.

11. Phalen GS and Kendrick JI. Compression neuropathy of the median nerve in the carpal tunnel. *J Am Med Assoc.* 1957; 164(5):524–530.

8C Peripheral Nerve Examination

Ulnar Nerve Palsy

Nikhil Agrawal and Chaitanya Mudgal

CONTENTS

Disclosures: Neither of the authors has a financial interest in any of the products, devices or drugs mentioned in this chapter.

INTRODUCTION

Ulnar nerve injuries are common and can result from a variety of mechanisms including trauma, compression neuropathy, ulnar artery aneurysms and much more. As a hand surgeon, or as a physician involved in the care of peripheral nerves, it is inevitable that you will encounter ulnar nerve pathology in your practice. Recognizing potential injury can be simple; however, there is nuance in distinguishing it from spinal cord injury or brachial plexus injury. In addition, when combined with other nerve, tendon or vascular injuries knowing the examinations specific for the ulnar nerve is vital. Furthermore, we will discuss how to better localize where the pathology is occurring. Regarding the diagnosis of compression neuropathy, a nerve conduction study in isolation is inadequate, and a good physical examination is essential [1]. The steps in a comprehensive physical examination are to carefully observe, palpate, check sensation, utilize provocative manoeuvres and perform a precise motor examination.

ANATOMY

The ulnar nerve fibres originate predominantly from the C8–T1 nerve roots and begin as a terminal branch of the medial cord. As it travels through the upper arm, it passes under a band of deep brachial fascia that has been deemed the arcade of Struthers. The nerve then moves between the medial epicondyle and the olecranon in a highly vulnerable position. The cubital tunnel retinaculum overlies the nerve and passes between the olecranon and the medial epicondyle [2]. This structure is also known as Osborne's band [3] (Figure 8C.1).

The intrinsic fascicular anatomy of the ulnar nerve at the elbow has been well described. The motor fascicles to the extrinsic muscles are deeper in the canal and are less vulnerable to direct compression. The sensory fascicles to the hand and motor fascicles to the intrinsic muscles are located medially and superficially within in the nerve and are therefore more vulnerable to compression. There are two separate motor fascicles to flexor carpi ulnaris (FCU) with one located deep and lateral and a second superficial and medial [4, 5].

The ulnar nerve then passes into the forearm between the humeral and ulnar heads of the FCU. It then continues just ulnar to the ulnar artery and deep to the FCU tendon. About 6–8 cm proximal to the wrist crease it gives off the palmar and dorsal sensory branches which provide sensation to the ulnar palm as well as the proximal little finger and ulnar half of the ring finger as well as the webspace [6]. As the remaining ulnar nerve enters the wrist, it passes through Guyon's canal (Figure 8C.2). A superficial branch innervates the palmaris brevis as well as sensation to the rest of the little finger and the ulnar half of the ring finger. The deep branch passes deep to the piso-hamate ligament and provides motor innervation to the hypothenar muscles, the ulnar two lumbricals, all seven interossei and finally the adductor pollicis. Depending on the zone of injury within the Guyon's canal, symptoms can be sensory only, motor only or combined motor and sensory symptoms.

OBSERVE AND PALPATE

Careful observation of a patient's upper extremity and hands is the first step to a comprehensive physical examination. However, even certain features of a patient's history

DOI: 10.1201/9781003125938-10

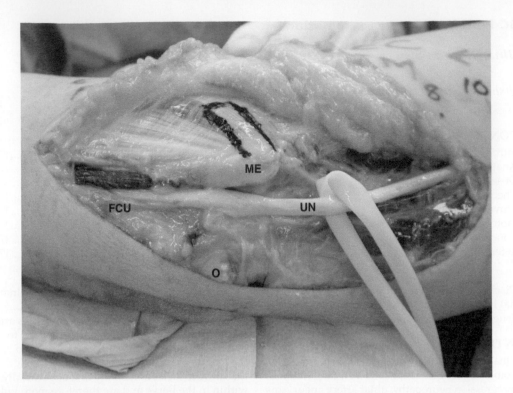

Figure 8C.1 The ulnar nerve (UN) is seen here at the level of the elbow after release of Osborne's band, the arcade of Struthers and exposure between the heads of the flexor carpi ulnaris (FCU). ME – Medial epicondyle O – Olecranon.

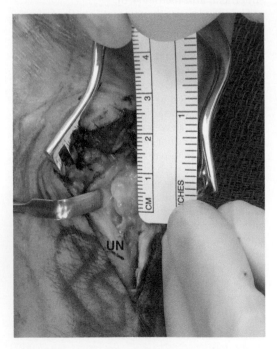

Figure 8C.2 Ulnar nerve (UN) compression in Guyon's canal by a 1 cm ganglion cyst.

can provide clues to ulnar nerve dysfunction. Most of these clues can be elicited by asking questions about intrinsic function in the hand. Deterioration of handwriting (the authors recognize that in the contemporary setting, most patients may use keyboards and handwriting alteration may be tough to elicit) specifically while signing any documents, is an indicator of intrinsic dysfunction. Furthermore, clumsiness in handling small objects or in playing musical instruments that require finger motion is also an indicator of intrinsic dysfunction. Indeed, this may explain why the ulnar nerve has been referred to in the past as "the musician's nerve."

Any scars from trauma or previous surgery must be noted for anatomical significance. In long-standing ulnar nerve palsy, the motor end plates will undergo necrosis and the intrinsic muscles of the hand will atrophy in a clinically predictable fashion. Dorsally, this is perhaps most striking at the first dorsal interosseous muscle (Figure 8C.3). Atrophy can also be noted in the volar intrinsic muscles (Figure 8C.4).

Observation of the resting posture of the hands can lead to an immediate diagnosis of high versus low ulnar nerve injuries. The intrinsic minus hand includes extension at

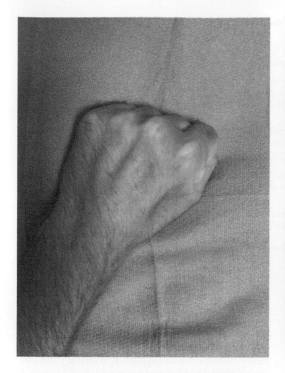

Figure 8C.3 Atrophy of the dorsal intrinsic muscles is most striking at the first dorsal interosseous muscle.

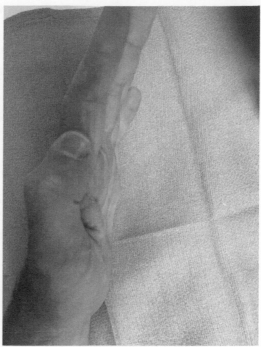

Figure 8C.4 Atrophy of the volar intrinsic muscles and the hypothenars can be clearly seen with careful observation.

the metacarpal phalangeal (MP) joints with slight flexion of the Proximal Interphalangeal (PIP) and Distal Interphalangeal (DIP) joints. This is called the ulnar claw. The flexion of the PIP and DIP joints is from the flexor digitorum superficialis (FDS) and flexor digitorum profundus (FDP) tendons. Therefore, when the nerve is injured proximal to the location of the FDP branches, the ring and little fingers will be resting in more extension than the index and middle finger. This is not in line with the normal digital cascade. This leads to educators explaining that the clawing is actually worse in distal injuries than in proximal ones. This latter phenomenon is called the "ulnar paradox." Furthermore, this paradox is manifest in high ulnar nerve injuries as they recover and the patient should be educated to expect worsening of an ulnar claw as the nerve recovers [7, 8].

More distally in the forearm, the ulnar side of the wrist should be examined and observed. A Tinel's sign here can be evidence of ulnar nerve compression in the canal. This is also a common site for a pseudoaneurysm of the ulnar artery from repetitive mechanical trauma in the area, termed "hypothenar hammer syndrome." The vascular enlargement manifests first as vascular compromise of the ulnar hand but can also exert a mass effect on the ulnar

nerve [9]. Other masses present within the canal, such as a ganglion can cause a similar mass effect on the nerve.

Also, while in the hand, the joints should be palpated to ensure good mobility and absence of contracture which can be seen in long standing ulnar nerve palsy. Testing for intrinsic tightness should be performed and will be covered in another chapter.

CHECK SENSATION

Sensation deficits in the little finger as well as the ulnar half of the ring finger is suggestive of ulnar nerve dysfunction. More subtle changes in sensation require checking of static two-point discrimination or the Semmes–Weinstein monofilament test. The Semmes–Weinstein monofilament test utilizes monofilaments of various thicknesses to determine what the thinnest diameter that a patient can feel.

These tests are immensely helpful when evaluating if an ulnar nerve palsy is improving after repair or a first- or second-degree Sunderland injury. A first-degree Sunderland injury is one in which axonal continuity is preserved and there is only a temporary conduction block. No Wallerian degeneration occurs and therefor the nerve will recover. In a second-degree Sunderland injury, Wallerian

Table 8C.1: Provocative Manoeuvres for the Ulnar Nerve Exam

Provocative Manoeuvre	How to Perform	Sensitivity	Specificity
Tinel's sign [12]	Four to six quick taps moving distally at the location of the nerve injury will send a pins and needles down into the little finger and the ulnar half of the ring finger	0.54–0.70	0.98–0.99
Pressure provocation test [12]	60 seconds of manual compression just proximal to the nerve's entry into the cubital tunnel	0.89	0.98
Elbow flexion test [12]	Flexion of the elbow for 60 seconds	0.75	0.99
Combined pressure and flexion test [12]	Keep the elbow flexed for 60 seconds while compressing just proximal to the nerve's entry into the cubital tunnel	0.46–0.98	0.95–0.99
Scratch collapse test [13, 14]	1. The patient is asked to have their elbows at neutral and externally rotate against the examiner's hands 2. The examiner scratches the skin over the ulnar nerve at the elbow 3. Repeat step 1	0.10–0.69	0.78–0.99

degeneration does occur, however the nerve can recover without surgical intervention due to the intact endoneurium. In these cases, recovery should be monitored closely utilizing these two-point discrimination and Semmes–Weinstein monofilaments [5, 10].

A key distinction for distinguishing between an ulnar nerve injury above or below the wrist is the presence of sensation in the ulnar palm. A lack of sensation signifies an injury more proximal to the branching of the sensory branches (6–8 cm proximal to the wrist crease). If there are sensory changes that do not fall into the expected ulnar nerve distribution, consider spinal cord pathology or an ulnar-medial nerve connection [11]. Sensation loss in the distribution of the dorsal cutaneous branch of the ulnar nerve indicates ulnar nerve dysfunction at a level proximal to their origin, most commonly at the cubital tunnel.

PROVOCATIVE MANOEUVRES

The ulnar nerve can be palpated at multiple locations along its course. This allows for a powerful Tinel's sign at various locations. Four to six quick taps moving distally at the location of the nerve injury will send a sensation of tingling or an "electric shock" or pins and needles down into the little finger and the ulnar half of the ring finger [12] (Table 8C.1).

The worsening of a compression neuropathy can be elicited by holding pressure over the nerve. Either by manual compression just proximal to its entry into the cubital tunnel, or by holding the elbow in flexion for 60 seconds or both. Manual compression is generally referred to as the pressure provocation test while flexing the elbow is aptly called the elbow flexion test. These tests can be combined by holding manual pressure while

the elbow is flexed. If a patient notes that their symptoms worsen, then there is suggestion that they have ulnar nerve pathology [12]. This is also a good time to evaluate for subluxation of the nerve over the medial epicondyle as the elbow is flexed from an extended position [10] (Video 8C.1).

The scratch collapse test has been offered as a more sensitive manoeuvre for the diagnosis of cubital tunnel syndrome. This test relies on allodynia of the skin that lies over the ulnar nerve. The test is performed in three steps. First the patient is asked to have their elbows at 90° of flexion with the forearm at neutral and are asked to externally rotate the arm at the shoulder, against the examiner's hands. Next the examiner scratches the skin over the ulnar nerve at the elbow. Finally, the first step is repeated. In a positive test, the patient's affected arm will collapse inward without being able to apply an outward external rotation force [13]. The studies evaluating the sensitivity versus electrodiagnostic studies or other clinical findings have found mixed results [14].

MOTOR EXAMINATION MANOEUVRES

Motor deficits will manifest if there is either a laceration of the nerve or in the setting of long-term compression neuropathy. Every physical examination of the hand includes an examination of finger and wrist flexion. The FCU will be weakened or paralyzed in ulnar nerve

 Video 8C.1 Ulnar nerve subluxation as seen in clinic and in the operating room.

www.routledge.com/9780367647162.

Table 8C.2: Motor Examination Manoeuvres for the Ulnar Nerve

Motor Examination Sign	How to Perform
Flexion of FDP to ring and little fingers	Hold PIPJ in extension and ask patient to flex at the DIPJ of that finger
Grasping motion	Ask the patient to grasp a rounded object such as a cup or ball and see if they can hold the IP joints in extension while flexion the MP joints
Wartenberg's sign	Have the patient keep the hand flat on a table and see if there is more room between the little and ring fingers than between the rest of the fingers
Cross finger	Have patient hold out both hands and ask them to cross the middle and index fingers back and forth
Egawa test	The middle finger then raised off the table and the patient is asked to move the finger from side to side
Froment's sign	Ask patient to grab a thick object like a thin binder or tabletop in the first webspace. A positive test is hyperflexion of the IP joint of the thumb
Jeanne's sign	Ask patient to grab a thick object like a thin binder or tabletop in the first webspace. A positive test is hyperextension of the MP joint of the thumb

injuries. This will manifest as pronounced radial deviation on wrist flexion. The FDP of the little and ring fingers need to be isolated from the FDS. In the event of a high ulnar nerve injury, the FDP of the little and ring fingers will be paralyzed (Table 8C.2).

The intricate dance between the intrinsic and extrinsic muscles allows the hand to be an incredibly versatile tool. With this, the hand will still be able to make a fist; however, the fashion in which it does so is incredibly hampered. When a patient with intrinsic muscle palsy creates a fist, they do so by utilizing the FDP and FDS muscles. Without being able to simultaneously extend the interphalangeal joints and flex the metacarpophalangeal joints, the fingers will curl. As such, the patient will be unable to firmly grasp large objects such as a ball or a cup. The unique anatomy of the lumbrical muscle directly inserting onto its antagonist, the FDP, make this motion simple and easy when the nerves are intact (Video 8C.2).

Simply observing the hand resting flat on a table will reveal Wartenberg's sign. This results in there being more space between the small and ring fingers than the other fingers i.e., the little finger appears abducted relative to the ring finger (Figure 8C.5). At first glance, it is unclear why this would occur considering that the hypothenar muscles including the abductor digiti minimi are innervated by the ulnar nerve. What Wartenberg correctly pointed out is that the extensor digitorum communis and extensor digiti minimi exert an abduction force due to their origin on the lateral epicondyle [15].

The simplest examination finding is to ask a patient to cross the index and middle fingers on either hand simultaneously. With this you are testing the abduction and adduction of the index and middle finger simultaneously. The

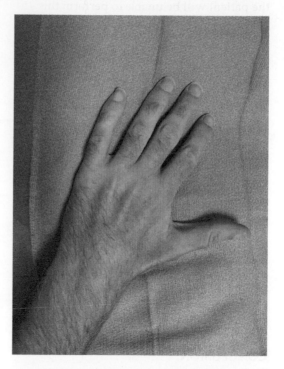

Figure 8C.5 Wartenberg's sign is the observation that there is an ulnar pull from the extrinsic extensors to the little finger resulting in more space between the ring and little fingers at rest. This must be compared to the opposite side.

 Video 8C.2 Without being able to simultaneously extend the interphalangeal joints and flex the metacarpophalangeal joints, the fingers will curl when trying to grab a large object

www.routledge.com/9780367647162.

more telling half of this examination is the passing of the middle finger above the index finger. This is specifically testing the abduction of the middle finger with adduction of the index finger (Video 8C.3). This is critical to know and perform. Crossing the index finger over the middle finger can be done easily by a patient with ulnar nerve dysfunction, by spuriously utilizing the extensor indicis proprius to create a false negative test [4].

An additional test to check the interossei muscles controlling the middle finger is to ask the patient to place the palm flat on a table. The middle finger is then raised off the table and the patient is asked to move the finger from side to side. This is the Egawa test. When the interossei are denervated, the patient will be unable to perform this manoeuvre [16].

Froment's sign specifically looks at the function of the adductor pollicis muscle. The examiner should ask the patient to tightly grasp an object between their index finger and thumb. When the examiner attempts to pull the object away, in a normal hand the patient will use the adductor pollicis and firmly hold on to the object without any associated flexion of the interphalangeal joint of the thumb. However, in a patient with ulnar nerve injury, the patient will oppose and flex the thumb as they will be unable to initiate contraction of the adductor pollicis. This is best observed by the flexion of the interphalangeal joint (IPJ) of the thumb when it is compared to the contralateral side [17]. The object should be the size of a narrow book, as a sheet of paper will result in most individuals using opposition and flexion on the normal side as well (Figure 8C.6) (Video 8C.4). Jeanne's sign is less often mentioned but refers to MP hyperextension when performing the manoeuvre.

CONCLUSION

The most common causes of ulnar nerve palsy encountered by the hand surgeon are from trauma and from compression neuropathy. Understanding the anatomy of the ulnar nerve will guide your physical examination. Begin by observing and palpating the patient's extremity. Then move onto checking

Video 8C.3   To perform the cross-finger test have patient hold out both hands and ask them to cross the middle and index fingers back and forth.

www.routledge.com/9780367647162.

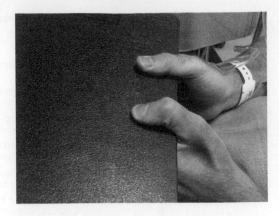

Figure 8C.6   Froment's sign is performed by asking the patient to tightly grasp an object between their index finger and thumb. When the examiner attempts to pull the object away, the patient will oppose and flex their thumb as they will be unable to use the adductor pollicis. In this photo the left hand displays the Froment's sign and also visible is the wasting of the first dorsal interosseous.

Video 8C.4   To elicit Froment's sign ask the patient to grab a thick object like a thin binder or tabletop in the first webspace. A positive test is hyperflexion of the IP joint of the thumb.

www.routledge.com/9780367647162.

sensation and performing physical examination manoeuvres. Utilizing a thorough physical examination, the diagnosis can the distinguished from spinal cord pathology or mixed nerve injuries. In addition, the difference between and high and low ulnar nerve palsy can be elucidated.

REFERENCES

1. Boone S, Gelberman RH and Calfee RP. The management of cubital tunnel syndrome. *Journal of Hand Surgery*. 2015;40(9):1897–1904. doi:10.1016/j.jhsa.2015.03.011

2. O'Driscoll SW, Horii E, Carmichael SW and Morrey BF. The cubital tunnel and ulnar neuropathy. *Journal of Bone and Joint Surgery - Series B*. 1991;73(4):613–617. doi:10.1302/0301-620x.73b4.2071645

3. Polatsch DB, Melone CP, Beldner S and Incorvaia A. Ulnar nerve anatomy. *Hand Clinics*. 2007;23(3):283–289. doi:10.1016/j.hcl.2007.05.001

4. Posner MA. Compressive ulnar neuropathies at the elbow: I. Etiology and diagnosis. *The Journal of the American Academy of Orthopaedic Surgeons*. 1998;6(5):282–288. doi:10.5435/00124635-199809000-00003

5. Posner MA. Compressive ulnar neuropathies at the elbow: II. treatment. *The Journal of the American Academy of Orthopaedic Surgeons*. 1998;6(5):289–297. doi:10.5435/00124635-199809000-00004

6. Uerpairojkit C, Kittithamvongs P, Puthiwara D, Anantaworaskul N, Malungpaishorpe K and Leechavengvongs S. Surgical anatomy of the dorsal cutaneous branch of the ulnar nerve and its clinical significance in surgery at the ulnar side of the wrist. *Journal of Hand Surgery: European Volume*. 2019;44(3):263–268. doi:10.1177/1753193418815800

7. Zaworski RE. Undiagnosed deep ulnar nerve paralysis resulting from stab wounds of the palm. *Journal of Trauma - Injury, Infection and Critical Care*. 1979;19(12):957–960. doi:10.1097/00005373-197912000-00004

8. Pfaeffle HJ, Waitayawinyu T and Trumble TE. Ulnar nerve laceration and repair. *Hand Clinics*. 2007;23(3):291–299. doi:10.1016/j.hcl.2007.06.003

9. Monacelli G, Rizzo MI, Spagnoli AM, Monarca C and Scuderi N. Ulnar artery thrombosis and nerve entrapment at Guyon's Canal: Our diagnostic and therapeutic algorithm. *In Vivo*. 2010;24(5):779–782. https://pubmed.ncbi.nlm.nih.gov/20952749/. Accessed 21 September 2020.

10. Sunderland SS. The anatomy and physiology of nerve injury. *Muscle & Nerve*. 1990;13(9):771–784. doi:10.1002/mus.880130903

11. Smith J, Siddiqui S and Ebraheim N. Comprehensive summary of anastomoses between the median and ulnar nerves in the forearm and hand. *Journal of Hand and Microsurgery*. 2019;11(01):001–005. doi:10.1055/s-0038-1672335

12. Novak CB, Lee GW, Mackinnon SE and Lay L. Provocative testing for cubital tunnel syndrome. *Journal of Hand Surgery*. 1994;19(5):817–820. doi:10.1016/0363-5023(94)90193-7

13. Cheng CJ, Mackinnon-Patterson B, Beck JL and Mackinnon SE. Scratch Collapse Test for Evaluation of carpal and cubital tunnel syndrome. *Journal of Hand Surgery*. 2008;33(9):1518–1524. doi:10.1016/j.jhsa.2008.05.022

14. Montgomery K, Wolff G and Boyd KU. Evaluation of the scratch collapse test for carpal and cubital tunnel syndrome—A prospective, blinded study. *Journal of Hand Surgery*. 2020;45(6):512–517. doi:10.1016/j.jhsa.2020.02.016

15. Wartenberg R. A sign of ulnar palsy. *Journal of the American Medical Association*. 1939;112(17):1688. doi:10.1001/jama.1939.62800170002011a

16. Goldman SB, Brininger TL, Schrader JW, Curtis R and Koceja DM. Analysis of clinical motor testing for adult patients with diagnosed ulnar neuropathy at the elbow. *Archives of Physical Medicine and Rehabilitation*. 2009;90(11):1846–1852. doi:10.1016/j.apmr.2009.06.007

17. Froment J. Prehension and the sign of the thumb in paralysis of the ulnar nerve. *Bull Hosp Joint Dis*. 1972;33(2):193–196. PMID: 4648258.

9 Wrist Examination: A Focused Approach

Shav Rupasinghe and Raj Murali

CONTENTS

"The difference between a helping hand and an outstretched palm is a twist of a wrist"

Laurence Leamer

INTRODUCTION

The function of the wrist is to position the hand in space, allowing it to interact with the environment to produce precise functions. Patients with wrist problems can present with a variety of symptoms and paucity of clinical signs. A thorough clinical history is extremely important and allows for a tailored examination. It is best to start the palpation from the less painful side of the wrist before moving to the more painful part. Signs and provocative tests can be difficult to perform and interpret, so a systematic approach is needed. The approach to wrist examination set out in this chapter will cover inspection, palpation, movement, power and special tests (Dutton et al., 2016).

Inspection

The examiner should sit opposite the patient with the patient's hands resting on a pillow on their knees.

General observation will involve the alignment of the joints and hand in relation to the unaffected side. Start with the hands in a pronated (palm down) position (Photo 9.1).

Obvious malignment can alert the examiner of underlying pathologies. Rheumatoid arthritis often presents with dorsal subluxation at the wrist with ulnar deviation of the digit. Volar bowing of the radius with a prominent ulnar head is found with Madelung's deformity. Scars may indicate previous operations, fractures, non- and mal-unions. Dorsal swelling is common in inflammatory arthritis and in ganglions affecting the wrist. With the hand supinated, the volar aspect of the wrist should be inspected for swelling, scars and muscle wasting (Photo 9.2).

Palpation

Most structures around the wrist are superficial and easy to palpate. A sound grasp of surface anatomy and a systematic approach is essential. Palpation should be directed towards discoloured, swollen or deformed structures which have been detected during the initial inspection.

The examiner should start with the dorsum of the wrist, moving to the volar aspect, radial and ulnar parts, in that order. It is often easier to group the patient's symptoms on history and then tailor the examination for a specific problem or pathology. Use the index finger and thumb and always look at the patient to see if palpation elicits pain.

With radial side pain, palpation should start on the dorsum with the thumb CMC joint (carpometcarpal joint), moving to the scaphoid, anatomical snuff box, Lister's tubercle, then the scapho-lunate ligament (1.5 cm distal to Lister's tubercle). The radial styloid should be palpated next, followed by the first dorsal compartment and APB (abductor pollicis brevis) /EPL (extensor pollicis longus) for signs of De Quervain's and intersection syndrome.

Finally, volar palpation of the radial styloid, scaphoid tubercle and distal radius should be done. Specific pathologies related to pain on palpation is listed.

Dorsal photo (the legend for the photo is below)

DOI: 10.1201/9781003125938-11

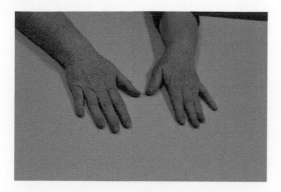

Photo 9.1 Dorsum of hand.

1) Base of first metacarpal arthritis	First CMC
2) Anatomical snuff box	Scaphoid fracture
3) Radial styloid	Fracture
4) First dorsal compartment	De Quervain
5) Lister's tubercle	
6) SLL	Scapholunate ligament injury
7) Scaphoid	Fracture/AVN/OA
8) Lunate	Fracture/AVN/OA

Volar photo (the legend for the photo is below)

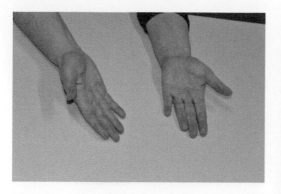

Photo 9.2 Volar aspect of hand.

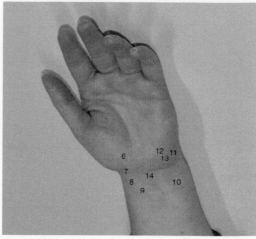

Volar

6)	Scaphoid tubercle	Fracture
7)	Radial styloid	Fracture
8)	Radial artery	Aneurysm
9)	FCR tendon	Tendonitis
10)	FCU tendon	Tendonitis
11)	Pisiform	Fracture
12)	Hamate hook	Fracture
13)	Guyon's canal	Ulnar nerve/mass
14)	Central wrist between PL and FCR tendon	Median nerve

The ulnar side of the wrist and its associated pathology should be examined at the same time. This will be covered in chapter 10.

Movement of specific joints related to pathology should be revisited. This should cover passive movement of the wrist in flexion, extension, radial and ulnar deviation to see if there is discrepancy with active movement performed previously.

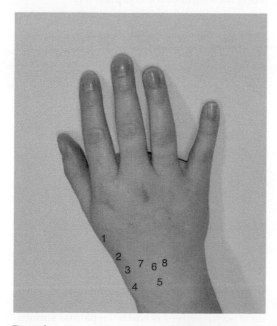

Dorsal   Pathology
                (with pain on
                palpation)

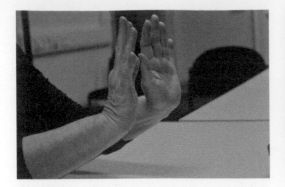

Photo 9.3 Extension of wrists.

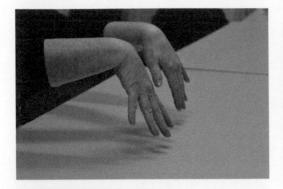

Photo 9.4 Flexion of wrists.

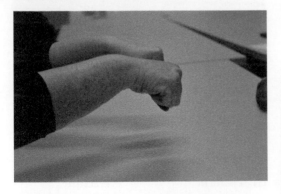

Photo 9.5 Flexion of wrists with fingers flexed showing reduced wrist flexion.

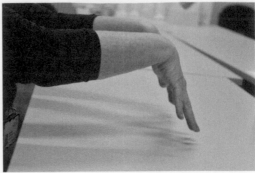

Photo 9.6 Flexion of wrists with fingers extended showing increased wrist flexion.

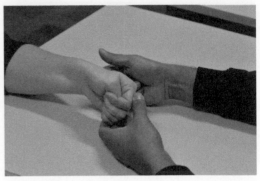

Photo 9.7 Finkelstein's test done with thumb in palm and wrist ulnar deviated, pain is felt along the length of the compartment.

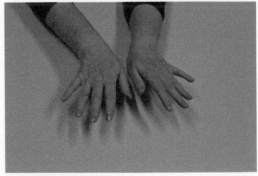

Photo 9.8 Ulnar deviation of wrists.

Movement

The range of motion of the wrist is a result of movement from the radiocarpal and mid carpal joints. A reduction in movement can be a result of a fracture or ligamentous injury involving any of these articulations (Tubiana et al., 1998). Flexion, extension, supination and pronation, along with wrist radial and ulnar deviation, should be examined (Photos 9.3, 9.4, 9.5, 9.6, 9.7, and 9.8).

Screening tests start with the patient placing both palms together and lifting their elbows

(prayer sign). This provides an easy comparison of extension (dorsiflexion). Flexion can be tested with the dorsum of each hand pressed together. This is a combined active and passive movement. Zero degrees is when the palmar surface of the hand and wrist are in line with the volar surface of the forearm. Each individual hand is then tested passively. Normal wrists have active

182

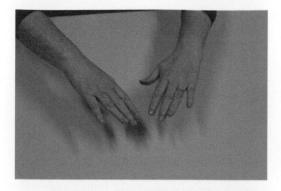

Photo 9.9 Active radial deviation of wrists.

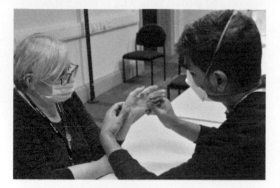

Photo 9.10 Radial deviation of wrists done passively.

 Video 9.1 Power testing. Testing muscle power.

www.routledge.com/9780367647162.

extension between 60 and 70°, and passively this can be increased to 90°. Flexion normally ranges from about 60 to 80°. This test must be done with the fingers in extension as flexion reduces the range of motion (Photos 9.5 and 9.6).

Radial and ulnar deviation is tested from the neutral position when the long axis of the third metacarpal lines up with the axis of the forearm. The patient is asked to bend the wrist to the radial and ulnar sides, best done with the arms by their side. Normal values of radial and ulnar deviation are 20 and 30 to 40° (Photos 9.9 and 9.10).

Forearm rotation should be assessed. Pronation and supination require a fully functioning distal radial ulnar joint. A screening of figure movement with opening and closing of the hand is useful to assess overall hand function.

Power

Power is tested with the fingers flexed and the hand in a fist position. The hand is then extended against resistance in the position of radial and ulnar deviation. This is then repeated with the hand flexed. Results should be compared with the non-affected side. Grading is done using the Medical Research Council's scale (MRC scale) of muscle power (Video 9.1).

Provocation and Instability Tests/Special Tests

There are many special tests addressing various pathologies. These tests should be done based on the differential diagnosis and previous examination findings and compared to the opposite heathy wrist for validity (Lastayo and Howell, 1995).

1) Scaphoid-lunate joint

Scapholunate instability
Clinical findings: Swelling and pain over the radial wrist with tenderness over the scapholunate ligament
Tests for a scaphoid-lunate ligament tear and instability:
Scaphoid shift test (Kirk–Watson test) (Watson et al., 1988a).
First described by H Kirk Watson, American hand surgeon, in 1988.
Sensitivity 82% Specificity 31% (Watson et al., 1988b).
Note that 20% of people have a normal positive test.
While holding the hand the examiner places their right thumb over the patient's scaphoid tubercle on the volar surface.
The index figure is placed on the dorsal surface. From a position of ulnar deviation and dorsiflexion of the wrist, the thumb presses the scaphoid tubercle on the volar surface, and the wrist is taken into radial deviation (Photo 9.11).

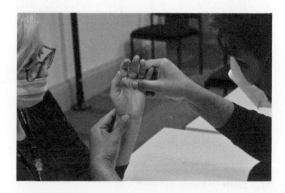

Photo 9.11 Scaphoid shift test: The test is started in a position of ulnar deviation. With pressure on the scaphoid the wrist is taken into radial deviation.

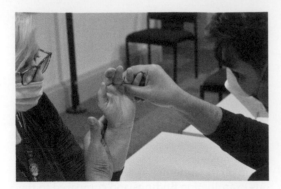

Photo 9.12 Scaphoid shift test: Pressure is released over the scaphoid.

 Video 9.2 Scaphoid shift test: Volar view.

www.routledge.com/9780367647162.

 Video 9.3 Scaphoid shift test: Dorsal view.

www.routledge.com/9780367647162.

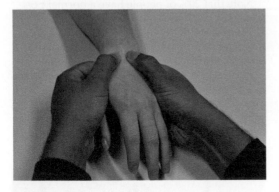

Photo 9.13 Scaphoid chuck test: Thumb and index finger of each hand are placed over scaphoid and lunate.

A positive test has the examiner feel the distal pole of the scaphoid sublux over the dorsal lip of the radius, causing pain to the patient. When the pressure is released, the scaphoid reduces relieving the pain (Photo 9.12).

In a normal wrist there is a minimal motion and pain (Videos 9.2 and 9.3).

Scaphoid chuck (ballottement test).

Unknown.

Sensitivity 64%, Specificity 44% (Kleinman, 2015).

 Video 9.4 Scaphoid chuck ballottement test.

www.routledge.com/9780367647162.

The patient's arm is flexed and the hand pronated. The examiner places his thumb and index finger on the volar and dorsal aspects of the scaphoid. With the other hand the thumb and index finger are placed over the lunate. The examiner then moves the scaphoid and the lunate in opposite directions. With a complete tear in the SL ligament there is excessive motion and pain (Photo 9.13) (Video 9.4).

2) Lunate-triquetral instability

Clinical findings: Swelling and pain over the ulnar side of wrist with tenderness over the lunate and triquetrum.

Tests for a lunate-triquetral ligament tear and instability:

Lunotriquetral ballottement test/Reagan shuck Test (Reagan et al., 1984).

Sensitivity 64%, Specificity 45%.

This is performed with the examiner using one hand to stabilize the wrist and the other thumb applying a radial force. This drives the triquetrum into the lunate causing pain in a positive result.

Lunotriquetral shear test (Kleinman shear test) (van de Grift and Ritt, 2016).

Sensitivity 61%, Specificity 40%.

This is similar to the scaphoid chuck test; however, the hands are placed over the lunate and the triquetrum. The examiner attempts to translate these bones in the opposite directions. Abnormal motion is detected in a tear, no movement is the normal finding.

3) Midcarpal instability

Clinical findings:

Pain and swelling along the mid carpal joint, with a reduction in movement.

Midcarpal Shift Test

This test is difficult and hard to interpret. The patient's hand and forearm are supported with one hand, the other hand's thumb is placed over the capitate. The wrist is ulnar deviated with a volarly and axial directed force on the wrist. In a positive test there is a palpable clunk, catching or jumping. Repeating the test with an upward force on the volar surface of the pisiform should reduce symptoms (Nagle, 2000).

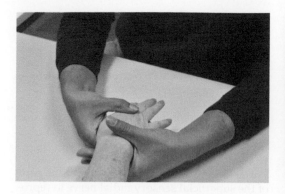

Photo 9.14   Midcarpal-radiocarpal draw test.

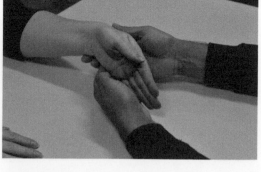

Photo 9.15   Finkelstein's test: Tested with fingers extended.

Video 9.5   Midcarpal-radiocarpal test.

www.routledge.com/9780367647162.

Video 9.6   Carpal instability test.

www.routledge.com/9780367647162.

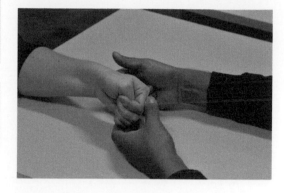

Photo 9.16   Finkelstein's test: Tested with thumb flexed across their palm.

Midcarpal-Radiocarpal Draw Test

This test is similar to the draw tests in the knee. In a positive test, excessive translation of the midcarpal-radiocarpal rows is felt. The examiner places one hand holding the distal forearm, the other hand is held at the level of the metacarpals. With a slight distraction force a volar then dorsal translation force is applied. This is then compared to the normal side. The test is repeated with the examiner placing one of their hands on the proximal carpal row and the other on the distal row. Excessive motion and movement are seen in an abnormal result (Photo 9.14) (Videos 9.5 and 9.6).

4) Tendopathies

Tendonitis of the First Dorsal Compartment

Clinical symptoms: Swelling over the first dorsal compartment with pain on palpation. Reduced ulnar deviation.

Finkelstein's test:

Described by Harry Finkelstein, American surgeon.

Sensitivity 51–91%, Specificity 33–88% (Goubau et al., 2014).

This is a provocation test for de Quervain's disease, which is tenosynovitis of the first dorsal compartment. Here the patient flexes their thumb across their palm. The hand is the ulnar deviated with patients elbow flexed and

Video 9.7   Finkelstein's test.

www.routledge.com/9780367647162.

forearm in neutral rotation. In a positive result pain is felts along the length of the compartment on the radial border of the wrist (Photos 9.15 and 9.16) (Video 9.7).

5) Compressive neuropathies

Carpal tunnel syndrome (Wiesman et al., 2003):

Compression of the median nerve at the wrist.

Clinical features: Altered sensation in radial three and a half digits with wasting of thenar eminence and weakness.

Carpal tunnel compression test (Durkan's test).

Described by JA Durkan, American orthopaedic surgeon.

Sensitivity 71 %, Specificity 22% (Durkan, 1991).

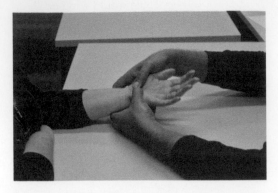

Photo 9.17 Carpal tunnel test: Compression of carpal tunnel with thumbs

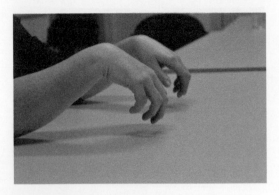

Photo 9.18 Phalen test.

 Video 9.8 Phalen test.

www.routledge.com/9780367647162.

The examiner uses his or her thumbs to press over the carpal tunnel holding for a period of 30 seconds. In a positive result the patient has pain and/or paraesthesia in the median nerve distribution (Photo 9.17).

Phalen test

Described by George S Phalen, an American orthopaedic surgeon.

Sensitivity 61%, Specificity 83%.

The patient is asked to hold their forearm vertically with elbows resting on the table. The wrist is allowed to volar flexion against gravity for 60°. A positive result is the same as above (Photo 9.18) (Video 9.8).

Tinel's test

Described by Jules Tinel, a French neurologist.

Sensitivity 67%, Specificity 91%.

With the patient's wrist supported in a neutral position, the examiner taps over the

medical nerve at the level of the distal wrist crease.

Wartenberg Syndrome (Lastayo and Howell, 1995).

Described by Robert Wartenberg, a German-American neurologist and professor, in 1932 (Aird, 1957).

Compression of the superficial branch of the radial nerve.

Symptom: Paraesthesia of first dorsal webspace.

Tinel's sign: The examiner taps over the path of the superficial sensory radial nerve to reproduce symptoms in a positive result.

Provocation test: Wrist flexion, ulnar deviation and pronation. The examiner asks the patient to do the action described for one minute.

Finkelstein's test: As described above, increased symptoms in 96% of patients due to traction on the nerve. (Note there is an association with de Quervain's disease in 20–50% of patients, the difference here is that pain is not aggravated by wrist pronation).

6) Ganglions

Ganglions are a common swelling found around the wrist and hand. Dorsal carpal swelling most commonly originates from the scapholunate articulation (60–70%). Volar swellings are often from the radiocarpal or STT joint.

These swellings are usually painless, firm and well circumscribed on palpation. They are often not fixed to deep tissue or overlying skin. Dorsal ganglions usually overlie the scapholunate ligament just distal to Lister's tubercle and can transilluminate if large.

A neurological examination of the hand should be performed in case of nerve compression. An Allen's test should also be done to rule out vascular compromise, especially with volar ganglions with their close association with the radial artery.

7) Vascular abnormalities

Allen's test (Allen, 1929).

Described by Edgar van Nuys Allen, Professor of Medicine at the Mayo Clinic in Rochester, in 1929.

The elbow is flexed and the forearm supinated. The examiner palpates the radial and ulnar pulses and places their thumbs on them with the rest of the hand supporting the wrist. The patient then opens and closes their hand multiple times making a fist. The radial and ulnar arteries are then compressed under the examiner's thumbs simultaneously. The examiner then releases one artery. The normal

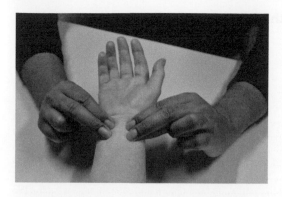

Photo 9.19 Allen's test: Compression of the radial and ulnar artery.

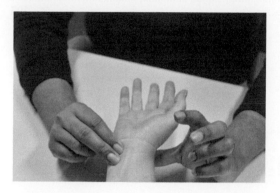

Photo 9.20 Allen's test: Release of the radial artery.

colour of the hand and figures should return in a few seconds. This is repeated with the release of the other artery. Any delay or difference may indicate an artery obstruction, and a difference also indicates which artery dominates blood supply to the hand. In 80% of individuals this is the ulnar artery (Photos 9.19 and 9.20).

CONCLUSION

When evaluating the wrist, a thorough history and examination is crucial. The examination should be systematic and involve the look, feel, move then special tests format of orthopaedic examinations. The provocation, instability and special tests should be done with regards to a working diagnosis. For completeness, the ulnar side of the wrist should also be examined, as discussed in another chapter.

REFERENCES

RB Aird and R Wartenberg. 1887–1956. *Arch Neurol Psych.* 1957;77(5):490–491.

EV Allen. Thromboangiitis obliterans: methods of diagnosis of chronic arterial lesions distal to the wrist with illustrative cases. *Am J Med Sci.* 1929;178(3):165–189.

JA Durkan. A new diagnostic test for carpal tunnel syndrome. *J Bone Joint Surg Am.* 1991;73:535–538.

M Dutton et al. *Orthopaedic, Examination, Evaluation and Intervention,* 4th Edition, Mcgraw-Hill, 2016, pp. 779–868.

J.F Goubau, L Goubau, A Van Tongel, P Van Hoonacker, D Kerckhove and B Berghs. The wrist hyperflexion and abduction of the thumb (WHAT) test: a more specific and sensitive test to diagnose de Quervain tenosynovitis than the Eichhoff's test. *J. Hand Surg (European Volume).* 2014;39(3):286–292.

WB Kleinman. Physical examination of the wrist: Useful provocative manoeuvres. *J Hand Surg.* 2015;40(7):1486–1500.

P Lastayo and J Howell. Clinical provocative tests used in evaluating wrist pain: a descriptive study. *J Hand Ther.* 1995;8:10–17.

DJ Nagle. Evaluation of chronic wrist pain. *J Am Acad Orthop Surg.* 2000;8:45–55.

DS Reagan, RL Linscheid and JH Dobyns. Lunotriquetral sprains. *J Hand Surg.* 1984;9:502–514.

R Tubiana et al. *Examination of the Hand and Wrist, CRC Press,* 1998, pp. 28, 156–170.

TC van de Grift and MJPF Ritt. Management of lunotriquetral instability: a review of the literature. *J Hand Surg (European Volume).* 2016;41(1):72–85.

HK Watson, D. Ashmead 4th, and MV Makhlouf. Examination of the scaphoid. *J Hand Surg Am.* 1988a Sep;13(5):657–60. [Watson's test]

HK Watson et al. Examination of scaphoid. *J Hand Surg.* 1988b;13A:657–60.

IM Wiesman, CB Novak, SE Mackinnon and JM Winograd. Sensitivity and specificity of clinical testing for carpal tunnel syndrome. *Can J Plast Surg.* 2003;11(2):70–72.

10 Examination of the Ulnar Side of the Wrist

Samuel Cohen-Tanugi and R Glenn Gaston

CONTENTS

Disclosures: The authors have no relevant commercial or financial disclosures and received no funding for this work.

Key points:

1. A broad differential diagnosis including traumatic and atraumatic etiologies of acute and chronic conditions is paramount to approaching ulnar wrist pathology.

2. Understanding surface anatomy is critical for proper diagnosis of ulnar wrist pain.

3. Specific provocative manoeuvres can help differentiate between competing diagnoses of ulnar wrist pain.

The ulnar side of the wrist is often considered a challenging anatomic region and a diagnostic conundrum, earning it the description of a "black box" [1–3]. Because pain in this area is ubiquitous, vague, and frustrating, it is also referred to as the "back pain" of hand surgery. However, it is the authors' belief that a systematic approach will yield a definitive solution. The first step is to maintain a broad differential diagnosis: All structures of the ulnar side of the wrist including the osseous anatomy, ligaments, tendons and neurovascular structures can be affected by distinct pathologies (Table 10.1). The next step is to "order" a history and physical examination: The physical examination, based on a solid understanding of the surface anatomy of the ulnar side of the wrist, and coupled to a pointed history can narrow the differential diagnosis even before advanced imaging is obtained. The physical examination follows a stepwise sequence, starting with observation, active and passive range of motion, and grip strength, all of which offer preliminary information. The highest yield diagnostic tool however is the systematic palpation of all structures

of the ulnar side of the wrist according to the examiner's knowledge of the surface anatomy. At this point in the clinical encounter, a particular diagnosis can be evaluated with specific provocative manoeuvres which help differentiate between similar complaints. Finally, if uncertainty remains between several pathologies, the use of anaesthetic and steroid injections in the office can be useful for diagnostic purposes and may even provide lasting relief.

CLINICAL HISTORY

The focus of this chapter is the physical examination of the ulnar side of the wrist. However, the clinical history is critical in initially narrowing the differential diagnosis as it provides crucial context. The history can be brief and should highlight a few key questions [4]. First, has the patient undergone previous surgeries to the hand and wrist? Next, are the patient's symptoms acute or chronic? Were they caused by a traumatic event? A knowledgeable clinician will recognize classic injury patterns associated with distinct activities. For instance, acute pain after a sport involving impact while gripping a bat or club suggests a fractured hook of the hamate, such as during a "fat shot" in golf, or a "check swing" in baseball [5]. Similarly, the two-handed backhand tennis swing has been associated with extensor carpi ulnaris (ECU) subsheath pathology [6]. As rock climbing gains wider popularity as a sport with the proliferation of indoor rock climbing facilities, a particular grip – the undercling grip – has been associated with hook of the hamate fractures [7]. Pain in the ulnar side of the wrist after a car accident in which the steering wheel is gripped can represent acute lunotriquetral (LT) ligament tear, as axial impact with the wrists in extension and radial deviation has

DOI: 10.1201/9781003125938-12

Table 10.1: Differential Diagnosis of Ulnar Wrist Pain by Location

Fourth to fifth CMC joints
  Fracture
    Base fourth or fifth MC
    Dorsal shear fractures of hamate)
  Dislocation
  Arthritis (typically post-traumatic)
  ECU insertional tendonitis
LT joint/ulnocarpal joint
  LT ligament tear
  Fracture
    Triquetrum (dorsal avulsion or body fracture)
    Lunate (body fracture or ligament avulsion)
  HALT (proximal hamate arthrosis and LT tear)
  Kienbock's (AVN lunate)
  Incomplete coalition LT joint
  Ulnar impaction
  TFCC tear
  Triquetro-hamate impingement
DRUJ
  Fracture
    Distal ulna
    Sigmoid notch radius
  Arthritis
  Instability
    TFCC deep fibre tears
    Ulnar styloid fracture
  ECU tendonosis/instability
PT joint
  Fracture
  Arthritis
  Instability
  Insertional or calcific FCU tendonitis
Vascular etiologies
  Hypothenar hammer syndrome (ulnar artery pseudo-aneurism)
  Cardiac emboli
  Raynaud's phenomenon or syndrome
  Peripheral vascular disease
  Thoracic outlet syndrome
Neurogenic Causes
  Guyon's canal (ganglion, hamate hook fracture, cycling, other mass effect)
  Cubital tunnel
  Neuroma
  C8–T1 cervical radiculopathy
  Neurogenic thoracic outlet
  Lower brachial plexopathy
  Pancoast tumour

been described as placing this structure at risk [8]. Acute pain that is atraumatic but following prolonged periods of strenuous work such as gardening or tool use points towards a tendinous etiology such as irritation of flexor carpi ulnaris (FCU) or ECU. The associated presence of warmth and redness should raise suspicion of inflammatory processes such as gout, infection or calcific tendonitis.

The clinician should note the language used to describe the pain, as certain descriptors have been correlated with particular etiologies. For instance, inflammatory pain is frequently hot and burning, whereas osteoarthritic pain is described more often as "persistent aches with episodes of sharp stabbing pain" and stiffness in the morning [9]. Finally, the clinician should take note of other relevant medical disease processes since systemic conditions can lead to pathology in the distal extremities. For example, autoimmune disorders (CREST, Sjogren's etc.) may be accompanied by Raynaud's phenomenon. Neurofibromatosis may involve the ulnar nerve anywhere along its course. Rheumatoid arthritis may present as tendonitis or tenosynovitis. Endocarditis may result in septic emboli in the small vessels of the hand. Gout is called the great mimicker and can certainly precipitate in the joints of the ulnar side of the wrist.

PHYSICAL EXAMINATION

Before delving into the physical examination of the ulnar side of the wrist, the clinician should remember that in addition to its diagnostic value, the physical examination constitutes an important ritual within the therapeutic relationship. It is no coincidence that, in his TED Talk "A Doctor's Touch," author and physician Abraham Verghese describes starting his physical examination with patients' hands: A particularly intimate part of the body and central to our identity as human beings.

The physical examination is conducted in a systematic manner every single time, with the examiner sitting across from the patient whose elbow is resting on a surface and flexed at 90° as if preparing for an arm-wrestling match (Figure 10.1). Both the examiner's hands are used to simultaneously stabilize the patient's forearm, wrist and hand while performing the examination. Before moving on, the patient should point to the area of maximal pain, which will be examined last.

The first step is observation. The appearance of the skin can reveal previous surgical incisions, skin or nail conditions (e.g., ecchymosis, gouty tophi, onycholysis), or differential perfusion of the digits (e.g., Raynaud's). Comparing

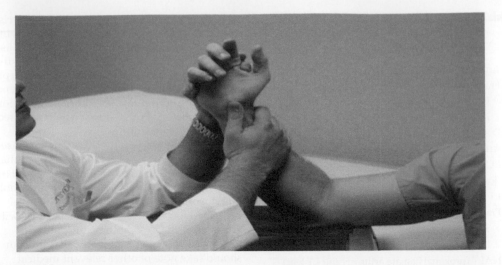

Figure 10.1 The proper position for conducting a physical examination of the ulnar wrist is demonstrated in the "arm wrestling" position.

the morphology of the hand and wrist to the unaffected extremity may show subtle deformities, such as a palmar sag of the carpus (chronic and complete LT ligament tear), a prominent ulnar head (*caput ulnae*, or chronic triangular fibrocartilage complex (TFCC) disruption) or swelling along the ulnar border of the distal forearm and wrist (tendinopathy or tenosynovitis). Wasting of the intrinsic muscles or altered position of the digits are often signs of ulnar nerve pathology (Figure 10.2).

Next, wrist range of motion should be assessed both actively and passively, it can be measured with a goniometer, and compared to the contralateral side. Pain with motion, either at the extremes or in the mid-range, stiffness or restricted motion and any mechanical symptoms such as clicking, popping or locking, should be noted.

The motor function of the ulnar nerve can be tested alongside active range of motion and should include key pinch and small finger

adduction. To test key pinch, the patient is asked to firmly grip a sheet of paper between the thumb and the radial side of the index and resist its pulling away by the examiner. Weakness of key pinch and associated thumb IP flexion caused by the recruitment of the median nerve innervated flexor pollicis longus (FPL) constitutes a positive Froment's sign and indicates weakness of the adductor pollicis and first dorsal interosseus (Figure 10.3). Similarly, Jeanne's sign – concomitant metacarpophalangeal (MP) hyperextension with key pinch – has been described in patients with ulnar nerve pathology. Wartenberg's sign designates the inability to maintain small finger adduction against the other fingers with the hand placed flat on the table, indicating overpowering of a weak third palmar interosseus by the unopposed extensor digiti minimi in the coronal plane. A complete sensory examination assesses both sensory (using a Seemes–Weinstein type monofilament) and innervation density (two-point

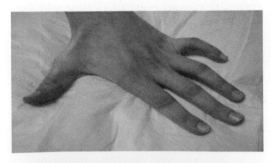

Figure 10.2 Clinical photograph of the classic ulnar nerve palsy hand with intrinsic atrophy and clawing of the ulnar digits.

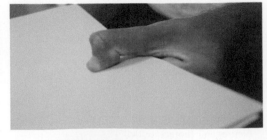

Figure 10.3 Clinical photograph of key pinch against a piece of paper demonstrating a positive Froment's sign (IP flexion) and mild Jeanne's sign (MP hyper-extension).

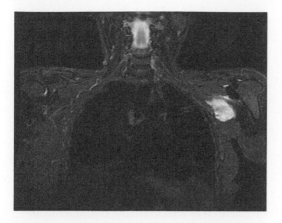

Figure 10.4(a) Chest MRI demonstrating a lower brachial plexus tumour that presented with complaints of ulnar-sided hand and wrist pain.

discrimination). Sensation in the ulnar nerve distribution of the small and ulnar side of the ring finger should be compared to that in the ipsilateral median nerve distribution as well as to the contralateral hand. If ulnar nerve symptoms are present, either sensory, motor or both, the examination must include a full neurological examination with particular attention paid to Guyon's canal as well as the cubital tunnel at the elbow, the lower cervical spine and the brachial plexus. Pathology of the ulnar nerve anywhere along its course from cervical nerve roots to the Guyon's canal may present as primary ulnar hand and wrist complaints (Figure 10.4a and 10.4b).

Grip strength testing using a dynamometer can be useful for several reasons. First, grip strength ratios of the injured to non-injured side has been found to correlate with the Disability of the Arm, Shoulder, and Hand (DASH) score while being quicker to perform and not relying on subjective questionnaires

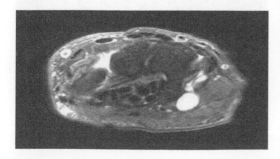

Figure 10.4(b) Axial wrist MRI demonstrating both a hamate hook non-union and a ganglion within the Guyon's canal in a patient presenting with ulnar wrist pain.

[10]. The normal ratio of dominant to non-dominant hands in healthy volunteers was found to be 0.97 [10]. Discrepancy beyond that should raise suspicion of injury. Grip strength testing has been proposed as a tool to gauge sincerity of effort, especially in instances in which disability may be tied to secondary gain. For instance, disability exaggeration has been reported to confound up to a third of workers' compensation cases [11]. However, while rapid exchange and five-station grip testing offer a thorough and systematic testing protocol, no study to date has been able to support the use of a grip-strength testing protocol to predict sincerity of effort [12].

The vascular examination began with observation of the skin, as digital ulcerations, splinter haemorrhages, or hand swelling/discoloration are signs of vascular pathology (Figure 10.5). Capillary refill in all digits should be assessed along with palpable pulses

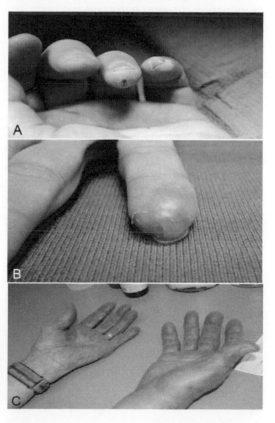

Figure 10.5 Clinical photographs of various vascular etiologies of patients presenting with ulnar-sided hand complaints: (a) Fingertip ulcerations from emboli secondary to hypothenar hammer syndrome. (b) Little finger ecchymosis from cardiac emboli. (c) Diffuse hand swelling from a subclavian DVT.

at the wrist. Differential perfusion can signify Raynaud's phenomenon or pathology of the ulnar artery at the Guyon's canal. Allen's test verifies that both the ulnar and radial artery are contributing to perfusion of the hand and is performed by placing the examiner's thumbs over the radial and ulnar artery simultaneously and asking the patient to make a tight fist, effectively exsanguinating the palm. When the patient opens up their hand the examiner releases pressure from either the ulnar or radial artery alone and assesses whether perfusion to the entire palm is restored. The manoeuvre is then repeated for the other artery. Pathology affecting the ulnar artery, such as aneurysm or thrombosis, or a congenital deficit in the anastomoses between the deep and superficial arches, will lead to lack of reperfusion when only the ulnar artery is released during Allen's test.

While preceding sections are all necessary components of a thorough history and physical examination, the most important and high-yield aspect step in diagnosing ulnar-sided wrist pain is knowledge of the palpable structures of the ulnar wrist to enable the examiner to accurately identify pathology with high specificity upon palpation. When palpating the patient's wrist, the examiner will essentially complete a full circuit of these structures, while saving the patient's self-reported point of maximal pain for last. Premature palpation of the painful structure may confound the rest of the examination.

The examiner must intimately know the anatomy of the wrist and be able to visualize where the structures lie under the skin – this is what is meant by "surface anatomy." Figure 10.6(a) and (b) are illustrations of what the examiner should be able to visualize in their "mind's eye" when looking at the patient's hand and wrist. The authors recommend that the reader practice palpating these structures on themselves while reading through the following paragraphs. Start by identifying the **pisiform (A4)**: It is the bony prominence immediately distal to the wrist flexion crease ulnarly. The **FCU (A5)** tendon inserts onto the pisiform and is easily palpated moving proximally along the ulnar volar wrist.

Next, place your thumb IP joint directly over the pisiform, aiming towards the ring finger. The tip of your thumb will land over the **hook of the hamate**, which will feel like a more subtle and deeper bony prominence.

The **ulnar head** is immediately palpable in the ulnar dorsal quadrant of the wrist and the **ulnar styloid** is the most dorsal and distal

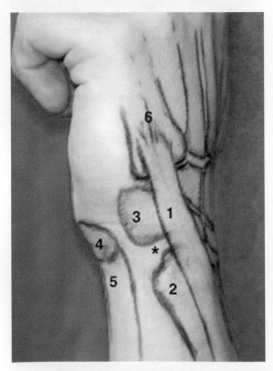

Figure 10.6a (1) ECU tendon. (2) Ulnar head. (3) Triquetrum. (4) Pisiform. (5) FCU tendon. (6) Fifth MC base. (*) Fovea.

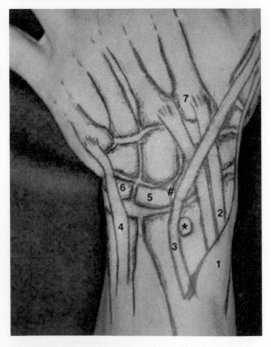

Figure 10.6b (1) Distal radius. (2) ECRB/ECRL. (3) EPL. (4) ECU. (5) Lunate. (6) Triquetrum. (7) First MC base. (*) Lister's. (#) SL interval.

aspect of the ulnar head. Starting on the ulnar styloid, let the tip of your examining finger slide volarly into a groove: This is the **fovea (A*)**, where the **TFCC** is located. The **ECU tendon (A1)**, which travels within the sixth dorsal compartment in its own separate subsheath, overlies the dorsal ulna and is most easily visualized with the forearm in full supination while abducting the fingers. Its course to its insertion on the base of the f metacarpal (A6) is in a straight line with the forearm pronated and oblique with the forearm in supination. Therefore, supination is best for visualizing the tendon and eliciting instability, while pronation is the preferred position for immobilization and protection of the ECU. Starting at the fifth metacarpal shaft dorsally, palpate proximally to the **fifth CMC joint**. Proximal to the joint is the dorsum of the **hamate** and radial to the fifth CMC joint is the **fourth CMC joint**.

Next, palpate Lister's tubercle over the dorsal distal radius. Move 1 cm on the ulnar until you fall off the edge of the radius into the distal radial-ulnar joint (DRUJ). From the DRUJ, move directly distal and fall into a small groove: This is the **LT interval**.

Once a distinct anatomic area of maximal tenderness is identified, the next step is to use specialized manoeuvres that have been described in the literature to aid in the diagnosis of specific pathologies.

Several provocative manoeuvres or "special tests" have been described to diagnose common pathologies and will be individually discussed below. These should be performed to confirm a suspected diagnosis or more confidently rule one out, rather than as screening tools on all patients.

Ulnocarpal Stress Test

The **ulnocarpal stress test** involves applying axial pressure to the patient's fist with their elbow held in flexion and the wrist in ulnar deviation, and then passively ranging the wrist in pronation and supination [13]. While described by Nakamura et al., as being 100% sensitive for pathology on the ulnar side of the wrist, the test was not able to differentiate between several etiologies of ulnar-sided wrist pain, including TFCC tears, LT tears, DRUJ arthritis and ulnar impaction syndrome and therefore is not considered specific. Nevertheless, it remains a valuable screening tool for ulnar wrist pathology [3, 13]. A variation of the ulnocarpal stress test is the "press test" described by Lester et al., as being 100% sensitive and highly specific for TFCC tears in patients with the appropriate pre-test clinical suspicion [14]. The "press test" simply involves the patient pushing themselves up from the seated position by gripping the sides of the seat portion of a chair. When the press test reproduces the pain that is bothering the patient it is considered positive. Although there are clear limitations in this article, the test is likely to be equivalent to the Nakamura's ulnocarpal stress test, and therefore unlikely to provide a higher specificity in distinguishing between the multiple etiologies listed by Nakamura.

Hook of Hamate Fracture

A fracture or non-union of the hook of the hamate should be suspected in any patient with focal tenderness to palpation over the hook of the hamate. The hook of hamate pull test, described by Wright et al., can aid in the diagnosis of hook of the hamate fractures which can produce otherwise vague pain and remain occult on standard plain radiographs. The test involves flexion of the fourth and fifth digits against resistance while the wrist is held in ulnar deviation [5]. With the hamate hook serving as a pulley for the ulnar digital flexors, the tendons' course around the hook becomes more oblique in ulnar deviation, causing increased pressure on the hook and more pain in the setting of injury. Pain with this manoeuvre marks a positive test, and radially deviating the wrist while maintaining flexion should lessen the patient's pain.

Pisiform–Triquetrum (PT) Arthritis

If an older patient has pain with direct palpation of the pisiform in the absence of trauma, PT arthritis should be considered as a diagnosis. PT arthritis is easily overlooked as a source of ulnar wrist pain and can confound the accurate testing of other structures, in particular the LT. The pisiform tracking test or PT grind test is performed with the patient's wrist in slight flexion, which relaxes the FCU tendon. The examiner then grasps the pisiform between index and thumb, while stabilizing the dorsal aspect of the wrist with the other hand. As pressure is applied onto the pisiform and into the PT joint, the pisiform is "shucked" radially and ulnarly. Pain and possibly crepitus should be present in patients with pathology at this joint [2].

Luno-Triquetral (LT) Ligament Tears

Kleinman has written extensively about the examination of LT tears [8]. Since partial LT tears are not discernible on X-rays, the physical examination is critical. Kleinman describes three manoeuvres: A "ballottement" test, a "shuck" test and his own "shear" test which he

7. Cole KP, Uhl RL and Rosenbaum AJ. Comprehensive review of rock climbing injuries. *J Am Acad Orthop Surg*. 2020; 28(12): e501–e509. doi:10.5435/JAAOS-D-19-00575

8. Kleinman WB. Physical examination of the wrist: Useful provocative maneuvers. *J Hand Surg Am*. 2015; 40(7): 1486–1500. doi:10.1016/j.jhsa.2015.01.016

9. Wagstaff S, Smith OV and Wood PHN. Verbal pain descriptors used by patients with arthritis. *Ann Rheum Dis*. 1985; 44(4): 262–265. doi:10.1136/ard.44.4.262

10. Beumer A and Lindau TR. Grip strength ratio: A grip strength measurement that correlates well with DASH score in different hand/wrist conditions. *BMC Musculoskelet Disord*. 2014; 15(1): 1–5. doi:10.1186/1471-2474-15-336

11. Mittenberg W, Patton C, Canyock EM and Condit DC. Base rates of malingering and symptom exaggeration. *J Clin Exp Neuropsychol*. 2002; 24(8): 1094–1102. doi:10.1076/jcen.24.8.1094.8379

12. Sindhu BS, Shechtman O and Veazie PJ. Identifying sincerity of effort based on the combined predictive ability of multiple grip strength tests. *J Hand Ther*. 2012; 25(3): 308–319. doi:10.1016/j.jht.2012.03.007

13. Nakamura R, Horii E, Imaeda T, Nakao E, Kato H and Watanabe K. The ulnocarpal stress test in the diagnosis of ulnar-sided wrist pain. *J Hand Surg Eur Vol*. 1997; 22(6): 719–723. doi:10.1016/S0266-7681(97)80432-9

14. Lester B, Halbrecht J, Levy IM and Gaudinez R. "Press test" for office diagnosis of triangular fibrocartilage complex tears of the wrist. *Ann Plast Surg*. 1995; 35(1): 41–45. doi:10.1097/00000637-199507000-00009

15. Szabo RM. Distal radioulnar joint instability. *Instr Course Lect*. 2007; 88(4): 884–894.

16. Ruland RT and Hogan CJ. The ECU synergy test: An aid to diagnose ECU tendonitis. *J Hand Surg Am*. 2008; 33(10): 1777–1782. doi:10.1016/j.jhsa.2008.08.018

17. Kleinman, William B. "Stability of the distal radioulnar joint." *Fractures and injuries of the distal radius and carpus*. The Cutting Edge, Philadelphia (PA), 2009. 261–274.

18. Tay SC, Tomita K and Berger RA. The "Ulnar Fovea Sign" for defining ulnar wrist pain: An analysis of sensitivity and specificity. *J Hand Surg Am*. 2007. doi:10.1016/j.jhsa.2007.01.022

11A Compression Neuropathies

Carpal Tunnel, Guyon's Canal, Cubital Tunnel Syndrome

J Terrence Jose Jerome

CONTENTS

CARPAL TUNNEL SYNDROME

Carpal tunnel syndrome (CTS) is a clinical diagnosis based on presenting symptoms, distinctive physical findings and supplemented with electrodiagnostic studies.

SURGICAL ANATOMY

The carpal tunnel has flexor retinaculum as the roof, scaphoid and trapezium on the radial side, hamate and triquetrum on the ulnar side and capsule, anterior radiocarpal ligaments as the floor. The flexor retinaculum has three parts and is composed mainly of transverse fibres. The proximal part, intermediate part and distal aponeurotic part (Figure 11A.1).

CONTENTS OF CARPAL TUNNEL

The carpal tunnel is open at its proximal and distal ends and maintains a characteristic fluid pressure level. The median nerve is accompanied by the four tendons of the flexor digitorum superficialis (FDS) muscle, the four tendons of the flexor digitorum profundus (FDP) and the flexor pollicis longus (FPL) tendon. The median nerve lies just beneath the flexor retinaculum. The FPL tendon is the most radial element, the median nerve most palmar. The diameter of the carpal tunnel syndrome is narrowest 2 cm from the leading edge where the median nerve gets compressed with all morphological signs of compressive neuropathy (Figure 11A.2).

In the axial (transverse) plane, the carpus forms the carpal tunnel, a palmar concavity enclosed by the transverse carpal ligament (also known as the flexor retinaculum). The narrowest portion of the carpal tunnel is located at the level of the distal carpal row. The distal carpal row bones are strongly bound to each other by stout transverse intercarpal ligaments (i.e., dorsal, palmar, intraarticular). They are essential to ensure the rigidity of the transverse carpal arch and to protect the carpal tunnel contents.

MEDIAN NERVE SUPPLY

The median nerve gives a recurrent motor branch at the distal end of flexor retinaculum to

DOI: 10.1201/9781003125938-13

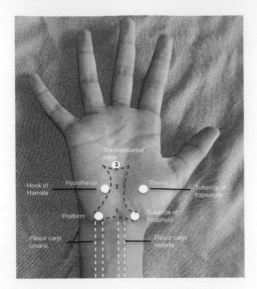

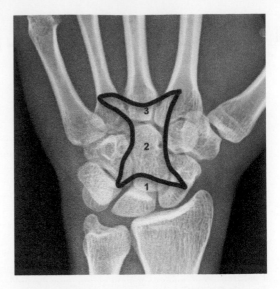

Figure 11A.1 Anatomy of the three portions of the flexor retinaculum. The distal portion of the flexor retinaculum (3) consists of a thick aponeurosis between the thenar and hypothenar muscles. The thenar muscles attach to the radial half of the classic flexor retinaculum, which is composed of the distal portion of the flexor retinaculum (3) and the transverse carpal ligament (2). Bony attachments of the transverse carpal ligament – pisiform, hamate, tubercle of the trapezium and tubercle of the scaphoid – are shown. The proximal portion of the flexor retinaculum (1) courses deep to the flexor carpi ulnaris and flexor carpi radialis. The flexor carpi radialis tendon is shown as it pierces the flexor retinaculum at the junction of the proximal and middle portions to enter its fibrosseous canal.

innervate the abductor pollicis brevis muscle, first two lumbricals and opponens pollicis muscles. The median nerve then divides into the digital nerves that provide sensation to the thumb and index finger, middle finger and radial half of the ring finger.

PRESENTING COMPLAINTS

1. Night-time pain, numbness, tingling sensation in the median nerve distribution in the hand (thumb, index finger, middle and radial side of the finger) and most of the time they present with frequent awakening from sleep. These symptoms get better with hand stretching, shaking (flick sign of Pryse–Phillips) and changing the position.

2. Exacerbation of numbness while driving, reading books, use of keyboard or mouse.

3. Pins and needles feeling, burning sensation, cold intolerance.

Figure 11A.2 Radiograph shows three portions of flexor retinaculum: (1) Proximal portion of flexor retinaculum. (2) Intermediate part characterized by its bony insertions – pisiform, hook of hamate on the ulna side, scaphoid tubercle and tubercle of trapezium on the radial side. (3) Distal fascial part extending between thenar and hypothenar muscles.

4. In severe cases, they may report aches in the thenar region, clumsiness, difficulty in holding, picking up and feeling objects.

5. Unilateral or bilateral symptoms.

Lundborg proposed an anatomo-clinical classification [1] useful for diagnosis and explained the reason for nocturnal symptoms. There are several factors behind the nocturnal increase in intracanal pressure.

1. Redistribution of the upper limb fluids in supine position.

2. Lack of muscle pump mechanism that contributes to the drainage of interstitial fluid in the carpal tunnel.

3. Tendency to place the wrist in flexion thereby increasing intracanalicular pressure.

4. Increased blood pressure in the second half of the night.

5. Fall of cortisol levels.

CLINICAL EXAMINATION

Idiopathic carpal tunnel syndrome occurs most often in women between 40 and 60 years, bilateral in 50 to 60% of cases. Secondary CTS may occur in conditions affecting the wall, and contents of carpal tunnel

Table 11A.1: Provocative Test for Compartment Syndromes

Nerve	Compression Site	Provocative Test
Median	Carpal tunnel	Pressure proximal to the carpal tunnel Phalen test Reverse Phalen test (hyperextension of the wrist)
	Proximal forearm	Pressure over the proximal forearm in the region of the pronator teres with the forearm in supination Resisted elbow flexion, pronation and finger flexion
Ulnar	Guyon's canal	Pressure proximal to Guyon's canal Reverse Phalen test
	Cubital tunnel	Elbow flexion and pressure proximal to the cubital tunnel
Radial (posterior interosseous)	Arcade of Fröhse	Pressure over the supinator Resisted supination Resisted middle finger and wrist extension
Radial (sensory)	Forearm	Pressure over the junction of the brachioradialis/ extensor carpi radialis tendon Forearm pronation with wrist ulnar flexion
Brachial plexus	Supraclavicular	Elevation of arms above the head Pressure over the brachial plexus in the interscalene region

PROVOCATION TESTS

The median nerve is felt distal to the flexion crease deep to the palmaris longus tendon (Table 11A.1).

1. Phalen test (67 to 83% sensitive, 47 to 100% specific)

The Phalen manoeuvre is performed with the wrist in maximum flexion [2] (Figure 11A.3(a, b)). Reverse Phalen is performed with the wrist in maximum extension (Figure 11A.3(c)). Reproduction of the numbness in the median nerve distribution within 60 seconds is considered positive (Video 11A.1).

2. Durkan compression test

The carpal tunnel compression test is performed by applying manual pressure over the transverse carpal ligament for 30 seconds [3] (Figure 11A.4).

3. Tinel's test

Tinel's sign is elicited by tapping along the median nerve at the level of the carpal tunnel and moving distal-proximo direction. The patient experience paraesthesia over the median nerve distribution. The test is considered positive with radiation of a tingling sensation into the affected nerve's sensory neural distribution. The sensitivity is 26 to 79% and specificity is 40 to 100% [2–4] (Figure 11A.5).

4. McMurthry's test and Paley's test

A manual pressure on the median nerve 1 to 2 cm proximal to the flexor crease causes pain or paraesthesia. Sensitivity is 89% and specificity is 45% [5] (Figure 11A.6).

5. Phdurkan test

The combination of carpal compression and wrist flexion decreases the space of the carpal tunnel and provokes the symptoms (reproduction of distal paraesthesia in the median nerve distribution) [6] (Figure 11A.7).

6. Scratch collapse test for evaluation of carpal tunnel syndrome

The test is performed with the patient facing the examiner, with arms adducted, elbows flexed and both hands outstretched with wrists at neutral position (Video 11A.2). The patient is asked to perform simultaneous resisted bilateral shoulder external rotation, keeping the arms abducted. The examiner gently pushes against both of the patient's forearms, asking him or her to sustain steady resistance. With fingertips, the examiner then scratches or swipes the skin overlying the course of the potentially compressed median nerve over the carpal tunnel at the volar wrist. A positive scratch collapse test is recorded for the median nerve if the patient demonstrates a momentary loss of external resistance tone on the affected side after "scratching" over the carpal tunnel. This loss of muscle resistance is quite brief, with the patient regaining strength essentially immediately with repeat resistance testing. However, the test could be repeated

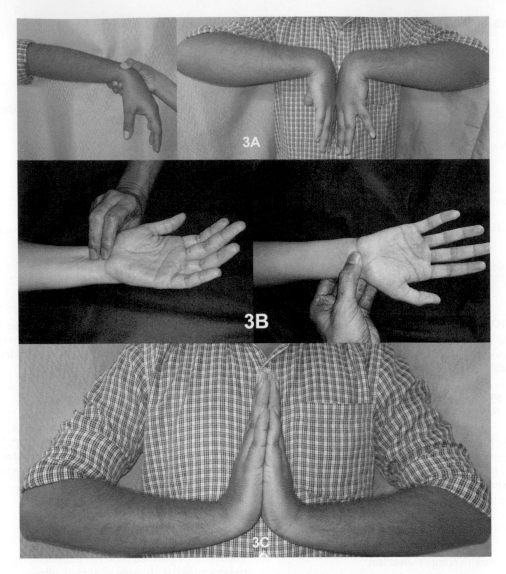

Figure 11A.3 (a) and (b) Phalen test is produced by wrist flexion held for up for 60 seconds. (c) Reverse Phalen is performed with the wrist in maximum extension. Different ways of doing it to reproduction of distal paraesthesia in the median nerve distribution which is considered as a positive test.

successfully without evidence of fatigue or habituation. The scratch collapse test is reliable, reproducible and has comparable sensitivity and specificity to the other existing tests [7].

 Video 11A.1 Movie of a 60-year-old lady with carpal tunnel syndrome performing active wrist flexion to confirm the distal paraesthesia in the median nerve distribution.

www.routledge.com/9780367647162.

A painful cutaneous stimulus causes a period of inhibition in tonic voluntary muscle activity in humans. This period of electrical silence is called a cutaneous silent period. The scratch collapse test uses the cutaneous silent period to briefly inhibit tonic shoulder external rotation as a response to noxious stimulus of the skin overlying a chronically constricted median nerve.

GENERAL AND MOTOR EXAMINATION

The examination should assess light touch or threshold testing and involve both palms. The bulk of the thenar muscles should be palpated

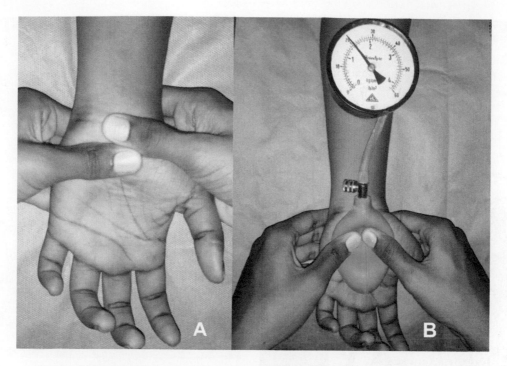

Figure 11A.4 (a) The carpal compression test is performed by the examiner exerting even pressure, with both thumbs, to the median nerve in the carpal tunnel (original description). (b) Also, direct compression of the median nerve running deep to the flexor retinaculum with a device that consists of a rubber atomizer-bulb connected to a pressure manometer from a sphygmomanometer. A pressure of 150 mm of mercury (20 kPa) is applied to the area of the carpal tunnel for as long as 30 seconds. Reproduction of paraesthesia in median nerve distribution is positive.

and any wasting of the abductor pollicis brevis (APB) should be documented (Figure 11A.8). The thumb is opposed to the little finger and strength is assessed (Video 11A.3). With loss of the thenar function, the patient may be able to oppose with the ulnar innervated deep head of the flexor pollicis brevis and flex the thumb across the palm to the little finger using the FPL tendon [8].

DIAGNOSIS

1. Nerve conduction studies and electromyography

The earliest and most sensitive electrical abnormality is a slower sensory conduction. A value of <45 m/s is considered carpal tunnel syndrome with median nerve compression. The prolonged distal motor latency between the wrist and the APB, onset of motor potential (>4 to 10 ms, normal value: <3.6 ms) and abnormal sensory conduction (3.9%) occurs in advanced stage. EMG has sensitivity of 54% and 97.5% specificity. Isolated sensory conduction velocity has 75–92% sensitivity and 97.5% specificity. Anatomical variations like Martin–Gruber and

Riché–Cannieu can interfere with the interpretation of electromyographic studies. ENMG can confirm the diagnosis, eliminate another disease (cervico-brachial neuropathy or TOS), detect associated polyneuropathy, specify single or multiple compression sites and assess the severity of nerve damage thus guiding the treatment plan [9–12].

2. Ultrasound

An increase in the cross-sectional area of the median nerve ≥10 mm² reflects increased volume proximal to stenosis, is the best diagnostic test with 87.3% sensitivity and specificity of 83.3%. The ratio of median nerve flattening facing the hamate is also a reliable criterion. Other signs such as notching, nerve oedema proximal to stenosis, flexor retinaculum bulge, decreased median nerve mobility during flexion-extension are helpful in diagnosing CTS. Ultrasound helps diagnosing the morphology content of the carpal tunnel such as persistent median artery thrombosis, bifid median nerve, FDS or lumbrical muscle in the canal [13].

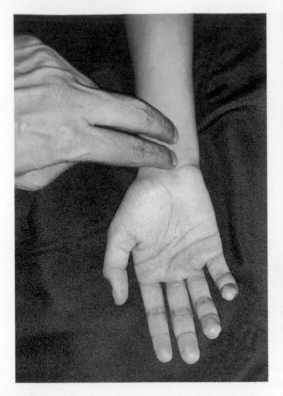

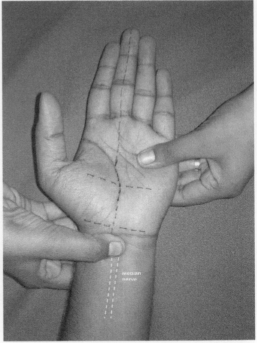

Figure 11A.6 McMurthy and Paley test: Manual pressure on the median nerve 1–2 cm proximal to the flexor crease causes pain or paraesthesia.

Figure 11A.5 Tinel's sign at the carpal tunnel was performed by percussion over the median nerve just proximal to the wrist crease and recorded as positive if associated with radiating paraesthesia distally in the median nerve distribution

3. Carpal tunnel view

A clear view of the hook of the hamate, the pisiform and the palmar ridge of the triquetrum can be obtained by profiling the carpal concavity of the wrist. It is difficult in acute cases to extend the wrist because of pain.

Posteroanterior and lateral views are useful to suggest acute or neglected perilunate dislocations with displaced lunate compressing the median nerve [4, 7, 8].

4. Magnetic resonance imaging (MRI)

MRI is useful in cases associated with secondary tenosynovitis, benign and malignant tumours, tuberculous, compound palmar ganglion, acute fracture dislocation of lunate, perilunate dislocations and neglected cases [4, 7, 8].

COMORBID CONDITIONS
Diabetes mellitus, hypothyroidism, excessive alcohol use, obesity, exposure to vibration, cold,

repetitive manual work and tobacco increases the carpal tunnel pressure.

POSTURES
The median nerve moves longitudinally 9.6 mm during flexion, 0.7 to 1.4 cm in wrist extension

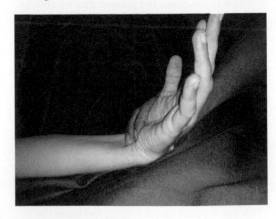

Figure 11A.7 A Phdurkan test is performed by manual compression of the carpal tunnel with the examiner's index and middle fingers and flexion of the wrist with the examiner's thumb and recorded as positive if associated with reproduction of distal paraesthesia in the median nerve distribution.

Video 11A.2 Scratch collapse test for carpal tunnel syndrome evaluation.

www.routledge.com/9780367647162.

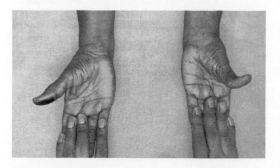

Figure 11A.8 Checking abductor pollicis brevis (APB) function. The patient has wasting of the thenar muscles in the right side (thumb marked).

 Video 11A.3 Movie of the same lady undergoing motor examination for the median nerve. She has weak abductor pollicis brevis, wasting of the thenar muscles and paraesthesia in the median nerve distribution.

www.routledge.com/9780367647162.

and can vary between 2.5 and 19.6 mm depending upon the shoulder, elbow, wrist and finger positions. Also, transverse movement of the median nerve occurs with wrist position or during finger flexion against resistance [14–18].

It is well accepted that wrist positions of moderate flexion and extension will increase pressure within the carpal canal, and this is hypothesized to contribute to carpal tunnel syndrome [15]. Similarly, elbow flexion will increase pressure within the cubital tunnel and thereby compromise the ulnar nerve.

DOUBLE CRUSH SYNDROME

Upton and Mac describe the concept of staged nerve compression [19].

1. Double crush syndrome: The proximal nerve compression makes it more sensitive to another more distal nerve compression by cumulative effects on antegrade axonal transport.

2. Reverse double crush syndrome: The distal nerve compression can promote the emergence of a more proximal nerve compression

syndrome (entrapment syndrome) by alterations in the retrograde axonal transport. For example, a proximal cervical disc prolapse with nerve compression causes radiculopathy or thoracic outlet syndrome associated with a carpal tunnel syndrome distally.

CONCLUSION

The diagnosis of CTS is established by history, physical examination with or without the aid of diagnostic questionnaires, electrodiagnostic studies and ultrasound. Nocturnal acroparaesthesia is the most sensitive symptom. No single provocative test is optimal and the use of multiple provocative tests in clinical practice is useful in diagnosing CTS.

EMG should follow clinical examination and is not essential for the diagnosis of a typical form of CTS. It is not necessary before a steroid injection. EMG is recommended in cases of doubt, prior to surgery and in occupational disease recognition.

PAIN EVALUATION SCORE SHEET

The pain evaluation questionnaire consists of pain adjectives, a body diagram, a questionnaire, and visual analogue scales scored from 0 to 10 for pain, stress and coping. Patients who select more than three adjectives, draw a pain pattern that does not follow a known anatomic pattern, or score more than 20 on the questionnaire are considered positive for that component. Patients who score positive in more than two components are considered for psychological or psychiatric evaluation before any surgical intervention [20, 21] (Figures 11A.9 and 11A.10).

CUBITAL TUNNEL SYNDROME

This chapter discusses the presentation, clinical examination and diagnosing modalities for diagnosing cubital tunnel syndrome.

SURGICAL ANATOMY

The cubital tunnel syndrome is a slack region with restricted mobility of the ulnar nerve [22]. The ulnar nerve passes posterior to the medial epicondyle and medial to the olecranon. The cubital tunnel is a taut fascial layer extending from the flexor carpi ulnaris muscle and the arcuate ligament of Osborne. The ulnar nerve passes through the tunnel and enters the forearm between the ulnar and humeral heads of the flexor carpi ulnaris [23]. The superficial position of the ulnar nerve in the cubital tunnel and increase in tension and traction during the elbow flexion cause the ulnar nerve to be susceptible to compression neuropathy. Also, the cubital tunnel area is decreased in elbow flexion thereby

Pain Questionnaire

Name:_____ Date:_____

Age:___ Sex: Male_ Female_ Dominant hand: Right_ Left_ Diagnosis:_____

1. Pain is difficult to describe. Circle the words that best describe your symptoms.

Burning	Throbbing	Aching	Stabbing	Tingling	Twisting	Squeezing
Cramping	Cutting	Shooting	Numbing	Vague	Stinging	Indescribable
Pulling	Smarting	Pressure	Coldness	Dull	Other:_____	

Level of symptoms: place a mark through the line to indicate the level of your pain, if zero is no pain and the end of the line is the most severe pain you can imagine having.

For Example:
No pain | Most severe pain

2. Mark your average level of pain in the last month
No pain | Most severe pain

3. Mark your worst level of pain in the last week
Right
No pain | Most severe pain

Left
No pain | Most severe pain

4. Where is your pain? (draw on diagram)

L R L R

5. Mark your average level of stress in the last month.
at home 0 ___ 10
at work 0 ___ 10

6. How well are you able to cope with that stress?
at home Very well ___ Not at all
at work Very well ___ Not at all

7. How did the pain that you are now experiencing occur?
a. Sudden onset with accident or definable event
b. Slow progressive onset
c. Slow progressive onset with acute exacerbation without an accident or definable event
d. A sudden onset without an accident or definable event

8. How many surgical procedures have you had **in order to eliminate the cause of your pain**?
a. None or one
b. Two surgical procedures
c. Three or four surgical procedures
d. Greater than four surgical procedures

9. Does movement have any effect on your pain?
a. The pain is always worsened by use or movement
b. The pain is usually worsened by use and movement
c. The pain is not altered by use and movement

10. Does weather have any effect on your pain?
a. The pain is usually worse with damp or cold weather.
b. The pain is occasionally worse with damp or cold weather.
c. Damp or cold weather has no effect on the pain.

11. Do you ever have trouble falling asleep or awaken from sleep?
a. No - Proceed to Question 12 b. Yes - Proceed to 11A & 11B

11A. How often do you have trouble falling asleep?
a. Trouble falling asleep every night due to pain
b. Trouble falling asleep due to pain most nights of the week
c. Occasionally having difficulty falling asleep due to pain
d. No trouble falling asleep due to pain
e. Trouble falling asleep which is not related to pain

11B. How often do you awaken from sleep?
a. Awakened by pain every night
b. Awakened from sleep by pain more than 3 times per week
c. Not usually awakened from sleep by pain
d. Restless sleep or early morning awakening with or without being able to return to sleep, both unrelated to pain

12. Has your pain affected your intimate personal relationships?
a. No   b. Yes

13. Are you involved in any legal action regarding your physical complaint?
a. No   b. Yes

14. Is this a Workers' Compensation case?
a. No   b. Yes

15. Are you presently receiving psychiatric treatment?
a. No   b. Yes   c. Previous psychiatric treatment

16. Have you ever thought of suicide?
a. No   b. Yes   c. Previous suicide attempts

17. Are you a victim of emotional abuse?
a. No   b. Yes   c. No comment

18. Are you a victim of physical abuse?
a. No   b. Yes   c. No comment

19. Are you a victim of sexual abuse?
a. No   b. Yes   c. No comment

20. Are you presently a victim of abuse?
a. No   b. Yes   c. No comment

21. If you are retired, a student, or a homemaker, proceed to Question 21B.
21A. Are you still working?
a. Working every day at the same job I had before pain developed
b. Working every day but the job is not the same as the job I had before pain developed; I now have reduced responsibility and physical activity
c. Working occasionally
d. Not presently working
21B. Are you able to do your household chores?
a. Do same level of household activities without discomfort
b. Do same level of household activities with discomfort
c. Do a reduced amount of household chores
d. Most household chores are now performed by others

22. What medications have you used in the past month?
a. No medications
b. List medications:_____
_____
_____

23. If you had three wishes for anything in the world, what would you wish for?
1._____
2._____
3._____

0% | 100%

Figure 11A.9 The pain evaluation questionnaire consists of pain adjectives, a body diagram, a questionnaire and visual analogue scales scored from 0 to 10 for pain, stress and coping.

increasing the intracanal pressure in the cubital tunnel. A 55% decrease in the cubital tunnel area and increase in pressure within the cubital tunnel is seen in elbow flexion with wrist extension or shoulder abduction (or with both) [24, 25]. The common sites for ulnar nerve compression in the arm, elbow and forearm are:

a) The arcade of Struthers

b) The intermuscular septum

c) The flexor carpi ulnaris fascia

PAIN EVALUATION SCORE SHEET

Name: _____   Date: _____

DOB: _____ Age: ____ Sex: M __ F __ Dominant Hand: R __ L __

Diagnosis: _____

1. Number of Descriptors: ___

2. Pain Level: on average ___   3. Pain level: worst right ___ left ___

4. Body Diagram: _____

5. Stress Level: home ___ work ___   6. Coping Level: home ___ work ___

7. a. 0 b. 0 c. 3 d. 4	8. a. 0 b. 2 c. 3 d. 4	9. a. 0 b. 2 c. 3	10. a. 0 b. 2 c. 3	11. a. 3 b. 0	11A. a. 0 b. 1 c. 2 d. 3 e. 4	11B. a. 0 b. 1 c. 3 d. 4

12. a. 0 b. 2	13. a. 0 b. 3	14. a. 0 b. 2 c. 2	15. a. 0 b. 4	16. a. 0 b. 2 c. 5	17. a. 0 b. 5 c. 3	18. a. 0 b. 5 c. 3

19. a. 0 b. 5 c. 3	20. a. 0 b. 5 c. 3	21A. a. 0 b. 0 c. 2 d. 3	21B. a. 0 b. 0 c. 2 d. 3	22. a. 0 b. 1 Valium c. 2 Narcotic d. 3 Psychotropic or antidepressant drugs	23. a. 0 No pain only wish b. 1 No pain one of wishes c. 2 Wishes only of personal nature d. 3 Wishes of nonpersonal nature (i.e., world peace)

Total: _____

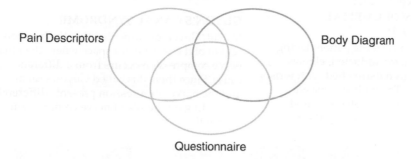

Pain Descriptors   Body Diagram

Questionnaire

Figure 11A.10 Pain evaluation score sheet.

d) The anconeus epitrochlearis

e) The Osborne ligament

f) Fascial bands within the flexor carpi ulnaris distally

ETIOLOGIES

a) Acute trauma

b) Chronic mechanical compression or ischemia

c) Tardy ulnar palsy (subsequent to lateral condyle non-union)

d) Posttraumatic scarring

e) Hansen disease

f) Anomalous musculature

g) Ulnar nerve subluxation

CLINICAL PRESENTATIONS AND FINDINGS

The patients present with paraesthesia, and numbness in the right and little fingers. In late cases they exhibit weakness, deformity and claw deformity in the ring and little fingers.

On detailed examination, the Tinel's sign is positive and motor weakness is confirmed by special tests like the Froment and Wartenberg signs. Many patients in the initial stages of nerve compression have no motor deficits. Careful sensory testing quantifies perceptible sensory loss in the volar aspect of the forearm, dorsum of the wrist, ring and little fingers.

A provocative test for cubital tunnel syndrome is combined elbow flexion with digital pressure of the ulnar nerve proximal to the cubital tunnel (Figure 11A.11). The patient reproduces the paraesthesia and numbness in the ulnar nerve distribution. This test is highly sensitive and specific for cubital tunnel syndrome.

A provocative test and alteration of threshold testing (vibration and Semmes–Weinstein monofilaments) are helpful in diagnosing the early stage of nerve compression. A two-point discrimination test is abnormal in late stages. McGowan described a classification for ulnar nerve neuropathy at the elbow based on the ulnar nerve motor loss only (sensory loss is not included in the classification) [26, 27]:

Grade I: Neuropathies have no muscle weakness.

Grade II: Neuropathies have muscle weakness with no atrophy.

Grade III neuropathies have muscle atrophy.

SCRATCH COLLAPSE TEST FOR EVALUATION OF CUBITAL TUNNEL SYNDROME

The test is performed with the patient facing the examiner, with arms adducted, elbows flexed and both hands outstretched with wrists at a neutral position. The patient is asked to perform simultaneous resisted bilateral shoulder external rotation, keeping the arms abducted. The examiner gently pushes against both of the patient's forearms, asking him or her to sustain steady resistance. With fingertips, the examiner then scratches or swipes the skin overlying the course of the potentially compressed ulnar nerve over the cubital tunnel at the elbow. A positive scratch collapse test is recorded for the ulnar nerve if the patient demonstrates a momentary loss of external resistance tone on the affected side after "scratching" over the cubital tunnel [28].

EMG AND NCV STUDIES

Electrodiagnostic studies confirm the diagnosis, localize the level of nerve compression and rule out upper motor neurone disease, peripheral neuropathy, cervical disc prolapses and other etiologies). Ulnar nerve motor conduction velocity across the elbow of less than 50 m/sec is considered confirmatory of cubital tunnel syndrome [25, 27].

DIFFERENTIAL DIAGNOSIS (SEVERE MOTOR LOSS WITH MINIMAL SENSORY CHANGES).

a) Motor neurone disease or Guillain–Barré syndrome

b) Cervical disk disease

c) Amyotrophic lateral sclerosis (rare but devastating problem)

GUYON'S CANAL SYNDROME

In 1861, Guyon documented that the hyothenar region of the wrist has a space where the ulnar nerve compression occurs from a different cause. Since then, it is called Guyon's canal and the nerve compression presents differently depending on the site of nerve compression within this canal.

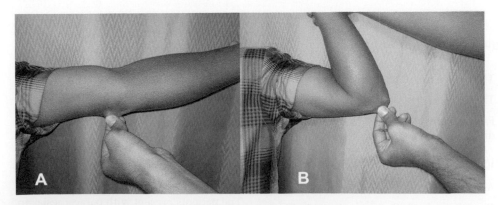

Figure 11A.11 (a) Elbow flexion increases the tension on the ulnar nerve. The skin is tight when elbow is flexed. (b) Elbow extension does not increase the tension on the nerve. The skin is loose when the elbow is extended.

Table 11A.2: Nerve Compression and Symptoms at Different Levels and Comparison with Cubital Tunnel Syndrome

Syndrome		Motor Loss	Sensory Loss	Remarks
Cubital tunnel		Intrinsic weakness, Froment's sign, clawing of the ring and little fingers	Numbness, paraesthesia in the medial aspect of the forearm, dorsum of the wrist, ulnar half of the ring finger, little finger (the ulnar nerve gives a dorsal sensory branch which supplies the dorsum of the wrist and the little finger)	This sensory loss differentiates the Guyon's canal compression from the cubital canal.
Guyon's canal	Zone I	Intrinsic weakness, Froment's sign, clawing of the ring and little fingers	Numbness and paraesthesia in the ring and little fingers	Unopposed action of the normal of flexor digitorum profundus produces claw deformity in low ulnar nerve palsy which is less obvious in high ulnar nerve palsy
	Zone II	Intrinsic weakness, Froment's sign, clawing of the ring and little fingers	Nil	
	Zone III	Nil	Numbness and paraesthesia in the ring and little fingers	

Motor deficits: Intrinsic muscle weakness, positive Froment's sign, clawing of the ring and little fingers.

ANATOMY OF GUYON'S CANAL

The ulna nerve courses through the Guyon's canal between the volar carpal ligament and the transverse carpal ligament. The floor is formed by the flexor retinaculum (inserted on the pisiform) and flexor carpi ulnaris expansion forms the roof. The ulnar nerve lies deep and medial to the ulnar neurovascular bundle. The ulnar nerve divides into superficial and deep branches after passing the flexor retinaculum. The neurovascular bundle is retracted medially to identify the motor branch of the ulnar nerve. The deep terminal branches divide under the fibrous band that stretches from the pisiform to the hook of the hamate, from which arise the abductor and flexor digiti minimi brevis.

The motor branch is identified by noting the oblique fascial pattern of the hypothenar muscle and 1 or 2 mm to the proximal edge of the hypothenar muscles. The nerve hooks around the hamate. The superficial branch innervates the palmaris brevis and then supplies sensory innervation to the little finger and the medial side of the ring finger. The deep branch innervates the hypothenar muscle, the medial two lumbricals, the interosseous muscles, the adductor pollicis muscle and half of the flexor pollicis brevis.

CLINICAL PRESENTATIONS

The clinical presentations depend upon the nerve compression level (Table 11A.2).

DIAGNOSIS

1. Ultrasound imaging

   Look for space occupying lesions (ulnar artery aneurysm, thrombosis), ganglion.

2. Electrodiagnostic studies

3. MRI

4. Radiographs

   Look for hook of the hamate fracture (acute, non-union), and pisiform fractures.

Differences between Guyon's canal and cubital tunnel syndrome (Table 11A.2).

REFERENCES

1. Lundborg G. *Nerve Injury and Repair.* Churchill Livingstone, London, 1988.

2. Phalen GS and Kendrick JI. Compression neuropathy of the median nerve in the carpal tunnel. *J Am Med Assoc,* 1957; 164(5): 524–530.

3. Durkan JA. A new diagnostic test for carpal tunnel syndrome. *J Bone Joint Surg Am*, 1991; 73(4):535–538.

4. Zhang D, Chruscielski CM, Blazar P and Earp BE. Accuracy of provocative tests for carpal tunnel syndrome. *J Hand Surg Global Online*, 2020; 2:121–125.

5. Paley D and McMurthry RY. Median nerve compression test in carpal tunnel syndrome diagnosis reproduces signs and symptoms in affected wrist. *Orthop Rev*, 1985; 14: 41–45.

6. Tetro AM, Evanoff BA, Hollstien SB and Gelberman RH. A new provocative test for carpal tunnel syndrome: assessment of wrist flexion and nerve compression. *J Bone Joint Surg Br*, 1998; 80(3): 493–498.

7. Cheng CJ, Mackinnon-Patterson B, Beck JL and Mackinnon SE. Scratch collapse test for evaluation of carpal and cubital tunnel syndrome. *J Hand Surg Am*, 2008; 33(9): 1518–1524. doi: 10.1016/j.jhsa.2008.05.022. PMID: 18984333.

8. Kenney RJ and Hammert WC. Physical examination of the hand. *J Hand Surg Am*, 2014; 39(11): 2324–2334.

9. Bouche P, Clinique E. (ed.). *Encyclopédie Médicochirurgicale*, Elsevier Masson SAS, Paris, 2008, 17-030-A-10.

10. Corlobé P. L'électromyogramme des syndromes canalaires. *Chir Main*, 2004; 23: S4–S14.

11. Witt JC, Hentz JG and Stevens JC. Carpal tunnel syndrome with normal nerve conduction studies. *Muscle Nerve*, 2004; 29: 515–522.

12. Seror P. Sonography and electrodiagnosis in carpal tunnel syndrome diagnosis, an analysis of the literature. *Eur J Radiol*, 2008; 67: 146–152.

13. Tai TW, Wu CY, Su FC, Chern TC and Jou IM. Ultrasonography for diagnosing carpal tunnel syndrome: A meta-analysis of diagnostic test accuracy. *Ultrasound Med Biol*, 2012; 38: 1121–1128.

14. Weiss ND, Gordon L, Bloom T, et al. Position of the wrist associated with the lowest carpal-tunnel pressures: Implications for splint design. J Bone Joint Surg, 1995; 77A(11):1695–1699.

15. Millesi H, Zoch G and Rath T. The gliding apparatus of peripheral nerve and its clinical significance. *Ann Chir Main Memb Super*, 1990; 9: 87–97.

16. Szabo RM, Bay BK, Sharkey NA and Gaut C. Median nerve displacement through the carpal canal. *J Hand Surg Am*, 1994; 19: 901–906.

17. Wright TW, Glowczewskie F and Wheeler DA. Excursion and strain of the median nerve. *J Bone Joint Surg Am*, 1996; 78: 1897–1903.

18. Nakamichi K, Tachibana S. Transverse sliding of the median nerve beneath the flexor retinaculum. *J Hand Surg Br*, 1992; 17: 213–216.

19. Upton AR and McComas AJ. The double crush in nerve entrapment syndromes. *Lancet*, 1973; 2: 359–362.

20. Hendler N, Viernstein M, Gucer P, et al. A preoperative screening test for chronic back pain patients. *Psychosomatics*, 1979; 20: 801–808.

21. Mackinnon SE, Dellon AL. *Surgery of the Peripheral Nerve*. New York, Thieme Medical, 1988 and Melzack R. The McGill pain questionnaire: Major properties and scoring methods. *Pain*, 1975; 1: 277–299.

22. Novak CB, Mehdian H and von Schroeder HP. Laxity of the ulnar nerve during elbow flexion and extension. *J Hand Surg Am*, 2012; 37A:1163–1167.

23. Apefelberg DB and Larson SJ. Dynamic anatomy of the ulnar nerve at the elbow. *Plast Reconstr Surg*, 1973; 51(1):76–81.

24. Pechan J and Julis I. The pressure measurement in the ulnar nerve. A contribution to the pathophysiology of the cubital tunnel syndrome. *J Biomech*, 1975; 8: 75–79.

25. Lowe JB, Novak CB and Mackinnon SE. Current approach to cubital tunnel syndrome. *Neurosurg Clin N Am*, 2001; 12(2): 267–284.

26. McGowan AJ. The results of transposition of the ulnar nerve for traumatic ulnar neuritis. J Bone Joint Surg, 1950; 32B(3): 293–301.

27. Novak CB, Lee GW, Mackinnon SE, et al. Provocative testing for cubital tunnel syndrome. *J Hand Surg Am*, 1994; 19A(5): 817–820.

28. Cheng CJ, Mackinnon-Patterson B, Beck JL and Mackinnon SE. Scratch collapse test for evaluation of carpal and cubital tunnel syndrome. *J Hand Surg Am*, 2008; 33(9): 1518–1524. doi: 10.1016/j.jhsa.2008.05.022. PMID: 18984333.

11B Compression Neuropathy

Radial Tunnel Syndrome

Vijay A Malshikare and J Terrence Jose Jerome

CONTENTS

INTRODUCTION

Radial tunnel syndrome (RTS) is analogous with carpal and cubital tunnel syndrome because of an absence of verifiable pathophysiology. Also, there is no reference standard for diagnosing radial tunnel syndrome. It is construed that this syndrome is a simple illness with lateral forearm pain. The objective of this chapter is an evidence-based approach to radial tunnel syndrome with clinical examination, diagnosis and differentiating conditions mimicking this syndrome.

ANATOMY

The radial tunnel begins anterior to the radiocapitellar joint and is approximately 5 cm in length. The tunnel extends from the radial head to the inferior (distal) border of the supinator muscle where compressive tendinous bands described as the arcade of Fröhse compress the nerve. The extensor carpi radialis longus and brevis and the brachioradialis muscles forms the lateral boundaries of the tunnel and medially by the biceps tendon and brachialis. The brachioradialis muscle which passes over the posterior interosseous nerve in a lateral to anterior direction forms the roof of the tunnel and radio capitellar joint capsule forms the posterior boundary of the tunnel. (Figure 11B.1) Table 11B.1 demonstrates the potential radial nerve compression sites (Figure 11B.2).

INCIDENCE

The authors have noted female to male occurrence of RTS at 9:1 compared to that in literature at 1:1 to 6:1 [1]. The patients are typically between 30 to 50 years at the time of diagnosis [1]. Right-hand dominance and previous surgical procedures for varying aetiology (carpal tunnel, trigger finger, cubital tunnel syndrome, de Quervain's tenosynovitis) are commonly noted as corroborative findings. The authors noted in their study that housewives involved in repetitive movements such as pronation-supination of the forearm while washing clothes, preparing Indian roti, cleaning vessels and working women with computer overuse in pronation are prone to develop RTS. Also, they noted that the lateral forearm pain is of long duration ranging from 1 to 5 years.

SIGN AND SYMPTOMS

Pain and tenderness are the vital signs and symptoms for diagnosing RTS. The location of pain and aggravating factors often remains a useful diagnostic tool.

Pain: This pain is located 5 cm distal to the lateral epicondyle, on the radial side of the forearm, radiating down the course of the radial nerve up to the dorsum of the wrist. Notably the pain does not go beyond the metacarpophalangeal (MCP) joint of the long finger. The authors have found in their large study that pain radiates proximally to the neck along the radial nerve course in a majority of their patients. The characteristic of pain is so excruciating, crushing and of a severely shooting nature that the patient cries for amputation of the limb. The pain also becomes severe when increased traction is applied to the nerve by extending the elbow, pronating the forearm or flexing the wrist.

DOI: 10.1201/9781003125938-14

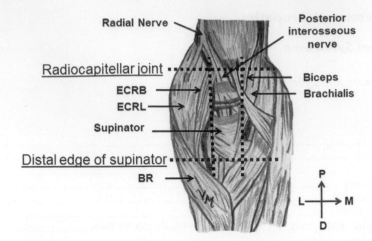

Figure 11B.1 Boundaries of the radial tunnel: The tunnel extends from the radial-capitellar joint to the distal edge of the supinator muscle. The extensor carpi radialis longus and brevis and the brachioradialis (BR) muscles form the lateral boundaries of the tunnel and medially by the biceps tendon and brachialis.

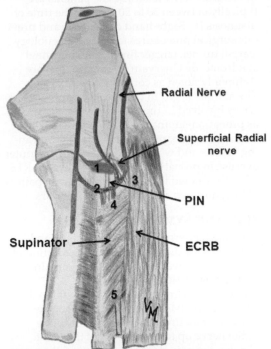

Figure 11B.2 The potential radial nerve compression sites: 1. Lateral elbow joint in the radial head. 2. Fibrous edge of the ECRB, 3. Leash of Henry, 4. The arcade of Frohse, 5. The distal edge of the radial tunnel.

The history and pain episodes are classic for diagnosis the RTS. The pain typically occurs at night and interferes with sleep, similar to common compression neuropathies in the earlier stages. Rest at night relieves the pain and patients postpone seeking medical advice. Also, restriction of activities, analgesics and changes of job transiently relieve the pain. Once the housewives start their chores and repetitive forearm activities, the pain appears and they become symptomatic. Also, at this duration they experience unexplained swelling of the forearm, tingling sensation in the forearm, numbness over the first web space and rarely pseudo-tetany of fingers.

CLINICAL EVALUATION

1. Localized tenderness:

The tenderness located 5 cm distal to the lateral epicondyle is a reliable sign for RTS (Figure 11B.3). (Video 11B.1).

 Video 11B.1 Demonstration of severe tenderness on the forearm. The patient has severe pain and discomfort.

www.routledge.com/9780367647162.

2. Movement:

The movements are usually normal in RTS except in chronic conditions, where there is terminal restriction of passive supination (Figure 11B.4).

Table 11B.1: Posterior Interosseous Nerve Compression Sites

Sites	Location	Possible Etiology for Compression
1*	Lateral elbow joint in radial head	Osteoarthritis or fibrous bands anterior to the radiocapitellar joint or synovitis of the radiocapitellar joint
2*	Leash of Henry	An arcade of anastomosing branches of the recurrent radial artery at the radial neck
3*	Fibrous edge of the ECRB (Extensor Carpi Radialis Brevis)	The leading (medial proximal) edge of the extensor carpi radialis brevis
4	The arcade of Fröhse	The proximal edge of the superficial layer of supinator muscle
5	Distal edge of radial tunnel	The distal edge of supinator muscle

* These are sites of compression where sensory involvement may be appreciated. It is because the posterior interosseous nerve, being a motor nerve, may provide pain stimuli with unmyelinated and small myelinated fibres.

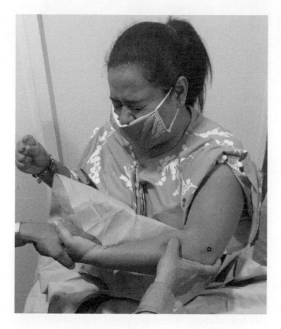

Figure 11B.3 Demonstration of the tenderness: 5 cm distal to the epicondyle (black circle)

3. Rule of Nine [2]:

Loh et al. (2) described the Rule of Nine Figure 11B.5 (Video 11B.2) as a valuable test for diagnosing RTS. Mark nine circles in three rows (3 × 3 grid) over the volar aspect of the proximal forearm. The size of the circles should match the size of a half dollar (3cm diameter). Apply pressure to the circles and note the symptoms and feedback. The feedback usually appreciated are statements such as "painful," "uncomfortable" or "nothing."
Significance of the test:

a. Three medial circles are control areas and expected to be free of pain and discomfort. In addition, the distal circle on the lateral

Video 11B.2 Video presentation of Rule of Nine test.

www.routledge.com/9780367647162.

column also represents a control area signifying absent radial nerve irritation.

b. Tenderness over the two proximal circles at the lateral column indicates radial nerve irritation.

c. Tenderness over the distal circles at the middle column indicates a high level of median nerve irritation.

4. Maudsley's third finger extension test

The patient is seated facing the examiner with elbow rested on a table at 90° flexion. The patient is instructed to extend the middle finger with the examiner applying resistance. Experiencing the excruciating pain or appreciation of severe pain and forearm stretch is a positive test for RTS [3] (Figure 11B.6, Video 11B.3).

5. Wrist extension test

The patient is seated facing the examiner with elbow rested on a table at 90° flexion. The patient is instructed to extend the wrist with the examiner applying resistance. Experiencing the excruciating pain or appreciation of severe pain, lateral epicondyle and forearm stretch is a positive test for RTS [4].

Video 11B.3 Finger extension test demonstration.

www.routledge.com/9780367647162.

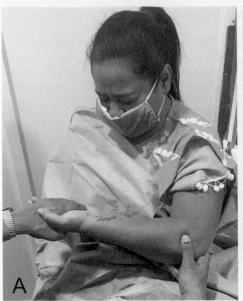
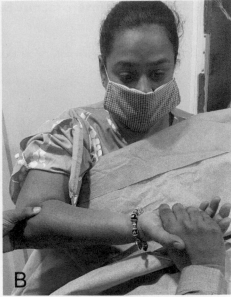

Figure 11B.4   (a) Passive supination terminal is restricted in chronic RTS. (b) Full passive supination of opposite forearm.

 Video 11B.4   Real-time Udvaahaka test in the affected hand.

www.routledge.com/9780367647162.

 Video 11B.5   Udvaahaka test in the unaffected hand.

www.routledge.com/9780367647162.

6. Udvaahaka test

The authors propose a special test called a Udvaahaka test, which is similar to a straight leg raise test where the nerve is stretched and the patient experiences a radiating pain. The test is performed in two stages and always compared with the opposite side (Video 11B.4).

The patient is seated facing the examiner with the elbow resting on a table at 90° flexion. The first part includes passive supination of the forearm with 90° elbow flexion where the patient experiences pain in the proximal forearm and along the course of radial nerve migrating proximally up to the nape of the neck. In the second part, by maintaining the forearm in the passive supinated position, the examiner lifts the shoulder and brings the patient's arm across his/her shoulder. This position stretches the radial nerve and precipitates the excruciating pain. Bring back to the pronation position relieves the compression and soothes the patient's pain (Figure 11B.7). The

authors always recommend this test to be done on the opposite side as bilateral RTS is a rare occurrence (Video 11B.5).

Note: Udvaahaka is the Sanskrit word for lift (escalator). When we press the button, lift moves; likewise, when we press the nerve in passive supination, pain escalates and the patient experiences severe pain and discomfort.

7. Diagnostic tests

Nerve block using a local anaesthetic (2% Xylocaine) in the radial tunnel partially or completely alleviates the pain.

DIFFERENTIAL DIAGNOSIS

Radial tunnel syndrome is a more controversial diagnosis relying mainly on the pain and tenderness over the proximal forearm (5 cm distal to the lateral epicondyle), there are certain conditions which mimic RTS. History evaluation, clinical examination and diagnostic tools help in differentiating them from RTS (Table 11B.2).

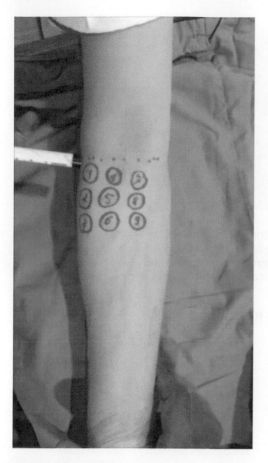

Figure 11B.5 The Rule of Nine tests: Volar side of the right proximal forearm, distal to elbow crease is divided to nine pressure points in three columns. Tenderness over two proximal lateral circles (1 and 2 circles) indicates radial nerve irritation, while tenderness over pressure points of 5 and 6 indicates proximal median nerve irritation. Three medial points are the control area.

ELECTROMYOGRAPHY (EMG) AND NERVE CONDUCTION STUDY (NCS) TESTS

Various authors have performed EMG and NCS tests for diagnosing RTS and noted normal study. Different active forearm manoeuvres (neutral, supination, pronation) could not find significant differences in motor latency.

ULTRASOUND IMAGING

USG is a valuable and increasingly used diagnostic tool for entrapment neuropathies. The authors have developed a neuromuscular ultrasound study to measure posterior interosseous nerve (PIN) diameter supination, mid prone and pronation of the forearm. This is called dynamic imaging, evaluating the nerve during movements. The normal diameter ranges between 1.30mm and 2.13mm at the antecubital fossa. The arcade of Frohse is the common site of the deep branch of radial nerve impingement followed by the fibrous medial border extensor carpi radialis and distal border of the supinator muscle. The nerve may be thickened (edematous, scarred) proximal to the arcade of Frohse and may become wrinkled proximal to the point of compression in the course of supination against resistance. A decrease in the diameter (anteroposterior) of the PIN confirms the nerve compression. This has to be compared with the same level of the contralateral nerve

In case of edema or a neuroma, ultrasound shows the irregular outline, decreased echogenicity and spindle-shaped focal thickening of the nerve. The authors measure the diameter above the arcade of Frohse, at and below the arcade of Frohse and compare it with the opposite side (Figure 11B.8).

Ultrasound visualizes various aetiologies causing nerve entrapments such as extensor

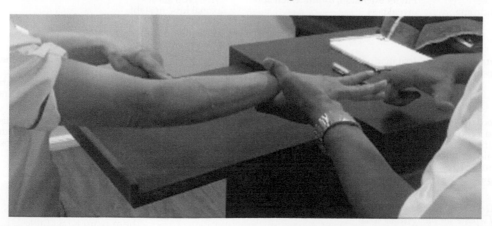

Figure 11B.6 Maudsley's third finger extension test: Pain during resisted extension of the middle finger is a valuable test in RTS diagnosis.

213

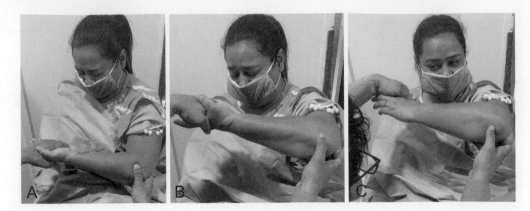

Figure 11B.7 Udvaahaka test: a new test based on the principle of the straight leg raise (SLR) test of the lower limb. (a) passive supination of the forearm increases pressure on PIN. (b) Elevate the shoulder while maintaining the supination exerts tension on the pressure nerve. (c) Passive pronation in the same position relives both tension and pressure. Note: Wincing of the face correlates with the severity of nerve compression.

Table 11B.2: Differential Diagnosis for RTS

Conditions	Features	Diagnosing Tool	Remarks
Brachial plexus neuritis/ injuries	Corresponding nerve root weakness and muscle paralysis Tinel's positive	EMG/NCS and MRI	
Rotator cuff tear or shoulder pathology	Pain in the shoulder with radiation to the elbow	Radiographs, clinical tests and MRI	
Lateral epicondylitis	Pain with resisted wrist extension; pain with gripping motion Focal point tenderness on the lateral epicondyle at insertion of the ECRB; exacerbated pain with resisted wrist extension with fully extended elbow, resisted extension of long fingers, and passive wrist flexion in protonation	Radiographs and MRI	5% has lateral epicondylitis with RTS (because of ECRB proximity to PIN)
Posterior interosseous nerve syndrome	Radial deviation of wrist (intact ECRL) Finger extension, thumb extension weakness	Absence of pain differentiates from RTS EMG/NCS shows axonal loss, unstable MUPs loss and fibrillation potentials, positive sharp waves	Pure motor weakness
Wartenberg syndrome	Irritation of superficial branch of the radial nerve Absence of sensation over the first webspace Positive Tinel's sign	EMG/ NCS	Cheiralgia paraesthetica (pain, dysesthesia radial dorsal forearm to thumb, index finger
Osteoarthritis and Synovitis of the radiocapitellar joint	Localized pain and restriction of the elbow movements	Radiographs, MRI	Rheumatoid arthritis presentations in other aspects of the limbs differentiates the condition
ECRB tear	Localized tenderness, gapping and weakness of wrist extension	USG and MRI	

USG – ultrasonography
PIN – posterior interosseous nerve
RTS – radial tunnel syndrome
MUP – motor unit potentials
NCS – nerve conduction study
EMG – electromyography

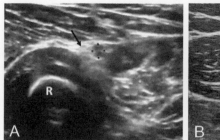
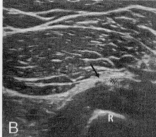

Figure 11B.8 Ultrasound (USG) diameter study and clinical correlation. (a) USG at the level of the arcade of Frohse in a normal patient shows well-demarcated circular PIN nerve. Also, the picture shows the transverse diameter in a red dot and longitudinal diameter in a blue dot. The black arrow represents the arcade of Frohse and R as radius. (b) USG of RTS patient at the level of the arcade of Frohse shows change at the transverse diameter level marked as 1 in yellow colour and 2 in the longitudinal diameter. Black arrow points towards the arcade of Frohse and R as radius.

carpi radialis brevis tears, masses/tumors, ganglion cysts, occult fractures, degeneration of the lateral compartment of the humeroradial joint, instability of the lateral radial ligament, vascular structures, surrounding tissues and iatrogenic causes.

MRI IMAGING

MRI show denervation edema of the supinator and forearm extensors. MRI could also demonstrate thickened ECRB edge, leash of Henry, tumors, ganglia, radiocapitellar synovitis, bicipital bursitis and radial head fractures and dislocations.

CONCLUSION

Pain on the dorsal forearm that worsens at night and arm fatigue are typical presentations of RTS. However, these symptoms are not specific to RTS and diagnosing RTS based on the presentation is difficult. RTS is dependent on clinical signs and symptoms.

REFERENCES

1. Moradi A, Ebrahimzadeh MH and Jupiter JB. Radial tunnel syndrome, diagnostic and treatment dilemma. *Arch Bone Jt Surg.* 2015; 3(3): 156–162.

2. Loh YC, Lam WL, Stanley JK and Soames RW. A new clinical test for radial tunnel syndrome-the Rule-of-Nine test: A cadaveric study. *J Orthop Surg.* (Hong Kong) 2004; 12: 83–86.

3. Roles NC and Maudsley RH. Radial tunnel syndrome: Resistant tennis elbow as nerve entrapment. *J Bone Joint Surg Br.* 1972; 54(3): 499–508.

4. Raimbeau G. Nerve compression syndromes of the upper limb. In: Allieu Y and Mackinnon SE, (eds), *Nerve Compression Syndromes of the Upper Limb*, 1st edition. New York: CRC press, 2002, pp. 149–160.

11C Compression Neuropathy

Thoracic Outlet Syndrome

Jorge G Boretto, Ignacio Rellán and Franco L De Cicco

CONTENTS

INTRODUCTION

Thoracic outlet syndrome (TOS) has two basic types: Vascular and neurogenic. The vascular type is further divided into arterial and venous subtypes, and the neurogenic type has been subdivided into "true" and "disputed." TOS is a straightforward diagnosis based on clinical examination supported by electrodiagnostic tests in vascular and "true" neurogenic types. The "disputed" type is electrically negative neurogenic TOS with an objective diagnosis disputing the clinicians with no definitive diagnostic criteria[1] (Table 11C.1).

TOS has an incidence of 1–2% in the general population because of being underdiagnosed, undertreated and poorly understood.[2, 3] The clinical presentations are similar to many shoulder and other differential diagnoses where patients had shoulder surgery and persisted to have the numbness, tingling sensation, dysesthesia and neurological symptoms. TOS is more frequently seen in women 3.5 to 4 times more than men and working-age adults are commonly involved. Awkward or static upper extremity positioning (holding arm in 45° of abduction) increases the TOS symptoms. Occupations involving repetitive lifting, uninterrupted arm movements with the hand above shoulder level (hairdressers, painters, nurses, clerical workers, grocery workers, switchboard operators) and static extremity postures have made TOS symptomatic.[4]

ANATOMY

TOS contains three important structures: The subclavian artery and vein and the brachial plexus (Figure 11C.1). The anatomy of the thoracic outlet is discussed in three spaces responsible for the compression of the neurovascular structures:

1. Interscalene triangle

This is the most common site for compression and is classically described as the first zone of the thoracic outlet. However, there is a more proximal space comprising the pleural suspensory apparatus. This suspensory apparatus runs from the cervical spine to the Sibson's fascia and is formed by three ligaments: 1) The vertebro-septal ligament, 2) The transverse-septo-costal ligament (the scalene minimus muscle) and 3) The costo-septo-costal ligament (Figure 11C.2).[5] While the first two have their origin in parts of the C7 vertebrae and the last one in the neck of the first rib, all three have their distal insertion in the suprapleural membrane (Sibson's fascia). The costo-septo-costal ligament also has a distal insertion over the medial border of the first rib creating a ring where the T1 root passes through.[5]

The scalene triangle is defined anteriorly by the anterior scalene muscle, posteriorly by the middle scalene muscle and inferiorly by the first rib. The insertion of these muscles of the first rib may vary and can cause a "V" or "U" formation by overlapping, thus creating a narrow space for the subclavian artery and the brachial plexus, since the subclavian vein runs anterior to the anterior scalene muscle (Figure 11C.3).[6] Cervical ribs, which are seen in 0.5 to 0.6% of patients suffering from TOS syndrome, may produce symptoms in 10 to 20% of cases. The cervical rib has been classified by Grüber in four types according to its size.[7] Roos first described nine different patterns of fibrous or muscular bands seen in clinical and cadaveric specimens and subsequently, he described five more variations which cause neurovascular compressions.[3] Juvonen et al.,[8] in a cadaveric

DOI: 10.1201/9781003125938-15

Table 11C.1: Characteristics of the Different Types of TOS

Types of TOS	Incidence	Pathology	Presentation	Provocation	Etiology
Arterial TOS	1 to 2%	Cervical rib. Anomalous first rib. Fracture.	Stenotic subclavian artery. Aneurysm. Thrombosis (fingertip ulceration, Raynaud's phenomenon, pain and claudication).	Sports activities.	Clavicle non-union, malunion, posttraumatic subluxation of the sternoclavicular joint, and rib fractures.
Venous TOS	2 to 3%	Hypercoagulable are at risk.	Sudden/ effort induced thrombosis (Paget-Schroetter syndrome), Supra and infraclavicular fullness. Venous collaterals around the shoulder, chest or breast.	Vigorous exercise or physical exertion. Throwing athletes and swimmers.	
"True" neurogenic TOS	Rare	Chronic nerve compression.	Pain, paraesthesia, hypothenar atrophy, decreased grip, and sensory deficits),usually in the C8-T1 distribution.		Rudimentary rib, fully developed cervical rib.
"Disputed" neurogenic TOS	Most commonly encountered		No objective findings (EMG/NCV, radiographs, doppler are normal).	Activity-related or positional exacerbation.	

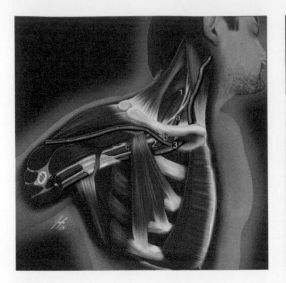

Figure 11C.1 (1) Brachial plexus. (2) Subclavian artery, (3) Subclavian vein. (a) Interscalene triangle. (b) Costoclavicular triangle. (c) Subcoracoid space.

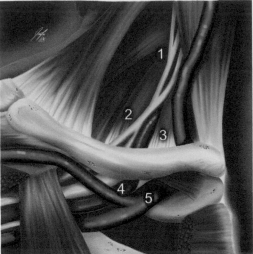

Figure 11C.3 (1) Brachial plexus. (2) Middle escalene. (3) Anterior escalene. (4) Subclavian artery. (5) Subclavian vein.

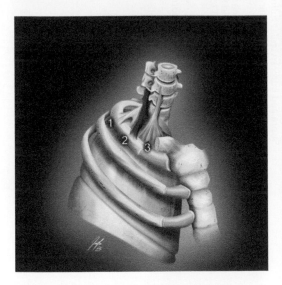

Figure 11C.2 (1) Costo-septo-costal ligament. (2) Transverse septo-costal ligament. (3) Vertebro-septo-costal ligament.

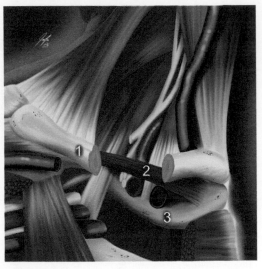

Figure 11C.4 (1) Clavicule. (2) Subclavian muscle. (3) First rib.

study, found that the Type III and Type V fibrous or muscular bands described by Roos were the most common encountered.

A wide range of anatomic variations predisposes to TOS in this triangle.[9]

2. Costoclavicular triangle

The costoclavicular space is formed anteriorly by the clavicle, subclavius muscle and costocoracoid ligament, posteromedially by the first rib and posterolaterally by the superior border of the scapula. Physiological narrowing of the space and a hypertrophied subclavius muscle may compress the brachial plexus producing TOS (Figure 11C.4). Although the clavicle and the subclavius muscle are the anatomical structures that are responsible for neurovascular compression, the Caldani's costo-coraco-clavicular ligament can also be involved in the compression. Physiological narrowing of the costoclavicular space is caused by poor posture with sagging shoulders or by shoulder abduction and retropulsion. The more hypertrophied subclavius muscle the more compression at the level of the brachial plexus and the subclavian vessels during the abduction and retropulsion. Pathological conditions that narrowed this space can be also the origin of neurovascular compression such as malunion of the clavicle.

3. Subcoracoid or pectoralis minor space

This space is less often encountered as a cause of the compression. This space is located below the coracoid process covered by the tendinous insertion of the pectoralis minor muscle. Overhead activities and arm abductions tense the pectoralis minor muscle and stretch the neurovascular bundle around the coracoid. External rotation of the scapula accelerates the compression. Also, the shoulder posture, repetitive strains, muscle imbalance and pectoralis minor contracture may contribute to TOS.

CLINICAL EXAMINATION

Clinical presentation is highly variable, depending on what part of the brachial plexus or the subclavian-axillary vessels have been compressed. Although vascular TOS is somewhat simpler for diagnosis, it is less common than the neurological TOS. A thoughtful and exhaustive history and physical examination are required to diagnose TOS and to exclude differential diagnoses (Table 11C.2).

POSITIVE HISTORY

Symptoms of neurological TOS can be overlapped with other more common neurological compression syndromes. Symptoms can develop spontaneously or following a trauma involving either the cervical spine or the shoulder. There are no specific pain characteristics that are unique to neurogenic TOS, and its location may also vary with no one specific location required for diagnosis.[10] However, according to the part of the brachial plexus involved, neurological TOS can be divided into lower brachial plexus TOS or upper brachial plexus TOS.

The lower is the most typical presentation affecting the lower roots of the brachial plexus (C8–T1+/−C7). The clinical presentation consists of pain of varying degrees at the neck that radiates to the arm through the forearm and into the hand over the ulnar nerve distribution. Numbness can be presented during the day in the ulnar aspect of the upper extremity or it wakes the patient during the night. In chronic advanced cases muscle atrophy can cause loss of dexterity of the fingers.

Upper plexus TOS (C5–C6+/−C7) causes pain in the side of the neck that radiates upward to the ear. The pain radiates posteriorly to the rhomboid area, anteriorly across the clavicle into the upper pectoral region, laterally through the trapezius and deltoid muscle areas, and down the outer arm. This pattern may simulate C5–C6 nerve root symptoms from a herniated disc. In advanced cases, the patient can develop thenar weakness.

Table 11C.2: Differential Diagnosis

Diagnosis	Symptoms	Clinical Examination
Cervical radiculopathy	• Pain radiating in a myotomal distribution. • Burning or sharp discomfort, associated with paraesthesia, that may radiate down the arm, forearm or hand, in the area of distribution of the nerve root involved (dermatome).	• Spurling test. • Shoulder abduction sign.
Shoulder: Rotator cuff tears, tendinitis	• Shoulder pain, weakness/ stiffness. • Functional impairment.	• Subacromial impingement test. • Hawkins–Kennedy test.
Lateral epicondylitis	• Lateral sharp elbow pain usually exacerbated by activities involving active wrist extension or passive wrist flexion with the elbow extended.	• Resisted extension of the wrist. • Mill's test.
Cubital tunnel syndrome	• Paraesthesia in the small and ulnar side of the ring finger, intrinsic atrophy and weakness.	• Tinel sign. • Elbow flexion test. • Froment's sign. • Wartenberg's sign.
Carpal tunnel syndrome	• Awakening at night with numbness and pain in the median nerve distribution of his or her hand that may progresses to daytime symptoms.	• Phalen test. • Tinel sign. • Durkan test.

The symptoms of thoracic outlet compression are induced or aggravated by exercise and by positional changes, such as overhead use of the hand.

INSPECTION AND PALPATION

Clinical examination should be focused not only in TOS diagnosis but also in all other differential diagnoses according to the symptoms (Table 11C.2). Physical examination of the TOS should start with inspection of the posture of the neck, the shoulders, spine and upper extremities. Look for the general appearance of the patients in standing and sitting positions. Muscle spasm or contracture is evaluated in the neck, pectoral region and interscapular region.

As any other compression neuropathy, provocative tests are the main manoeuvres in the clinical examination. Provocative tests are used to identify the sites of compression. In general, provocation tests that are elicited by position or pressure are held for a total of one minute and are positive with sensory complaints in the specific sensory distribution of that nerve. Positional manoeuvres may be performed by increasing tension (traction) on the nerve, or increasing pressure around the nerve, since both traction and pressure produce intraneural microcirculation disorders.[11]

PROVOCATIVE TESTS

1. Tinel's sign

Percussion over the brachial plexus with reproduction of symptoms indicate the point of maximum neurologic involvement.

2. Brachial plexus compression

Compression in the supraclavicular fossa, known as Morley's sign (tenderness in the supraclavicular fossa), may have a diagnostic value when it is clearly asymmetrical and especially when it reproduces the patient's usual, more distal pain.[4, 7, 12, 13]

3. The Roos test

The patient holds the arms in the abducted, externally rotated position and pumps the hands open and closed quickly and repetitively for three minutes. It is called a 90° abduction external rotation test, elevated arm stress test (EAST) and stick-up test. A positive test reproduces the symptoms or rapid fatigue of the extremity (Video 11C.1). This test is sensitive for patients with TOS and the severity

of compression correlates to the degree of symptoms. Note the radial pulse during each test [4, 5].

4. Upper-limb tension test

This test is Sander's modification of the test described by Elvey.[9] This test has three sequential steps, and it reproduces symptoms by placing maximal stretch on the brachial plexus. To perform this test, the patient is seated with the arms abducted 90° with the elbows straight. Secondly, the patient dorsiflexes both wrists. Finally, the patient tilts the head to one side, ear to shoulder and then the head is tilted to the other side. While the first and second positions elicit symptoms on the ipsilateral side, the third position elicits symptoms on the contralateral side (Video 11C.2).

In cases of patients with severe pain at rest (infrequently) the test could be performed passively as it was described by Elvey. In the original test, the arm is abducted 90° with the elbow flexed 90°.

5. The Adson test

When positive, this test was described in 1927 as a pathognomonic sign of scalenus anticus syndrome.[14] The patient takes a long deep breath, elevates the chin, and turns it to the affected side. This is done as the patient is seated upright, with their arms resting on their knees (Video 11C.3). From its original description, several studies have raised concerns about its specificity.

Video 11C.1 Roos test. See the description in the text.

www.routledge.com/9780367647162.

Video 11C.2 Upper limb tension test. See the description in the text.

www.routledge.com/9780367647162.

Video 11C.3 Adson test. See the description in the text.

www.routledge.com/9780367647162.

Table 11C.3: TOS Diagnostic Modalities

Diagnostic Study	Findings	Sensitivity	Specificity
Radiographs	• Cervical ribs • Clavicle fractures, cervical degenerative disc disease • Prominent C7 transverse processes • Low-lying shoulder girdle • Chest wall abnormalities	N/A	N/A
Computed tomography	• Confirmation of spine-related impingement • Space-occupying soft tissue lesions	N/A	N/A
Magnetic resonance imaging	• Confirmation of spine-related impingement • Space-occupying soft tissue lesions • Syringomyelia • Multiple sclerosis • Expensive and is generally not necessary in TOS	N/A	N/A
Colour duplex sonography	• Most usefully venous TOS • Stenosis, thrombosis, flow abnormalities	92%	95%
Photoplethysmography (i.e., pulse volume recordings)	• Suggest arterial compression	N/A	N/A
Angiography (gold standard for arterial TOS)	• Compression, stenosis	N/A	N/A
EMG & NCS	• Rule out other peripheral compression neuropathies	N/A	N/A

EMG: electromyogram. **NCS:** nerve conduction studies. **N/A:** not available.

6. The Wright test

The radial and ulnar pulses are palpated at each wrist with the hands in the lap, and then the radial pulse is monitored with the arm in the 90° abduction – external rotation position, with the head neutral or turned to the opposite direction.

DIAGNOSTIC STUDIES

A summary of available diagnostic studies, findings, sensitivity and specificity (when reported) can be found in Table 11C.3.

Chest and cervical spine X-rays should be the first ancillary tests ordered as they can provide useful information regarding previous clavicle fractures, the presence of cervical ribs, cervical degenerative disc disease, prominent C7 transverse processes, low-lying shoulder girdle or chest wall abnormalities.

Computed tomography (CT) and magnetic resonance imaging (MRI) are useful for confirmation of spine-related compressions, to evaluate for neural compression or to rule out tumours or other space-occupying soft tissue lesions (e.g., a Pancoast tumour). However, excluding these potential diagnoses, MRI is an expensive diagnostic test and is generally not necessary for patients under study for TOS.

Colour duplex sonography has been successfully reported for the diagnosis of venous TOS though its clinical diagnostic significance in arterial TOS has not been determined to date. In the context of proper physical examination findings, angiography has an important role in vascular TOS confirmation.

ELECTRODIAGNOSTIC STUDIES

The most basic and often analyzed electrodiagnostic studies (EDXs) in TOS are electromyography (EMG) and nerve conduction studies (NCS). However, there is much controversy surrounding the role of EMG and NCS in TOS, mainly because of its multiple etiologies and changing definitions of TOS. Additionally, there is a lack of standardization in these studies when used in a patient seeking diagnosis for TOS. Moreover, while some physicians favour either the EMG or the NCS data more heavily, or sometimes exclusively in arriving at their diagnosis, others seem to take a more balanced approach.

Traditionally, EMG findings tend to become positive only late in the course of pathology when permanent nerve damage has already occured.[15, 16] However, other authors have stated that nerve fibres derived from T1, and to a lesser degree from C8, may show changes in neurogenic TOS.[17] In this scenario, NCS has been suggested to be more useful in the earlier-symptom patients.[18, 19] However, most experts on this disease do not find electrodiagnostic studies useful in a TOS population.[20] Despite this, its most important diagnostic role in TOS patients is its usefulness in ruling out other peripheral compression neuropathies such as carpal tunnel syndrome, cubital tunnel syndrome, polyneuropathy, motor neurone disease or radiculopathy.[20, 21]

Somatosensory evoked potentials (SSEP) tests for nerve dysfunction by measuring conduction latencies and amplitudes following peripheral sensory stimulation through the brachial plexus and spinal cord with more proximally placed recording electrodes. However, the value of the test remains controversial as there are to date no studies showing its utility in TOS patients.[22-24]

REFERENCES

1. Meyer R. Thoracic outlet compression syndrome. In: Wolfe SW, Hotchkiss RN, Pederson WC, Kozin SH and Cohen MS, (eds), *Green's Operative Hand Surgery*. Elsevier, Philadelphia, PA, 2017, pp. 959–978.

2. Atasoy E. Thoracic outlet compression syndrome. *Orthop Clin North Am.* 1996;27(2):265–303.

3. Roos DB. The thoracic outlet syndrome is underrated. *Arch Neurol.* 1990;47(3):327–328.

4. Laulan J, Fouquet B, Rodaix C, Jauffret P, Roquelaure Y and Descatha A. Thoracic outlet syndrome: Definition, aetiological factors, diagnosis, management and occupational impact. *J Occup Rehabil.* 2011;21(3):366–373.

5. Poitevin LA. Thoraco-cervico-brachial confined spaces an anatomic study. *Ann Chir Main.* 1988;7(1):5–13.

6. Atasoy E. Thoracic outlet syndrome: Anatomy. *Hand Clin.* 2004;20(1):7–14, v.

7. Merle M and Jacques B. Syndromes de la traversée cervico-thoracobrachiale. In: Merle M, ed. *Chirurgie de La Main. Affections Rhumatismales, Dégénérative. Syndromes Canalaires*. Elsevier Masson, 2007Issy, 335–370.

8. Juvonen T, Satta J, Laitala P, Luukkonen K and Nissinen J. Anomalies at the thoracic outlet are frequent in the general population. *Am J Surg.* 1995;170(1):33–37.

9. Sanders RJ, Hammond SL and Rao NM. Diagnosis of thoracic outlet syndrome. *J Vasc Surg.* 2007;46(3):601–604.

10. Panda N and Donahue DM. Evaluation of patients with neurogenic thoracic outlet syndrome. *Thorac Surg Clin.* 2021;31(1):55–59.

11. Allieu Y, Chammas M and Roux JL. Syndromes canalaires et des défilés (canal carpien exclu). In: Encycl Méd Chir (Editions Scientifiques et Médicales Elsevier SAS, Paris, tous droits réservés), ed. *Appareil Locomoteur.*; 1997:15–005 - A - 10.

12. Morley J. Brachial pressure neuritis due to a normal first thoracic rib: Its diagnosis and treatment by excision of rib. *Clin J.* 1913;22:461.

13. Merle M, Borrelly J, Villani F and Parra L. Bilan de la chirurgie des défilés cervico-thoraco-axillaires. *Bull Acad Natl Chir Dent.* 2011;10(1):84–94.

14. Adson AW and Coffey JR. Cervical rib: A method of anterior approach for relief of symptoms by division of the scalenus anticus. *Ann Surg.* 1927;85(6):839–857.

15. Brantigan CO and Roos DB. Diagnosing thoracic outlet syndrome. *Hand Clin.* 2004;20(1):27–36.

16. Tolson TD. "EMG" for thoracic outlet syndrome. *Hand Clin.* 2004;20(1):37–42, vi.

17. Tsao BE, Ferrante MA, Wilbourn AJ and Shields RW. Electrodiagnostic features of true neurogenic thoracic outlet syndrome. *Muscle Nerve.* 2014;49(5):724–727. doi:10.1002/mus.24066

18. Urschel HC Jr. Management of the thoracic-outlet syndrome. *N Engl J Med.* 1972;286(21):1140–1143.

19. Urschel HC Jr and Kourlis H. Thoracic outlet syndrome: A 50-year experience at Baylor University Medical Center. *Proc.* 2007;20(2):125–135.

20. Colbert SH. Thoracic Outlet Syndrome. In: Mackinnon SE and Andrew S, (eds), *Nerve Surgery*. Thieme Medical Publishers, New York, 2015, pp. 311–337.

21. Sanders RJ. Thoracic outlet syndrome. *J Neurosurg Spine.* 2008;8(5):497; author reply 497–498.

22. Komanetsky RM, Novak CB, Mackinnon SE, Russo MH and Padberg AM. Somatosensory evoked potentials fail to diagnose thoracic outlet syndrome. *J Hand Surg*. 1996;21(4):662–666. doi:10.1016/s0363-5023(96)80022-0

23. Yilmaz C, Kayahan IK, Avci S, Milcan A and Eskandari MM. The reliability of somatosensory evoked potentials in the diagnosis of thoracic outlet syndrome. *Acta Orthop Traumatol Turc*. 2003;37(2):150–153.

24. Rousseff R, Tzvetanov P and Valkov I. Utility (or futility?) of electrodiagnosis in thoracic outlet syndrome. *Electromyogr Clin Neurophysiol*. 2005;45(3):131–133.

12 Brachial Plexus Examination

Janice He, Bassem Elhassan and Rohit Garg

CONTENTS

INTRODUCTION

Brachial plexus injuries are devastating injuries and cause significant disability. An accurate physical examination is critical in making a diagnosis. Physical examination forms the backbone of decision-making by determining the level of injury, presence of functioning muscle groups, donors and recipients for treatment. To be able to perform a thorough physical examination, one needs to have a complete understanding of the anatomy of the brachial plexus and upper extremity. The purpose of this chapter is to outline the anatomy and physical examination of brachial plexus injuries.

ANATOMY

Organization

The brachial plexus is organized into roots, trunks, divisions, cords and branches. The roots and trunks are supraclavicular while the divisions, cords and branches are infraclavicular. The brachial plexus is formed by five spinal nerves, most commonly C5 to T1. However,

pre-fix – involving C4–C8 – and post-fix – involving C6–T2 do occur. The spinal nerves each emerge from the neuroforamen and the C5 and 6 together form the upper trunk, the C7 continues as the middle trunk and C8 and T1 form the lower trunk. These three trunks then each form anterior and posterior divisions. These divisions then combine to form the cords. The cords are described by their relation to the axillary artery, after it emerges from under the clavicle. The posterior divisions all coalesce to form the posterior cord. The anterior divisions of the upper and middle trunk merge to form the lateral cord, and the anterior division of the lower trunk continues to form the medial cord. Each cord then gives off the terminal branches. The lateral cord splits into two terminal branches, the musculocutaneous nerve and a contribution to the median nerve. The medial cord also splints into two terminal branches, the ulnar nerve and the other contribution to the median nerve. The posterior cord terminates as the radial and axillary nerves. In addition to the terminal branches,

DOI: 10.1201/9781003125938-16

there are nerves that originate from all the sections of the brachial plexus described above. Understanding the innervation from these nerves and the terminal branches can help guide the physical examination and determine the level of injury and treatment options.

INTERMEDIATE BRANCHES
Branches at the Level of Roots

The dorsal scapular nerve and long thoracic nerve originate at the level of roots. The dorsal scapular nerve branches from C5 prior to its merging with C6 to form the upper trunk. It innervates the rhomboid major and minor and the levator scapulae. These cause scapular retraction and elevation respectively. The long thoracic nerve has contributions from C5 to C7 at the root level. This innervates the serratus anterior which provides scapular protraction.

Branches at the Level of Trunks

The branches at this level come only from the upper trunk. These branches, the suprascapular nerve and subclavian nerve, go on to innervate muscles around the shoulder. The suprascapular nerve branches from the upper trunk after C5 and C6 have merged. It provides innervation to the supraspinatus and infraspinatus and provides shoulder abduction and external rotation. The subclavian nerve innervates the subclavius muscle which helps to stabilize the clavicle during movement of the shoulder and arm.

There are no nerve branches at the level of middle and lower trunk. Similarly, there are no nerve branches at the level of divisions.

Branches at the Level of Cords

All three cords give branches before proceeding as the terminal branches, which are detailed below. The lateral cord gives off the lateral pectoral nerve and the medial cord gives off the medial pectoral nerve, which together innervate the pectoralis major, which forward flexes, adducts and internally rotates at the shoulder. The medial cord also provides medial brachial cutaneous nerve and medial antebrachial cutaneous nerve which provide sensory innervation to the medial aspect of arm and forearm respectively.

The posterior cord gives off the upper subscapular nerve, the thoracodorsal nerve and the lower subscapular nerve. The upper and lower subscapular nerves innervate the upper and lower portions of the subscapularis respectively, which provides shoulder internal rotation. The lower subscapular nerve also innervates the teres major which is a shoulder adductor. The thoracodorsal nerve innervates the latissimus muscle, which helps to adduct, extend and internally rotate the shoulder (Table 12.1).

TERMINAL BRANCHES

The musculocutaneous nerve is a terminal branch arising from the lateral cord and

Table 12.1: Intermediate Branches of the Brachial Plexus

Branch	Roots	Innervated Muscles	Actions
Branches at the Level of the Roots			
Dorsal scapular nerve	C5	Rhomboid major Rhomboid minor Levator scapulae	Scapular retraction Scapular elevation
Long thoracic nerve	C5, C6, C7	Serratus anterior	Scapular protraction
Branches at the Level of the Trunks			
Suprascapular nerve	C5, C6	Supraspinatus Infraspinatus	Shoulder abduction Shoulder external rotation
Branches at the Level of the Cords			
Upper subscapular nerve	C5, C6	Subscapularis (upper portion)	Shoulder internal rotation
Lower subscapular nerve	C5, C6	Subscapularis (lower portion) Teres major	Shoulder internal rotation Shoulder adduction
Thoracodorsal nerve	C6, C7, C8	Latissmis dorsi	Shoulder adduction Shoulder internal rotation Shoulder extension
Lateral pectoral nerve	C5, C6	Pectoralis major (clavicular head)	Shoulder forward flexion Shoulder internal rotation Shoulder adduction
Medial pectoral nerve	C7, C8, T1	Pectoralis major (sternal head)	Shoulder forward flexion Shoulder internal rotation Shoulder adduction

contains contributions from C5 to C7. Prior to becoming a terminal sensory nerve, it gives off branches to innervate the coracobrachialis, the biceps brachii and a large portion of the brachialis, which has a dual innervation. Thus, the musculocutaneous nerve helps to power both elbow flexion and forearm supination. Its terminal branch, the lateral antebrachial cutaneous nerve provides sensibility to the anterolateral aspect of the forearm.

The median nerve is formed by terminal contributions from both the lateral and medial cords and has contributions from C5 to T1. The median nerve proper, along its course, innervates the pronator teres, flexor carpi radialis, palmaris longus and flexor digitorum superficialis. The anterior interosseous branch of the median nerve innervates the flexor pollicis longus and the radial half of the flexor digitorum profundus. The recurrent motor branch provides innervation to the muscles of the thenar eminence. Thus, the median nerve plays important roles in forearm pronation, wrist flexion, digital flexion, thumb flexion, thumb palmar abduction and thumb opposition. The palmar cutaneous branch provides sensation over the thenar eminence. Its terminal branches form the common and proper digital nerves that provide sensibility to the radial four fingers.

The ulnar nerve is the terminal continuation of the medial cord and has contributions from C8 and T1. The ulnar nerve innervates the flexor carpi ulnaris, the ulnar half of the flexor digitorum superficialis, the dorsal and palmar interosseus, the ulnar two lumbricals, hypothenar muscles and adductor pollicis. The dorsal cutaneous branch supplies the dorsal skin over the ulnar half of the hand and the terminal cutaneous branch provides sensation to the ulnar two fingers. The ulnar nerve plays an important role in wrist flexion, digital flexion, digital abduction and adduction and little finger opposition. Perhaps even more importantly, the ulnar nerve is also essential in providing the coordination of hand motor function.

The radial nerve is one of the terminal branches of the posterior cord and has contributions from C5 to T1. It innervates the triceps brachii, anconeus, a portion of the brachialis, brachioradialis, extensor carpi radialis longus and brevis and supinator. The posterior interosseous nerve branches from the radial nerve and innervates the extensor carpi ulnaris, extensor digitorum communis, extensor digiti minimi, extensor indicis proprius, extensor pollicis longus and brevis and abductor pollicis longus. Thus, the radial nerve has important functions

in elbow, wrist and finger extension and forearm supination.

The axillary nerve is the other terminal branch of the posterior cord and has contributions from C5 and C6. It innervates the deltoid and the teres minor. In some variations, it may also provide a branch to the long head of the triceps. The posterior branch of the axillary nerve terminates as the superior lateral cutaneous nerve of the arm and provides sensation to the skin overlying the lower aspect of the deltoid muscle. The axillary nerve has a role in shoulder abduction as well as external rotation (Table 12.2).

COMMON PATTERNS OF INJURY
Upper Trunk Injury

Often called Erb's palsy, this injury commonly occurs at Erb's point, which is the junction of C5 and C6 to form the upper trunk. This injury is characterized by deficits of shoulder motor function (deltoid, rotator cuff musculature), elbow flexion (biceps brachii, brachialis, brachioradialis) and forearm supination (biceps brachii, supinator). Patients have normal elbow extension and normal wrist and hand function.

C6–7 Injury

In many patients, the upper plexus injury involves both the upper trunk as well as C7. These patients have the same deficits as those with upper trunk injury described above, plus deficits in elbow extension, wrist extension and variably digital extension and flexion. The extent of digital weakness may vary depending on the patient's anatomy.

Lower Trunk Injury

Patients with lower trunk injuries have deficits in the C8–T1 injured muscle groups. They present with weakness in the hand intrinsics, as well as variable weakness of the extrinsic digital flexors and extensors.

Pan Plexus Injury

Patients with pan plexus injury have a flail extremity, with disability of shoulder, elbow and hand function.

GENERAL EXAMINATION

Examination of the brachial plexus must be done serially to evaluate for changes in the examination if there is any recovery. A thorough examination must consist of range of motion of all joints in the upper extremity, inspection, sensory and motor examination and special signs of upper cervical neurologic injury.

Table 12.2: Terminal Branches of the Brachial Plexus

Branch	Roots	Innervated Muscles	Actions
Musculocutaneous nerve	C5, C6	Coracobrachialis Biceps brachii Brachialis (partial)	Elbow flexion Forearm supination
Median nerve	C5, C6, C7, C8, T1	Pronator teres Flexor carpi radialis Palmaris longus Flexor digitorum superficialis Flexor digitorum profundus (partial) Flexor pollicis longus Pronator quadratus Abductor pollicis brevis Flexor pollicis brevis Opponens pollicis Lumbricals (partial)	Forearm pronation Wrist flexion Digital flexion Thumb palmar abduction Thumb flexion Thumb opposition
Ulnar nerve	C8, T1	Flexor carpi ulnaris Flexor digitorum profundus (partial) Dorsal interosseus Palmar interosseus Lumbricals (partial) Palmaris brevis Abductor digiti minimi Flexor digiti minimi Opponens digiti minimi Adductor pollicis	Wrist flexion Digital flexion Digital extension at the IP joints Digital abduction and adduction small finger opposition Hand coordination
Radial nerve	C5, C6, C7, C8, T1	Triceps brachii Anconeus Brachialis (partial) Brachioradialis Extensor carpi radialis longus Extensor carpi radialis brevis Supinator Extensor carpi ulnaris Extensor digitorum Extensor digiti minimi Extensor indicis proprius Extensor pollicis longus Extensor pollicis brevis Abductor pollicis longus	Elbow extension Forearm supination Wrist extension Digit extension Thumb abduction and extension
Axillary nerve	C5, C6	Deltoid Teres minor Triceps brachii, long head (variable)	Shoulder abduction Shoulder external rotation

Range of Motion

Range of motion examination is important as supple joints will not only provide patients with good upper extremity function should they have neurologic recovery, but also determine whether a patient is a good candidate for reconstructive procedures. Patients can develop significant joint stiffness if they have decreased use or no use of their extremity during their workup or observation period. An examination should include:

1) Shoulder motion in flexion, extension, adduction, abduction, internal rotation and external rotation

2) Elbow motion in flexion and extension

3) Forearm pronation and supination

4) Wrist flexion and extension

5) Digital flexion and extension, abduction and adduction

Inspection

Inspection of the patient's extremity is useful to assess for muscle bulk, resting posture, skin quality and for special signs of neurologic injury. Loss of muscle bulk and decrease in sweat production are signs of neurologic injury to the spinal level corresponding to that muscle or dermatome.

To assess for muscle bulk, the patient should be inspected with their shirt removed. A gown open to the front or back can be provided for modesty. The injured extremity should be compared to the uninjured contralateral extremity. Differences in muscle contour can be noted between the two limbs.

Atrophy of the deltoid, supraspinatus, infraspinatus and the intrinsic muscles of the

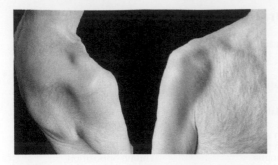

Figure 12.1 Atrophy of the deltoid, supraspinatus and infraspinatus: The scapular spine and clavicle are more prominent when there is atrophy of the deltoid, supraspinatus and infraspinatus. The patient's posterior view shows that there is hollowing above and below the scapular spine signifying supraspinatus and infraspinatus atrophy respectively. From the anterior view, there a concavity below the acromion and clavicle indicative of deltoid atrophy.

hand are especially easy to detect on physical examination (Figure 12.1). Deltoid atrophy will manifest itself as loss of bulk over the shoulder. The injured shoulder may appear lower than the uninjured side. Atrophy of the supraspinatus and infraspinatus can be seen as a hollowing out of the musculature overlying the scapula with increased prominence of the scapular spine. Inspection of the hand should include inspecting the bulk of the thenar muscles as well as the interossei. The thenar musculature should form a convex surface but can become concave in cases of atrophy. Atrophy of the interossei will manifest itself as hollowing out of the spaces between the metacarpals with increased prominence of the metacarpal bones. Clawing of the ring and little fingers is indicative of intrinsic dysfunction.

Inspection should also take note of the skin quality of the limb. Neurologic injury impairs sweat production and dermatomes corresponding to the level of injury may have drier skin compared to uninjured dermatomes, especially in cases of more chronic injury.

Inspection can also demonstrate special signs of neurologic injury that suggest pre-ganglionic injury (Table 12.3). Specifically, the loss of bulk of the paraspinal musculature of the neck and rhomboids implies injury to the dorsal rami and dorsal scapular nerve (C5), which are associated with pre-ganglionic plexus injury. Horner syndrome, consisting of ptosis of the ipsilateral eyelid and miosis of the ipsilateral eye corresponds to cervical sympathetic injury, which is also associated with pre-ganglionic injury.

Sensory Examination

Sensory examination should consist of light touch testing to dermatomal distributions in the upper extremity. Sensory examination may be normal in many instances as there is crossover in innervation between dermatomes.

Motor Examination

Motor examination should include strength testing of muscle groups innervated by the brachial plexus, as well as for the spinal accessory nerve, which is a useful extra-plexus donor. This strength examination assesses a patient's current function, tracks recovery and evaluates the suitability for nerve and tendon transfers. It is useful to think of motor strength in terms of the MRC muscle power assessment scale (see Table 12.4). In this scale, a score of 0 denotes no muscle contraction and 5 denotes normal muscle power.

Accurate assessment of motor strength depends on the amount of power the patient has. For patients in whom the examiner is expecting limited muscle contraction, the examiner should place his or her hand over the muscle group to feel whether the muscle contracts. If there is a flicker of muscle contraction, the patient scores a 1 for that muscle. If the examiner is expecting some muscle movement, he or she should stabilize the patient proximal to the muscle group tested and ask the patient to fire that muscle. This can be done both in the plane or gravity or against gravity depending on the patient's strength. If the patient is able to produce active movement within the

Table 12.3: Signs of Pre-Ganglionic Brachial Plexus Injury

Finding	Implication
Paraspinal muscle atrophy	Dorsal rami injury
Rhomboid atrophy	Dorsal scapular nerve injury
Scapular thoracic abnormal motion (STAM)	Possible Long thoracic nerve injury
Horner syndrome	Cervical sympathetic injury
Hemidiaphragm paralysis	Phrenic nerve injury
Pseudomeningocele	Dural injury

Table 12.4: Medical Research Council Muscle Power Scale

Score	Description
0	No muscle contraction
1	Muscle contraction but no movement
2	Able to produce active movement in plane with gravity
3	Able to produce active movement against gravity
4	Active movement against resistance
5	Normal power

plane of gravity, then the patient scores a 2 for that muscle group and if the patient is able to produce active movement against gravity, then he or she scores a 3. To differentiate between a 4 or a 5 in muscle power, the examiner should place his or her hand over the muscles tested and provide resistance. A score of 5 connotes normal power while a score of 4 means that the patient can produce some movement against resistance, but less than normal. A strength of 4 or more out of 5 is required for a muscle group to be used as a donor.

It is important to systemically test every muscle group and make note of the strength in each. This provides significant information in elucidating the pattern of brachial plexus injury. Additionally, it determines the possible donors for nerve or tendon transfers. There are some muscles where accurate determination of MRC grade is challenging or impossible by physical examination. For these, it is helpful to note whether there is palpable movement, and whether the power is normal or weak.

Neck

A neck examination is necessary to assess the status of the spinal accessory nerve, which is an important extra-plexal donor. The sterno-cleidomastoid is innervated by the accessory nerve and is a major neck rotator. The examiner should ask the patient to turn their face to one side, then place a hand over the chin and as the patient to turn his or her head in the opposite direction against resistance. The other major muscle innervated by the spinal accessory nerve is the trapezius muscle. The patient is asked to shrug their shoulders with and without resistance to test the trapezius muscle, which can also be visualized and palpated (Figure 12.2).

Chest and Back

It is important to examine the serratus anterior (long thoracic nerve), rhomboids (dorsal scapular nerve), latissimus dorsi (thoracodorsal nerve) and pectoralis major (medial and lateral pectoral nerves). Manual testing and exact MRC grading can be challenging for muscles of

the thoracic wall, but function of these muscles can nevertheless be determined.

The serratus anterior can be tested by three different examination manoeuvres. Protraction against resistance is an important examination manoeuvre especially in patients with brachial plexus injuries. The examiner stabilizes the trunk of the patient and provides resistance on the anterior shoulder while the patient is asked to protract the scapula (Figure 12.3(a)). If there is serratus weakness, then the inferior border of the scapula would wing off the thoracic wall and retract instead of protract. Be aware that patients with serratus weakness may try to protract by activating their pectoralis minor muscles, which leads to protraction and excessive anterior tilt of the scapula. In this case, the patient protracts vertically instead of

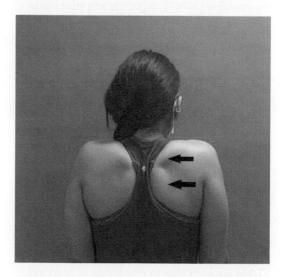

Figure 12.2 Trapezius muscle testing: The trapezius muscles can be visualized when the patient is asked to shrug his or her shoulders. The dimple formed is in between the middle and lower trapezius with the trapezius muscle forming a V. The upper arrow is pointing towards the upper trapezius, with the middle trapezius just below. The lower arrow is pointing to the lower trapezius.

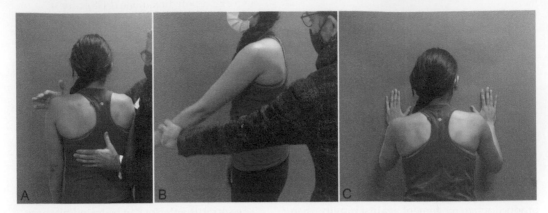

Figure 12.3 Serratus anterior testing: (a) Shows resisted scapular protraction, (b) shows resisted forward flexion at the shoulder. In patients with serratus weakness, the scapula will wing off the thoracic wall with this manoeuvre, (c) demonstrates the push up test. All three tests evaluate for scapulothoracic abnormal motion (STAM).

horizontally which can give a wrong impression about the function of the serratus.

The serratus anterior provides the most stability to the scapula in the beginning of shoulder flexion with the elbow in extended posture. This can be used to test the serratus strength. With the elbow extended, patient is asked to initiate shoulder forward flexion and the examiner provides resistance to this motion. If there is weakness of serratus anterior, then the examiner would notice the scapular blade winging off the thoracic wall (Figure 12.3(b)). Thirdly, the push up test is a classic manoeuvre that is described extensively however this might not be as practical for a patient with brachial plexus injury. This test uses the same principle as scapular protraction against resistance. The patient is asked to push up against the wall while the examiner inspects for scapular thoracic abnormal motion (STAM) (Figure 12.3(c)).

STAM at rest with evidence of increased prominence of the distal scapula or increased anterior tilt of the shoulder might be due to trapezius weakness, clavicle fracture/shortening or hyperactivity of pectoralis muscles. STAM from serratus anterior palsy becomes apparent only with scapular motion or manoeuvres described above.

Dorsal scapular nerve injury may also produce mild STAM, but typically pronounced STAM could be due to long thoracic or spinal accessory nerve palsy. To test the rhomboids, which are innervated by the dorsal scapular nerve, the examiner should ask the patient to bring his or her shoulder blades together and place their hand behind their back. The rhomboids can be palpated on the medial border of the scapula during this motion.

To test the pectoralis major, the patient's shoulder is placed flexed and internally rotated.

The examiner provides downward resistance against the forearm. This tests for the strength of the clavicular head of the pectoralis major (lateral pectoral nerve), which can be easily visualized with this manoeuvre (Figure 12.4(a)). To test the sternal head (medial pectoral nerve),

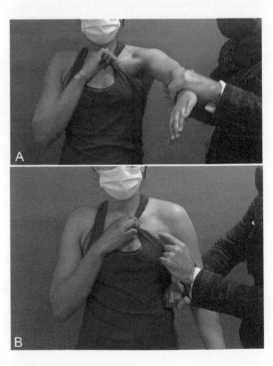

Figure 12.4 Pectoralis major testing: The clavicular head of the pectoralis major can be tested with the manoeuvre shown in (a) and the muscle can be visualized easily in this position. In (b), the examiner can palpate the sternal head when asking the patient to adduct the arm against resistance.

the patient's arm is held with shoulder in slight flexion and abduction and the examiner provides resistance on the medial arm while the patient attempts to adduct the arm (Figure 12.4(b)). In male patients, the sternal head can be easily visualized in this manoeuvre. The pectoralis is one of the muscles in the upper extremity that has innervation from all the roots and hence testing of this muscle can be useful in differentiating between pan plexus and partial plexus injury.

To test the latissimus dorsi, the patient can be asked to cough while the latissimus is palpated in the posterolateral chest wall. Alternatively, the patient's arm is placed in slight extension at the shoulder with the elbow straight. With the arm in this position, the patient adducts against resistance while the examiner palpates the latissimus on the chest wall (Figure 12.5).

Shoulder and Arm

In addition to the chest wall muscles described above, the shoulder motor examination should include the deltoid (axillary nerve) and rotator cuff muscles (axillary nerve, suprascapular nerve, upper and lower subscapular nerves). This portion of the examination should also be performed in a standing position.

The deltoid has three muscle groups – anterior, middle and posterior. It is challenging to isolate the anterior deltoid. To test the middle deltoid (axillary nerve), the examiner places a hand on the lateral aspect of the elbow, the patient is asked to abduct the arm in the lateral plane. Abduction strength or flicker in the deltoid muscle can be appreciated. It can be tough to isolate the deltoid from the supraspinatus as both abduct at the shoulder. To isolate the middle deltoid, the shoulder is placed in an abducted and internally rotated position. If patients have deltoid paralysis, then they will not be able to maintain this position (Figure 12.6). To isolate the posterior deltoid, the examiner elevates and brings the arm into full extension at the shoulder and the patient is then asked to maintain the arm in that position. If the posterior deltoid is weak, the patient will be unable to maintain the position and the arm will drop. This is known as deltoid extension lag sign [1] (Figure 12.7(a)). Alternatively, the patient is asked to flex the elbow and bring the hand behind his or her back while maintaining the elbow to the level of the shoulder. The patient will be unable to maintain this position if the posterior deltoid is weak, and this is known as the swallow tail sign [2] (Figure 12.7(b)).

The supraspinatus is tested by testing abduction strength in the plane of the scapula. Both the supraspinatus and infraspinatus are innervated by the suprascapular nerve. The infraspinatus is tested by resisted external rotation of the shoulder with the arm fully adducted. External rotation testing with the shoulder in an abducted position has contribution from

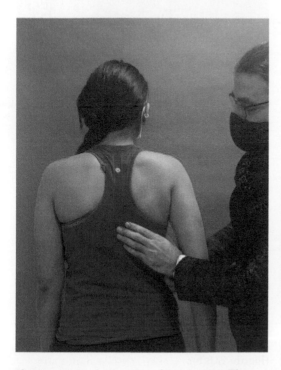

Figure 12.5 Latissimus dorsi testing: The examiner is palpating the latissimus dorsi on the posterolateral chest wall while asking the patient to adduct the arm.

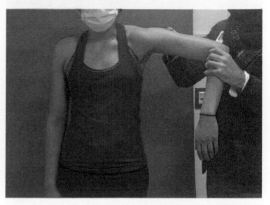

Figure 12.6 Middle deltoid testing: The abduction contribution of the supraspinatus is largely eliminated in this position. There is middle deltoid weakness if the patient is unable to hold this position, with the shoulder abducted and internally rotated.

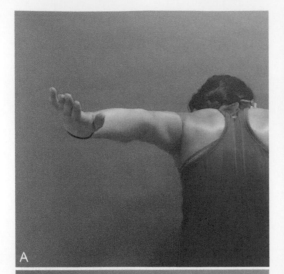

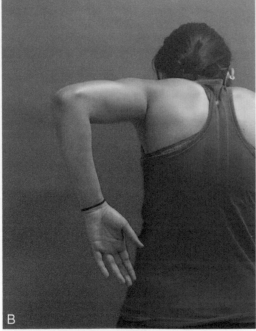

Figure 12.7 Posterior deltoid testing: The posterior deltoid extension lag sign is seen in (a) and the swallow tail sign is seen in (b). Patients with posterior deltoid weakness will not be able to maintain either of these positions.

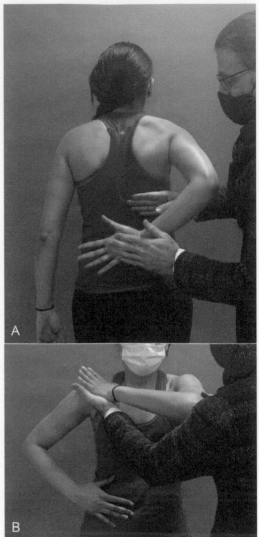

Figure 12.8 Subscapularis testing: The lift-off test as seen on the left and the bear hug test as seen on the right are two of the manoeuvres frequently used for testing subscapularis strength.

both the infraspinatus (suprascapular nerve) and teres minor (axillary nerve).

To test the subscapularis (upper and lower subscapular nerves), the patient is asked to place their palm on their abdomen and bring his or her elbow forward in the scapular plane. The examiner should provide resistance against the hand while the patient tries to touch his or her abdomen. Alternatively, the lift-off test can also be used to test subscapular function by having the patient place their hand behind his or her back, lift off the hand from the back and providing resistance to test strength (Figure 12.8(a)). Additionally, the bear hug test can also be used to test the upper subscapularis. Here the patient is asked to flex the elbow and shoulder and push his or her hand against their chest while the examiner provides resistance (Figure 12.8(b)).

Elbow and Forearm

Elbow flexion and extension, and forearm rotation should be tested. Elbow flexion strength has contributions from three muscles: The biceps brachii (musculocutaneous nerve), brachialis (dually innervated by the musculocutaneous and radial nerves) and brachioradialis (radial nerve). To test elbow flexion, the patient's arm should be adducted and elbow flexed to 90°. The examiner should stabilize the patient's elbow with one arm while providing resistance with the other. The brachialis has the greatest contribution to elbow flexion when the forearm is in a pronated position. The biceps brachii is the major flexor with the forearm supinated. The brachioradialis is a major flexor with the forearm in a neutral to slightly pronated position. It is challenging to isolate the individual effect of each of these muscles and thus it is important to palpate the biceps and brachioradialis (Figure 12.9) for contraction while testing elbow flexion and to test with the forearm pronated, neutral and supinated. The brachialis is unable to be palpated. If the patient is unable to flex against gravity, the arm can be abducted to 90° such that elbow flexion is within the plane of gravity. It is important to assess the contraction of the biceps and brachioradialis muscle to assess their function. The brachioradialis has contributions from the C5–C6 roots and hence

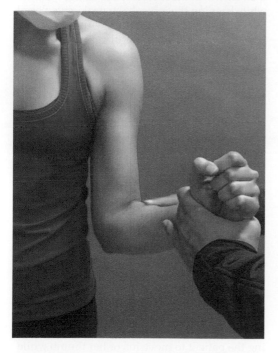

Figure 12.9 Brachioradialis testing and palpation: The brachioradialis must be palpated in the forearm while testing elbow flexion in a neutral to semi-pronated position. Palpation is key to determining muscle function as there are multiple elbow flexors.

the presence or absence of its function can differentiate between an upper plexus injury from an isolated musculocutaneous palsy.

Patients can often compensate very well for elbow flexion even with upper trunk injuries, producing a limited amount of elbow flexion through "trick motion" [3]. Thus, it is important to scrutinize the patient's elbow flexion very carefully. For example, patients can use the flexor pronator mass, which originates from the medial epicondyle and inserts on the volar forearm and fingers to produce elbow flexion. Patients must flex their wrist and fingers while pronating their forearms to allow elbow flexion. This is known as the Steindler effect. Additionally, patients can also utilize their supinator-extensor mass, which originates on the lateral epicondyle and inserts on the dorsal forearm and fingers, to product elbow flexion by extending their wrist and fingers. This is known as the reverse Steindler effect.

The triceps brachii (radial nerve), is the major elbow extensor. To test the triceps, the arm should either be abducted to 90° so that elbow motion is within the plane of gravity or be abducted overhead such that elbow extension is against gravity. The examiner stabilizes the elbow with one hand while providing resistance with the other. If the elbow extension is examined in the same position as elbow flexion, the examiner can overestimate the elbow extension strength due to the assistance of gravity.

The pronator teres (median nerve) and pronator quadratus (anterior interosseous branch of median nerve) are the main pronators of the forearm. The supinator (radial nerve) and biceps brachii (musculocutaneous nerve) are the major supinators of the forearm. To test forearm rotation, the patient's arm is adducted to his or her side and the forearm is placed in neutral. The examiner stabilizes the elbow with one hand while grasping the patient's hand with the other as if to shake hands. This second hand is used to provide resistance while the patient is asked to pronate and supinate. It is easy to trick forearm pronation by using compensatory muscles and gravity. Of these muscles, the pronator teres is palpable. The examiner should place the patient's forearm in maximum supination and patient is asked to pronate and at the same time examiner is feeling for contraction along the pronator teres.

Wrist

The wrist flexors include flexor carpi ulnaris (ulnar nerve), flexor carpi radialis (median nerve) and palmaris longus when present (median nerve). The flexor carpi ulnaris is also an ulnar deviator and the flexor carpi radialis

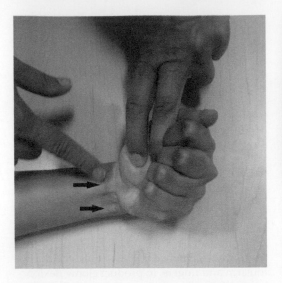

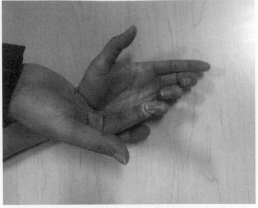

Figure 12.11 Flexor digitorum profundus testing: The individual digital flexors can be tested with resisted flexion at the PIP and DIP joints.

Figure 12.10 Wrist flexor testing: When the wrist is flexed, the flexor tendons can be visualized. The flexor carpi radialis (top arrow) and the flexor carpi ulnaris (bottom arrow) are the two major wrist flexors with contributions from palmaris longus when present.

is a radial deviator. Wrist flexion strength can be tested by stabilizing the patient's forearm and asking the patient to flex (Figure 12.10). Palpation of individual muscle tendons is done to assess their respective function.

Extensor carpi radialis longus and brevis (radial nerve) and extensor carpi ulnaris (radial nerve) are wrist extensors. Wrist extension can be tested similarly to wrist flexion, except asking the patient to extend. It is important to have the patient make a fist when assessing wrist extension to avoid trick wrist extension by using finger extensors.

Hand

While testing the individual muscles of the hand may not always be necessary to determine the pattern of brachial plexus injury, as many of the muscles are innervated by the same terminal nerves, a detailed motor examination may be very useful for planning purposes for tendon and nerve transfers.

Flexor digitorum profundus (median nerve to index and middle, ulnar nerve to ring and little fingers) and flexor digitorum superficialis (median nerve) are the two digital flexors. The profundus flexes at the distal interphalangeal joints while the superficialis flexes at the proximal interphalangeal joints. To test digital flexor strength, the examiner must stabilize the joint proximal to the one being tested and ask the patient to then flex at either the proximal or distal interphalangeal joint (Figure 12.11).

The digital extensors are the extensor digitorum communis, extensor indicis and extensor digiti minimi (all radial nerve). To isolate the action of the extrinsic extensors from the action of the hand intrinsic muscles, the examiner must ask the patient to flex all the fingers, and then extend at the metacarpophalangeal joints while keeping the interphalangeal joints flexed.

The hand intrinsic muscles, with the exception of the thenar musculature and the radial two lumbricals are innervated by the ulnar nerve. The palmar and dorsal interossei (ulnar nerve) act as digital abductors and adductors respectively. First, the dorsal interosseous can be tested by assessing radial abduction of index finger (Figure 12.12). In addition, crossing of middle over index can also assess presence of interossei function.

The thumb can flex, extend, radially abduct and palmarly abduct. The flexor pollicis longus (median nerve) is the flexor at the thumb interphalangeal joint. The extensor pollicis longus (radial nerve) is the extensor at the interphalangeal joint and also allows the thumb to retropulse. Thumb radial abduction is primarily the action of the abductor pollicis longus (radial nerve) and adduction is the action of the adductor pollicis (ulnar nerve). The thenar muscles (median nerve) are responsible for thumb palmar abduction and opposition. These can all be tested by stabilizing the patient's wrist and asking the patient to move his or her thumb while providing resistance (Figures 12.13 and 12.14).

SUMMARY

In summary, a thorough neurologic examination is necessary to establish the diagnosis of brachial plexus palsy and to plan for potential

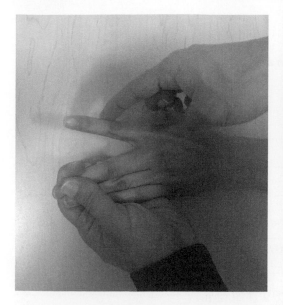

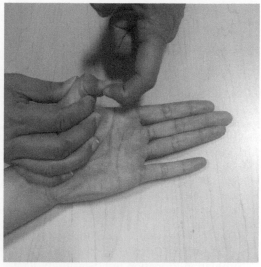

Figure 12.12 First dorsal interosseus testing: The first dorsal interosseous can be palpated in the first webspace and tested with resisted abduction of the index finger.

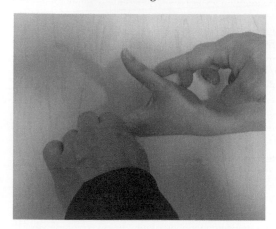

Figure 12.13 Abductor pollicis brevis testing: The abductor pollicis brevis is supplied by the recurrent motor branch of the median nerve and can be tested with resisted palmar abduction.

reconstructive procedures. Fully understanding the nervous anatomy and undertaking the examination in a systematic fashion – by examining the range of motion, inspecting the patient for skin quality and muscle bulk,

Figure 12.14 Flexor pollicis longus testing: The thumb flexor can be tested by stabilizing the thumb, asking the patient to flex the thumb IP joint against resistance.

testing sensation and performing a manual motor examination encompassing the entire upper limb from the chest wall down to the digits – is the key to understanding the patient's injury.

REFERENCES

1. Hertel R, Lambert SM and Ballmer FT. The deltoid extension lag sign for diagnosis and grading of axillary nerve palsy. *Journal of Shoulder and Elbow Surgery*, 1998, 7(2): 97–99.

2. Nishijima N, Yamamuro T and Onha M. The swallow-tail sign: A test of deltoid function. *The Journal of Bone and Joint Surgery, British volume*, 1995, 77(1): 152–153.

3. Suh N, Wagner E, Spinner RK, Bishop AT and Shin AY. Trick elbow motion in patients with brachiaplexus injuries. *The Journal of Hand Surgery*, 2014, 39(11): 2312–2314.

13 Elbow/Forearm Examination

Vaikunthan Rajaratnam, Timothy Teo Wei Wen and Usama Farghaly Omar

CONTENTS

DOI: 10.1201/9781003125938-17

ACUTE EMERGENCY SETTING

As most upper limb pathology involves injuries and emergency conditions it is important to be able to assess the patient with these acute conditions of the elbow and forearm. It calls for a targeted history while simultaneously providing reassurance comfort and pain relief.

It is important to ascertain the nature of the injury that has occurred or the emergent situation. The overriding principles in the assessment of an injured limb would be to ascertain the anatomy and the extent (volume) of the structures that have been damaged. This requires further assessment in the form of the nature of the damage – clean incisive nature as in a sharp object or untidy nature because of blast injuries or crushing injuries.

This assessment is executed via a targeted history and inspection. During the rapid assessment of the limb, the volume of tissue that has been damaged and the viability of the remaining tissue must be analyzed to facilitate targeted reconstruction. The use of digital photography is essential for recording the extent of the injury as part of the medical record documentation. Remember also that the assessment may not be complete and accurate when conducted without adequate anaesthesia/analgesia and full evaluation is usually competed under anaesthesia. In some instances, it is better to wait for demarcation of viability and presentation of infection prior to definitive management. It is best to avoid complex reconstruction or the introduction of foreign materials (like grafts and implants) in such situations.

The injury factors that are crucial for this assessment include:

- The time of the injury

- The type of injury and the type forces involved

- The nature of the contact surface and its temperature and contact time with the limb

The patient factors that need consideration in the planning of the reconstruction include:

- The age and comorbidities

- The occupation and the expectations to return to a similar occupation

- The recreational expectations

- The financial implications of the time off work and cost of treatment

- Residual deformity and disability

Injuries of the forearm and elbow are painful and produce intense emotional fear and anxiety in the patient and their family. The immediate concerns are the possibility of the loss of the limb and later long-term disability. It is important therefore in the evaluation process that the patients be reassured and provided with adequate comfort, pain relief and emergency first aid treatment. In cases with open wounds and active bleeding the application of a compressive bandage over a moist dressing over the open wound is a crucial first aid measure as shown in Figure 13.1. Most bleeding will stop with adequate compression and elevation. Avoid the use of a tourniquet unless necessary as a life saving measure.

It is important at this stage for the patient and the attending surgeon to build a trusting relationship as most of these complex injuries require long term treatment requiring trust and confidence between the patient and the surgeon. Understanding the vocational and recreational background of the patients helps the surgeon to manage the demands, expectations and needs of the patient. The psychosocial aspects of the patient must also be quickly evaluated to allow for appropriate strategies in the long-term management of these patients. There is significant psychological impact on patients with upper limb injuries warranting early intervention [1].

Once this targeted history has been obtained, the next phase is to assess the nature of the injury that has occurred and to understand the patient's expectation and concerns of the injury. This requires a targeted and rapid physical and functional assessment of the forearm and elbow. The main objective of an immediate assessment of an injured forearm and elbow is to assess the extent of anatomical structures involved and the volume of tissue affected. The structures that need to be evaluated are as follows:

- The skin

- The bones and joints

- The nerves

- The muscles and tendon tissue

- Vessels

There are various scoring systems that are available to objectively evaluate major extremity traumas. However, all these are just guidelines

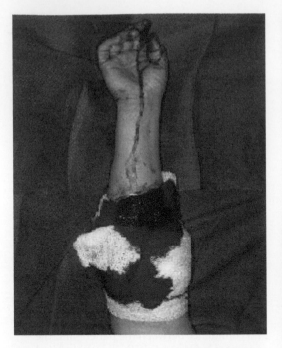

Figure 13.1 Control of active bleeding with compressive bandage.

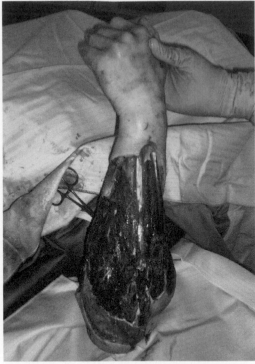

Figure 13.2 Extensive composite tissue loss with loss of skin subcutaneous tissue and deep fascia, exposing extensor muscle mass and extensor tendons with some segmental loss of the ECU tendon.

in predicting the outcome of major injuries to the forearm and elbow, but the management of the individual patient requires other factors that need to be accounted for, including the patients' expectations, concerns and surgeons' expertise and also looking at the psychosocial aspects of the situation [2].

INSPECTION

Looking at the attitude of the limb can provide clues to the type of structures that have been damaged and the extent of the injury. Classically, injuries in the forearm and elbow can produce specific attitudinal changes in the hand which provide an indication of the possible structures that are damaged as in Figure 13.2.

THE LOSS OF CASCADE OF THE FINGERS

This indicates the loss of the integrity of the long flexors or extensors of the fingers and depends on the site of the maximum trauma shown in Figure 13.3. The injury can be in the form of a laceration or contusion and the location can provide clues by its proximity to the anatomy of the structures that can be involved. This requires a thorough understanding of the anatomy of the region.

ABNORMAL POSITION OF THE DIGITS

Ulnar nerve lesion at the wrist level results in the loss of only the intrinsic muscles of the hand and thus the loss of the intrinsic action – which is flexion of the metapcarophalangeal joint (MCPJ) and extension of the proximal interphalangeal joint (PIPJ). This then produces

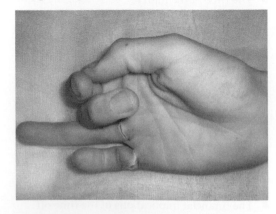

Figure 13.3 Loss of cascade of the ring and little finger secondary to flexor tendon injury.

a claw hand – described as hyperextension of the MCPJs and flexion of the proximal inter-phalangeal joint (those innervated by the ulnar nerve i.e., little and ring finger).

If injuries occur around the elbow with involvement of the ulnar nerve, it is easily affected as it lies superficial as the nerve winds around the medial epicondyle. It will present with the classical ulnar paradox. In this situa-tion the high lesion of the ulnar nerve around the elbow results in the paralysis of the flexor digitorum profundus (FDP) to the ring and little fingers. This will reduce the severity of the deformity due to loss of flexion of the distal interphalangeal joint (DIPJ). The paradox is that with increased volume of tissue involved the deformity is less when the expectation is that there should be a worse deformity [3].

The Simian hand or ape-like hand, is because humans have three large creases: The distal traverse palmar crease, the proximal transverse palmar crease and the thenar transverse crease Figure 13.4). The ape does not have an oppos-able thumb and thus lacks the thenar crease and the thumb lies in the same plane as the palm. With the loss of opposition of thumb due to paralysis of the abductor muscles of the thumb, the simian hand sign is seen as a classi-cal sign of combined lesion involving the motor branch of the median nerve with the associated

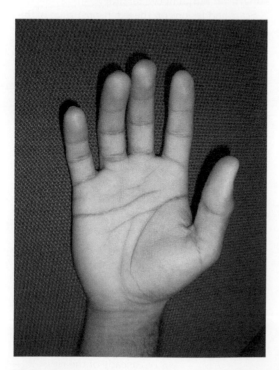

Figure 13.4 The normal hand with the three creases in the palm.

ulna nerve injury, and produces a full "main en griffe," or the full claw hand involving both the median and ulnar digits [4].

THE BENEDICTION SIGN

With a high median nerve palsy, where the lesion is proximal to the level of the flexor digitorum superficialis arch results in paraly-sis of the flexor pollicis longus and the flexor digitorum profundus and sublimis to the index finger. This results in the resting hand having lost the cascade to the thumb and index finger with loss of interphalangeal flexion and the index finger and thumb are in extended posi-tion, resembling the posture of the hand during benediction of a Catholic priest [5].

FLEXION CONTRACTURES OF THE DIGITS

The classical contractures in the finger present with the flexion of the MP and PIP joints with no hyper extension of the metacarpal phalan-geal joint indicating contracture of the flexor mass in the forearm. The causes of this can be due to adhesion scar contractures or following flexor tendon injuries in the forearm or second-ary to Volkmann's contracture producing con-tractures with the pathognomonic feature of an increase in the flexion deformity of the digits when the risk is extended indicating that the shortening of the flexor tendon mass proximal to the wrist [6].

SCARS

Accurate knowledge of the surface anatomy of the elbow, forearm and hand is crucial in determining the anatomical impact of an injury (Figure 13.5). The position of scars or incision wounds and their angle of entry in penetrating wounds can aid in the prediction of the struc-tures that could be injured as in Figure 13.6.

SURFACE ANATOMY

In understanding the surface anatomy of the forearm, the superficial markings of the flexor carpi radialis (FCR) and palmaris longus (PL) provide significant landmarks to map the vari-ous important structures. In between the FCR and PL lies the median nerve. On the radial side of the FCR will be the radial artery and the other structures are shown in Figure 13.7.

On the extensor surface the bony landmarks are shown in Figure 13.8.

Next to the radial styloid is the first dorsal compartment with the extensor policies brevis and the abductor policies longus. It is important to note that this site of location is where the superficial radial nerve can be damaged and easily missed in acute trauma situation and can

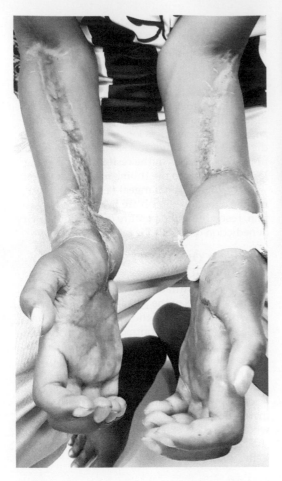

Figure 13.5 Post release of Volkmann's contractures affecting both forearms.

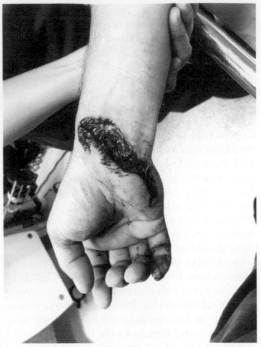

Figure 13.6 Possible injury to median and ulnar nerves with ulnar artery injury and associated flexor tendon injuries.

present late as disabling painful neuroma. Scars around the base of the thumb especially about 5 cm proximal to the radial styloid volar plate can be associated with injuries to the palmar cutaneous branch of the median nerve and presented once again with delayed neuropathy pain.

Scars and incision over the medial aspect of the elbow must be carefully evaluated for damage to the underlying ulnar nerve or the media cutaneous nerve of the forearm. On the radial side, penetrating injuries over the lateral epicondyle the elbow may be associated with posterior interosseous nerve palsy as in Figure 13.9.

Scars over the extension compartment of their elbow and forearm can indicate lesions to the extensor mechanism (Figure 13.10) and the superficial radial nerve. This is close to the extensor retinaculum over the wrist area especially in the middle and can be associated with the division of the extensor pollicis longus. Extensive scarring around the elbow joint in the extensor surface area can involve the radial

nerve producing intractable pain along the superficial radial nerve territory.

Scars and lesions on the extensor surface of the forearm 5 cm proximal to the ulna styloid can be associated with injuries to the dorsal cutaneous branch of the ulnar nerve and again present with disabling neuroma pain if neglected.

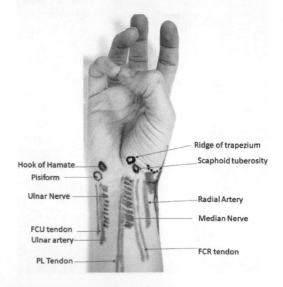

Figure 13.7 Surface markings of the anatomy of the volar surface of wrist.

Labels: Hook of Hamate, Pisiform, Ulnar Nerve, FCU tendon, Ulnar artery, PL Tendon, Ridge of trapezium, Scaphoid tuberosity, Radial Artery, Median Nerve, FCR tendon

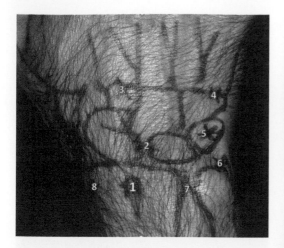

Figure 13.8 (1) Lister Tubercle. (2) Scapholunate ligament. (3) 2nd CMC. (4) 5th CMC. (5) Triquetrum. (6) Ulnar styloid. (7) DRUJ. (8) Radial styloid.

Bruising and swelling in the forearm and elbow may indicate underlying bony injuries and haemorrhage – especially in the forearm. The presence of extensive swelling in the flexor surface associated with bruising and a flexion attitude of the fingers may indicate impending compartment syndrome in the forearm. This can be confirmed by palpation of the flexor muscle mass producing intense pain and tenderness with excessive pain on passive stretching of the fingers associated with decreased sensation in the distribution of the median nerve. A high index of suspicion of compartment syndrome must be considered in the presence of swelling, bruising and intense pain in the forearm. An emergent decompression of the forearm muscles must be considered [7].

Posterior inspection of the elbow with obliteration of the para olecranon fossae may be an indication of fluid in the elbow joint secondary to infection, haemorrhage or fractures. The loss of the isosceles triangle formed by the medial and lateral tips of the epicondyle and the tip of the olecranon could indicate the loss of the congruity of the elbow joint or fractures around the elbow as in Figure 13.11.

In the next pages the special tests of elbow and forearm examination will be discussed. The way to perform each test is shown in Video 13.1.

SPECIAL TESTS

Hook Test	(Sensitivity 81–100%/ Specificity 100%)
Patient position	Seated, passive supination forearm, 90° elbow flexion

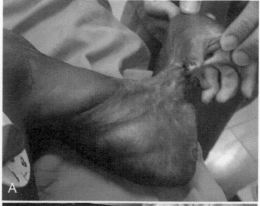

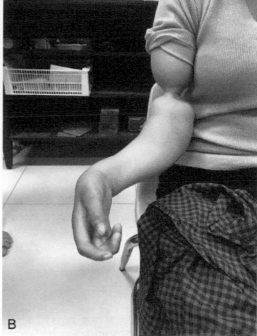

Figure 13.9 (a) Deformities of the elbow and wrist due to scar contractures. (b) Producing circumferential scar deformity due to congenital constriction band syndrome.

Examiner position	Index finger on antecubital fossa
Test	Hook index finger under intact biceps tendon from lateral side
Assessment	No cord-like structure to hook a finger indicates total distal biceps rupture; painful test indicates partial rupture

PFP Test	(Sensitivity 95%/Specificity 100%)
Patient position	Seated, 90° elbow flexion

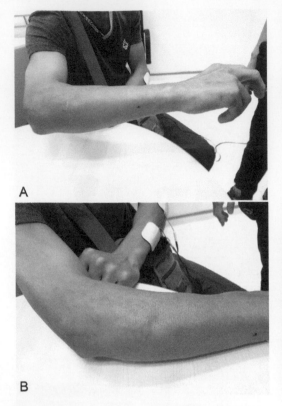

A

B

Figure 13.10 (a) Dropped finger (ring and little) deformity secondary to injury at the extensor part of forearm wad of muscles. (b) Scar over extensor surface of the proximal forearm

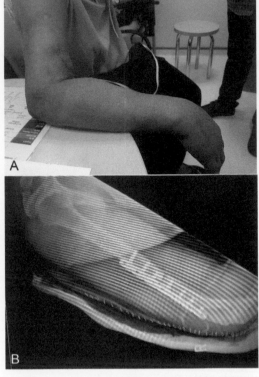

A

B

Figure 13.11 (a) Inability to extend wrist – "dropped wrist" deformity after distal humerus fracture, indicating a high radial nerve injury. (b) Plain X-ray showing lateral view of the arm with plated fracture of the humerus.

Examiner position	Hand on m. biceps, fixate wrist
Test	Palpate m. biceps while pro-/supinating forearm passively
Assessment	No proximal excursion of biceps in supination and distal migration in pronation indicates total distal biceps rupture

Supination-Pronation

Test	(Sensitivity 100%)
Patient position	Standing, shoulders abducted 90°, elbows flexed 60–70°
Examiner position	Stand in front of patient, observe contour biceps
Test	Ask patient to actively supinate and pronate forearms by turning hands
Assessment	Lack of migration of the biceps muscle indicates total biceps rupture

 Video 13.1 Elbow and forearm special tests.

www.routledge.com/9780367647162.

Biceps Squeeze Test	(Sensitivity 100%/ Specificity 67%)
Patient position	Seated, forearm resting comfortably, 60–80° elbow flexion
Examiner position	Hand on distal biceps tendon, other around muscle belly
Test	Pronate forearm slightly, squeeze both hands firmly
Assessment	No supination of the forearm indicates total distal biceps rupture

BA Flex Test **(Sensitivity 100%/ Specificity 90%)**

Patient position: Seated, 0° elbow extension, active wrist flexion, forearm supinated

Examiner position: One hand on wrist, index finger on antecubital fossa

Test: Flex elbow passively to 75°, palpate medial/lateral/central parts of the antecubital fossa

Assessment: No sharp edge medially – BA rupture and could indicate total distal biceps rupture

BCI **(Sensitivity 88–92%/ Specificity 50–100%)**

Patient position: Seated, 90° elbow flexion

Examiner position: Fixate wrist, index finger on antecubital fossa

Test: Passively extend the elbow, supinate forearm. Mark flexion crease in antecubital fossa. Mark start of biceps curve. Measure distance between marks

Assessment: Absolute BCI value >6 cm indicates total distal biceps rupture

BCR **(Sensitivity 96%/Specificity 80%)**

Patient position: Seated, 90° elbow flexion

Examiner position: Fixate wrist, index finger on antecubital fossa

Test: Repeat steps of BCI test on contralateral arm, calculate ratio between BCIs in both arms

Assessment: BCR > 1.2 indicates total distal biceps rupture

Total Distal Triceps Rupture
Triceps Squeeze Test

Patient position: Seated, forearm hanging comfortably over the back of a chair, 90° elbow flexion

Examiner position: Hand on distal triceps tendon, other around muscle belly

Test: Squeeze both hands firmly

Assessment: No extension of the elbow indicates total triceps rupture

Posteromedial Impingement Syndrome
Arm Bar Test

Patient position: Standing, shoulder in full internal rotation (thumb pointing downwards) and 90° anteflexion, elbow extended, index finger resting on examiners' shoulder

Examiner position: Hand on distal humerus

Test: Apply pressure on distal humerus to fully extend patients' elbow.

Assessment: Distinctive posteromedial pain indicates posteromedial impingement syndrome

Valgus Overload Test/Posteromedial Impingement Test

Patient position: Seated or standing, 20–30° elbow flexion

Examiner position: Fixate upper arm and grasp wrist

Test: From starting position the examiner forcibly extends the elbow while applying valgus stress

Assessment: Distinctive posteromedial pain indicates posteromedial impingement syndrome

MCL Insufficiency
Moving Valgus Stress Test **(Sensitivity 100%/ Specificity 75%)**

Patient position: Seated, 90° shoulder abduction, maximum elbow flexion

Examiner position: Stabilize humerus and hold wrist

Test: Apply valgus stress until shoulder reaches maximum external rotation. Maintain valgus stress and quickly extend elbow to 30°

Assessment: Distinctive pain, max. between 120° and 70° flexion ("shear angle") indicates MCL insufficiency

Valgus Stress Test **(Pain: Sensitivity 65%/Specificity 50%, Laxity: Sensitivity 19%/ Specificity 100%)**

Patient position: Seated, 70° elbow flexion, supinated maximally

Examiner position: Stabilize humerus and hold forearm

Test: Apply valgus stress

Assessment: Distinctive pain or laxity (compare with other elbow) indicates MCL insufficiency

Milking Manoeuvre

Patient position	Seated, shoulder 90° anteflexion, elbow >90° flexion, forearm supinated, fingers in fist, thumb pointing lateral
Examiner position	While maintaining patient's position, stabilize humerus and grab thumb
Test	Apply downwards and valgus stress on patients' thumb
Assessment	Distinctive pain indicates MCL insufficiency

PLRI

Table-Top Relocation Test   (Sensitivity 100%)

Patient position	Standing in front of a table, hand placed over lateral edge of the table, elbow pointing laterally, and forearm supinated
Examiner position	Standing next to patient
Test	(1) Ask patient to perform press-up with symptomatic arm. (2) Repeat with examiners' thumb on radial head. (3) Remove thumb with patient maintaining position in step 2.
Assessment	(1) Distinctive pain and positive apprehension at 40° elbow flexion. (2) Symptoms relieved. (3) Reproducing pain + positive apprehension.

Stand-Up Test/
Chair Push-Up Test   (Sensitivity 88%)

Patient position	Seated, both elbows 90° flexion, holding armrests with shoulder abduction and forearm supinated
Examiner position	Standing/sitting close to patient
Test	Ask patient to arise chair by pushing down
Assessment	Pain that slowly extends while patient rises indicates PLRI

Push-Up Test   (Sensitivity 88%)

Patient position	Lie with chest on the floor, elbows flexed at 90°, shoulders abducted, forearm supinated
Examiner position	Standing/sitting close to patient
Test	Ask patient to perform push-up
Assessment	Apprehension or radial head dislocation indicates PLRI

Lateral Pivot Shift Test   (Awake: Sensitivity 38%; Anaesthesia: Sensitivity 100%)

Patient position	Supine, shoulder anteflexion about 100° and full external rotation, forearm fully supinated, elbow maximally extended
Examiner position	Grasp patients' forearm and wrist
Test	Apply a combination of supination, valgus stress and axial compression to the elbow while flexing the elbow
Assessment	At approx. 40° flexion apprehension or dislocation of radial head (dimple in skin) indicates PLRI

Lateral Epicondylitis
Cozen's Test

Patient position	Seated, elbow extended, forearm maximal pronation, wrist radially abducted, hand in a fist
Examiner position	Stabilize elbow while palpating lateral epicondyle, other hand placed on dorsum of the hand
Test	Ask patient to move the wrist to dorsal flexion and move the wrist towards palmar flexion
Assessment	Pain on the lateral epicondyle indicates lateral epicondylitis

Polk's Test Lateral

Patient position	Seated, elbow flexion about 100°, pronation of the forearm
Examiner position	Close/next to patient, carrying an object of approx. 2.5 kg/5 lb
Test	Ask patient to grab and lift the object
Assessment	Pain on the lateral epicondyle indicates lateral epicondylitis

Maudsley's Test /
Middle Finger Resistance Test

Patient position	Seated, extended elbow, forearm and palmar side of the hand on table
Examiner position	Stabilize forearm on table, finger on tip of middle finger
Test	Ask patient to lift middle finger while the examiner pushes the finger down to the table
Assessment	Pain on the lateral epicondyle indicates lateral epicondylitis

Mill's Test

Patient position	Seated, elbow extended, forearm pronated
Examiner position	Stabilize elbow while palpating lateral epicondyle, grab wrist
Test	Move the wrist passively in palmar flexion
Assessment	Pain on the lateral epicondyle indicates lateral epicondylitis

Grip Strength Test	**(5–8–10% decrease: Sensitivity 83–80–78%/Specificity 80–85–90%)**
Patient position	Seated, holding hand dynamometer with adducted shoulder, neutral rotation, forearm and wrist in neutral position
Examiner position	Seated next/close to patient
Test	Ask patient to squeeze the dynamometer as strong as possible (pain may occur) in 90° elbow flexion and secondly in full extension
Assessment	5%%–8%–10% decrease in grip strength between flexion and extension indicates lateral epicondylitis

Medial Epicondylitis

Epicondylitis Medialis
/Golfer's Elbow Test

Patient position	Seated, elbow extended and fully supinated
Examiner position	Place one hand on the patient's ventral side of the hand, stabilize the elbow with other hand
Test	Ask patient to move to hand to palmar flexion against your resistance
Assessment	Pain on the medial epicondyle indicates medial epicondylitis

Polk's Test Medial

Patient position	Seated, elbow flexion about 100°, supination of the forearm
Examiner position	Close/next to patient, carrying an object of approx. 2.5 kg/5 lb
Test	Ask patient to grab and lift the object
Assessment	Pain on the medial epicondyle indicates medial epicondylitis

These clinical tests have been described in literature; however, they lack robust evidence in terms of reliability and validity evaluation. As with all other musculoskeletal assessment, sufficient knowledge of clinical anatomy is mandatory to interpret test results.

They cannot be relied on fully for a clinical diagnosis and must be taken in context with the rest of the clinical presentation and supplementary investigations.

- All tests described here were performed in a specialist clinical setting with a high pre-test probability, so diagnostic accuracy cannot be generalized to a general practice.

- Descriptions for the execution of the tests demonstrated in the videos can be used to perform the tests in a similar manner.

- Diagnostic accuracy that has been published must be interpreted accordingly, based on limitations of the methodology.

Point-of-care ultrasound (POCUS)

Musculoskeletal POCUS is used to diagnose and guide treatment of many joint and soft tissue conditions as shown in Figure 13.12. It is as accurate as magnetic resonance imaging in the diagnosis of complete rotator cuff tears performed by a physician at the bedside and is standard practice in obstetric, emergency and musculoskeletal medicine.

Despite known diagnostic and procedural values, the prevalence of POCUS in ED was found to be lower than what was expected. The prevalence was shown to be proportional to the level of clinical expertise among the operators. Training and utility of POCUS among physicians and trainees should be further advocated and supported.

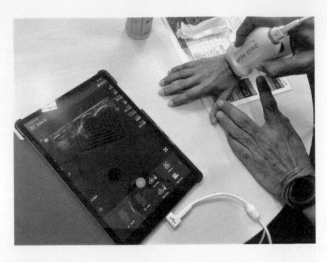

Figure 13.12   Use of handheld ultrasound in diagnosis of dorsal wrist ganglion.

Signs No:	Signs Title	Learning Objectives
#1	Scars	Be able to comprehensively describe: • The scar • Its effects on the limb • Its cosmetic implications
#2	Deformity	Be able to comprehensively describe: • The deformity • Its anatomy and pathology • Its implications on function/cosmesis
#3	Swelling	Be able to comprehensively describe: • The swelling • The anatomical origins and pathological nature • Its effects on the limb (neurovascular) • Regional lymphadenopathy
#4	Palpation	Be able to: • Locate and describe the tenderness • Interpret the anatomy and pathology of the tenderness • Perform provocative and relieving test to ascertain the anatomy of the lesion
#5	Movement	Be able to: • Move the nearby joints / structures actively, passively and perform special diagnostic movements • Describe normal and abnormal movements • Determine the cause of abnormality
#6	Special test and manoeuvres	Be able to: • Select and perform specialized test • Confirm the diagnosis • Describe the anatomical and pathological basis of the test

REFERENCES

1. Becher S, Smith M and Ziran B. Orthopaedic trauma patients and depression: A prospective cohort. *J Orthop Trauma.* 2014;28: e242. doi:10.1097/BOT.0000000000000128

2. Demir IA and Karsidag S. Scoring systems in major extremity traumas. *Limb Amputation.* 2019 [cited 16 October 2020]. doi:10.5772/intechopen.85290

3. deSouza R-M and Choi D. Peripheral nerve lesions. *Surg Oxf.* 2012;30: 149–154. doi:10.1016/j.mpsur.2011.12.006

4. Prabhakar S, Dhatt SS and Hooda A. Examination of the peripheral nervous system. In: Dhatt SS and Prabhakar S, (eds), *Handbook of Clinical Examination in Orthopedics: An Illustrated Guide.* Singapore: Springer, 2019. pp. 5–25. doi:10.1007/978-981-13-1235-9_2

5. Futterman B. Analysis of the Papal Benediction Sign: The ulnar neuropathy of St. Peter. *Clin Anat.* 2015;28: 696–701. doi: 10.1002/ca.22584

6. Kistler JM, Ilyas AM and Thoder JJ. Forearm compartment syndrome: Evaluation and management. *Hand Clin.* 2018;34: 53–60. doi:10.1016/j.hcl.2017.09.006

7. Kalyani BS, Fisher BE, Roberts CS and Giannoudis PV. Compartment syndrome of the forearm: A systematic review. *J Hand Surg.* 2011;36: 535–543. doi:10.1016/j.jhsa.2010.12.007

14 Examination of the Shoulder

Theodore Guild and Neal Chen

CONTENTS

INTRODUCTION: THE BASIS FOR EXAMINATION OF THE SHOULDER

The goal of this chapter is to provide a didactic and concise introduction to the clinical examination of the shoulder. Evaluation of any patient with a shoulder-based complaint necessarily begins with a thorough history of the patient's symptoms, including location, onset, duration, aggravating and alleviating factors, quality, timing and associated symptoms or trauma. Investigation of the cervical spine is integral to evaluation of the shoulder, as issues with the cervical spine may often masquerade as shoulder symptoms. It is also important to ascertain the patient's handedness and take a thorough social history including recreational and professional activities and responsibilities. Overall, taking a thorough history is the most important part of evaluating any patient with shoulder pathology, and the clinical examination should be used sequentially to confirm and provide supplementary evidence for diagnosis.

The shoulder is comprised of both the acromioclavicular and glenohumeral joints, as well as the muscles of the rotator cuff – subscapularis, teres minor, supraspinatus and infraspinatus – teres major, pectoralis minor and major, biceps and triceps brachii, coracobrachialis, latissimus dorsi and the deltoid. The ligamentous and tendinous structures of the shoulder include the labrum, glenohumeral joint capsule, long head of biceps tendon and subscapularis tendon, as well as the superior transverse scapular, coracoacromial, acromioclavicular and coracoclavicular ligaments – all of which may contribute to shoulder pathology.

The intimate relationships between these bony, connective and muscular components of the region, in addition to the proximity of the brachial plexus and other major neurovascular structures to the shoulder, make accurate diagnosis of shoulder pathology more nuanced. As there is no single pathognomonic test for each specific shoulder pathology, obtaining a thorough clinical history on which to base your examination of the shoulder is paramount.[1] The patient's history changes the likelihood that a given examination manoeuvre, or series of manoeuvres, will lead to an accurate diagnosis. As such, the goal of this chapter is to provide the necessary clinical examination skills to augment a thorough historical and radiographical workup of the shoulder.

PATIENT POSITIONING

To allow for optimal inspection, palpation and testing of the shoulder, the patient should be placed into a gown for examination. Examination of the shoulder begins with the patient in the standing or seated position, with adequate space around them for the examiner to assess the shoulder both anteriorly and posteriorly. The patient should have enough room about them to freely move their shoulder in all planes without hesitation. When testing anterior and posterior stability of the shoulder, the patient is positioned in the supine position on the examination table.

INSPECTION

Examination of the shoulder begins with inspection. The entirety of the skin about the neck and shoulder, including the axilla, is visually reviewed for evidence of trauma – both acute and prior – including open wounds, ecchymosis, scars or gross deformity. Scapular winging should be noted, in particular whether it is medial or lateral. The examiner should note any evidence of previous surgery, including location, status and size of surgical scars. Finally, any changes to the skin itself such as rashes or concerning lesions should be noted.

DOI: 10.1201/9781003125938-18

Any time that the skin is inspected, screening of abnormal cutaneous lesions should be performed according to the ABCDE criteria – Asymmetry, Border irregularity, Colour variegation, Diameter (X > 6 mm) and Evolution, with remarkable lesions being referred for further dermatologic evaluation.[2]

Muscle bulk is next assessed with direct visualization. Wasting of the musculature within the supraspinatus and infraspinatus fossae, trapezius, deltoid and pectoralis major is assessed. Peripheral neuropathies of the shoulder may be difficult to detect on clinical examination alone. Nerves such as the suprascapular nerve lack sensory components or reflexes, and symptoms may be difficult to discern from additional shoulder pathology such as rotator cuff tears.[3] If there is concern for neuropathy based on further examination, an Nerve Conduction Velocity/ Electromyograph (EMG) may be obtained to further the diagnostic workup.

PALPATION

Direct palpation for assessment of muscle bulk and wasting follows visual inspection. Softening or decreased breadth of the muscle belly as compared to ipsilateral or contralateral muscles may indicate mechanical or neurologic pathology. The acromioclavicular joint is palpated as well, to assess for tenderness, instability or gapping. Although, there is no optimal single test – or set of physical examination manoeuvres – that significantly increases the post-test probability of screening for or confirming acromioclavicular joint pathology.[4] The long head of the biceps should also be palpated, which is found just medial to the greater tuberosity in the bicipital groove on the anterior shoulder. Tenderness to palpation of the long head of the biceps is the most common isolated physical examination finding in patients with biceps tendonitis and may be combined with the uppercut test – which is performed by having the patient flex the elbow to 90° and perform resisted flexion and adduction of the shoulder towards the contralateral shoulder – to increase the accuracy of diagnosis of biceps tendon pathology.[5]

Vascular examination of the upper extremity including checking capillary refill in the fingers and palpating for ulnar and radial pulses should be performed. Neurologic evaluation of axillary, median, radial and ulnar distributions is completed to conclude this portion of the exam.

SHOULDER JOINT RANGE OF MOTION

Passive range of motion of the shoulder is performed first. The shoulder is assessed in passive forward flexion (FF), extension, abduction,

internal rotation (IR) and external rotation (ER) with the arm at the patient's side as well as with it abducted to 90°. Any clicking, crepitation, or block to movement during these manoeuvres should be noted by the examiner. The active range of motion is then measured with the patient reproducing the previously listed movements, which are compared to their passive values and values from the contralateral shoulder. The active range of motion manoeuvres may be again repeated against resistance to gauge strength in the associated muscle groups. While there is variation among reported "normal" range of motion values for the shoulder, a review by Anderton et al., reports the following average "normal" range of motion for each shoulder function: Forward flexion: 165° (117–180°), extension 54° (28–80°), abduction 171° (117–189°), internal rotation 74° (30–110°), external rotation 83° (40–117°).[6] In general, if the passive range of motion is greater than the active range of motion, the primary pathology is likely to be a muscle or nerve disorder. If both passive and active ranges of motion are limited, a mechanical limitation caused by bony or soft tissue pathology is more likely the culprit.

The Apley Scratch Test is used to evaluate both internal and external rotation of the shoulder. First, the patient is asked to touch the contralateral shoulder with their hand, which is then repeated on the contralateral side. The patient next abducts and externally rotates their shoulder, reaching behind their head, to touch the superior aspect of their contralateral scapula. In the final part of the manoeuvre, the patient internally rotates and adducts the ipsilateral arm to reach behind them and touch the inferior pole of the contralateral scapulae. Increased pain, difference in ability of each arm to perform the test manoeuvres or abnormal scapular motion are all considered positive tests.[7]

PROVOCATIVE EXAMINATION MANOEUVRES

When guided by a thorough history, provocative manoeuvres of the shoulder joint can be used to further support the etiology of a patient's symptoms.

1. *Hawkins–Kennedy test:* This test is used to assess supraspinatus pathology or subacromial impingement. The patient's shoulder is abducted to 90°, elbow flexed to 90° and the arm is internally rotated by the examiner at the wrist while maintaining the shoulder in abduction by supporting the elbow (Figure 14.1). A positive test is pain with this manoeuvre. Based on metanalysis by Hegedus et al., there is 80% sensitivity, and 56% specificity of this test.[1]

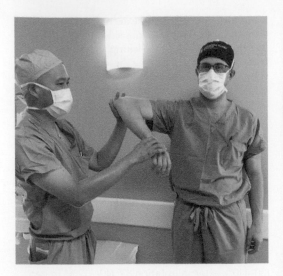

Figure 14.1 Hawkins–Kennedy test.

2. *Cross arm adduction test:* This test is used to assess for acromioclavicular joint pathology. The patient forward flexes their arm to 90° and adducts the arm across their chest (Figure 14.2). If there is pain with this motion, the test is considered positive. The test has a reported sensitivity of 77% and specificity of 79%.[8]

3. *Neer's sign:* This test is used for the evaluation of subacromial impingement. The patient's arm is full pronated, with the thumb pointing downwards and the shoulder is forward flexed overhead while the examiner stabilizes the scapula (Figure 14.3). A positive result is pain with this manoeuvre, or inability to completely raise the

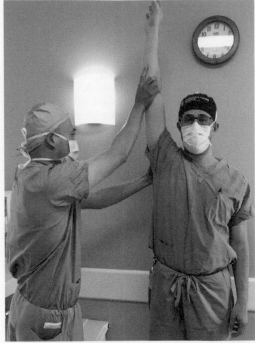

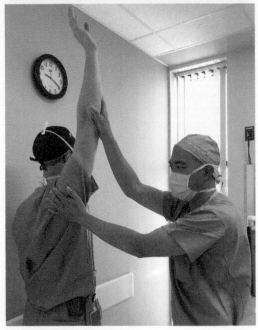

Figure 14.3 Neer's sign.

arm overhead. The sensitivity of this test is reported as 72%, and the specificity is 60%.[1]

4. *Jobe's (empty can) test:* A test used for assessment of the supraspinatus, the patient's arm is forward flexed to 90°, fully pronated so that the thumb is facing down, and abducted to the plane of the scapula – approximately 30° from neutral (Figure 14.4).

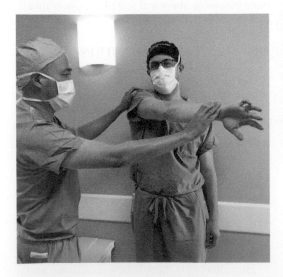

Figure 14.2 Cross-arm adduction test.

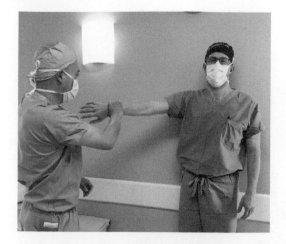

Figure 14.4 Jobe's (empty can) test.

The examiner then applies a downward force at the patient's wrist, with the test being considered positive if there is pain or the patient is unable to resist the examiner's force. The sensitivity of this test is reported to be 96%, with a specificity of 31%.[9]

5. *Hornblower's sign*: This test is used to evaluate teres minor. The patient's arm is forward flexed and abducted to 90°, and the patient is asked to hold that position (Figure 14.5). If the patient has pain with this manoeuvre or the patient is unable to hold the position and the arm drifts into internal rotation, the test is considered positive. The sensitivity of this test has been reported as 100%, with a specificity of 93%.[10]

6. *Belly-press and lift-off tests*: Both tests are used to evaluate the integrity of the subscapularis. In the belly-press test, the patient's arm is internally rotated over their abdomen, and they are asked to pull in internal rotation towards their abdomen while the elbow is stabilized by the examiner (Figure 14.6). The test is positive if the patient has weakness or pain with the manoeuvre. The lift off test is performed with the arm placed into internal rotation behind the patient. The patient is then asked to push back against the hand of the examiner (Figure 14.7). This exam manoeuvre is considered positive if the patient has pain or inability to perform the exam. The sensitivity of the belly-press test has been reported as 57% with a specificity of 83%, while the lift-off test has a sensitivity of 35% and specificity of 97%.[11]

7. *O'Brien's active compression test*: This test is used to evaluate the glenoid labrum, and for Superior Labrum Anterior-Posterior (SLAP) lesions. The patient forward flexes their shoulder to 90° and adducts the arm 10° from neutral. With the hand held in full pronation (thumb down), the examiner places a downward force on the wrist (Figure 14.8). The patient then fully supinates the arm (thumb up) and a downward force is once again applied by the examiner. The test is positive if the patient has pain in the shoulder with downward force during pronation only. The sensitivity of this test is 67%, with a specificity of 37%.[1]

EXAMINATION OF SHOULDER STABILITY

1. *Load and shift test*: The patient is positioned either seated or standing, arm relaxed at their side. Standing behind the patient, stabilize their scapula with your contralateral hand, and grip the humeral head of their

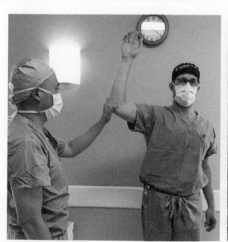
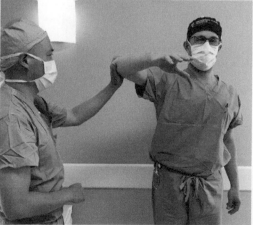

Figure 14.5 Hornblower's test, with a positive finding on the right.

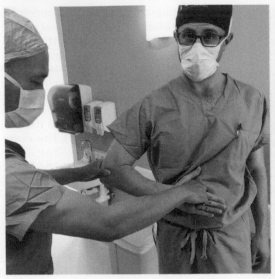

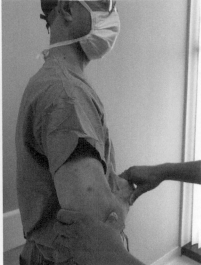

Figure 14.6 Belly-press test.

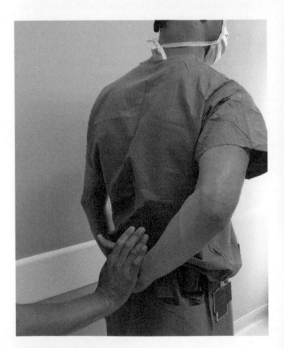

Figure 14.7 Lift-off test.

shoulder between your ipsilateral hand's thumb and fingers. Apply a gentle anterior-posterior force to the shoulder, inducing sub-luxation of the joint. Alternatively, the test may be performed with the patient supine on an examination table or stretcher. The arm is abducted to 90°, and the examiner stabilizes the elbow with one hand while using their other hand to grasp the humeral head and apply a gentle anterior-posterior

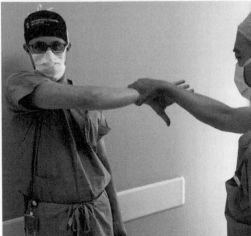

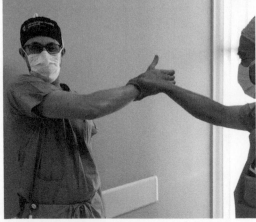

Figure 14.8 O'Brien's active compression test.

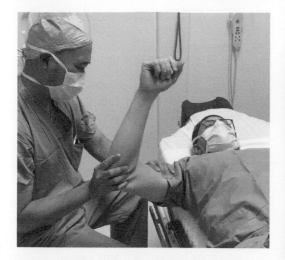

Figure 14.9 The load and shift test.

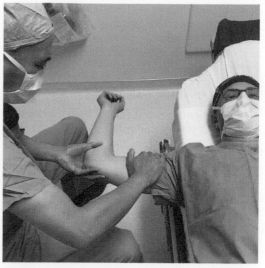

Figure 14.11 The relocation test.

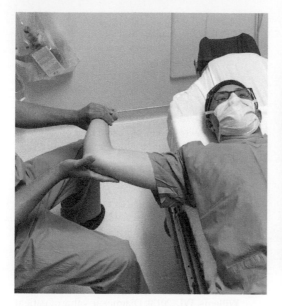

Figure 14.10 The anterior apprehension test.

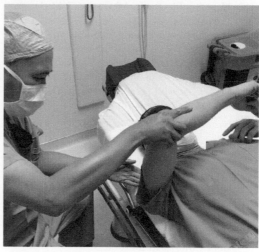

Figure 14.12 The posterior apprehension test.

force on the proximal humerus (Figure 14.9). The test is considered positive if it reproduces the patient's symptoms of instability, or if there is increased laxity as compared to the contralateral side. The sensitivity of this test is 72%, with a specificity of 90%.[12]

2. *Anterior apprehension test and relocation test:* The patient is instructed to lay supine on an examination table or stretcher with their shoulder at the edge of the bed. The patient's arm is abducted and externally rotated 90° (Figure 14.10). The test is positive if there is reproduction of symptoms of instability or discomfort in the anterior shoulder with gentle external rotation of the arm. This

test has a reported sensitivity of 66% and a specificity of 95%.[1] The relocation test is performed by placement of the examiner's hand on the anterior shoulder with a posterior directed force and is considered positive if there is a resolution of the symptoms stated above (Figure 14.11). The sensitivity of this test is 65% while the specificity is 90%.[1]

3. *Posterior apprehension test:* This test is used to assess for posterior glenoid or labral pathology. This test may be performed with the patient seated or supine. The shoulder is forward flexed to 90°, and a longitudinal force is placed from the elbow down the axis of the humerus into the shoulder. The patient's arm is then slowly adducted while under

load, and the test is considered positive if there is a palpable clunk as the shoulder adducts and the humeral head translates posteriorly due to a deficient posterior glenoid or labrum (Figure 14.12). The sensitivity and specificity of this test is reported as 90%, with a specificity of 85%.[13]

4. *Sulcus sign*: This test is used to assess for laxity of the rotator cuff interval. With the patient standing, position their arm at their side, pull longitudinal traction downward. The test is considered positive if there is a sulcus or dimpling of the skin that develops inferior to the acromion. Tzannes et al., reported a sensitivity of 72% and specificity of 85% with more than 1 cm of inferior translation, and a sensitivity of 28% and specificity of 97% with more than 2 cm of translation.[14]

REFERENCES

1. Hegedus, EJ, Goode, AP, Cook, CE, Michener, L, Myer, CA, Myer, DM and Wright, AA. (2012). Which physical examination tests provide clinicians with the most value when examining the shoulder? Update of a systematic review with meta-analysis of individual tests. *British Journal of Sports Medicine*, 46(14), 964–978. doi:10.1136/bjsports-2012-091066

2. Tsao, H, Olazagasti, JM., Cordoro, KM, Brewer, JD, Taylor, SC, Bordeaux, JS, Chren, MM, Sober, AJ, Tegeler, C, Bhushan, R and Begolka, WS. (2015). Early detection of melanoma: Reviewing the ABCDEs American Academy of Dermatology Ad Hoc Task Force for the ABCDEs of melanoma. *Journal of the American Academy of Dermatology*, 72(4), 717–723. doi:10.1016/j.jaad.2015.01.025

3. Vad, VB, Southern, D, Warren, RF, Altchek, DW and Dines, D. (2003). Prevalence of peripheral neurologic injuries in rotator cuff tears with atrophy. *Journal of Shoulder and Elbow Surgery*, 12(4), 333–336. doi:10.1016/S1058-2746(03)00040-5

4. Krill, MK, Rosas, S, Amoo-Achampong, K, Kwon, K, Nwachukwu, BU and McCormick, F. (2018). A concise evidence-based physical examination for diagnosis of acromioclavicular joint pathology: A systematic review. *The Physician and Sportsmedicine*, 46(1), 98–104. doi:10.1080/00913847.2018.1413920.A

5. Rosas, S, Krill, MK, Amoo-Achampong, K, Kwon, K, Nwachukwu, BU and McCormick, F. (2017). A practical, evidence-based, comprehensive (PEC) physical examination for diagnosing pathology of the long head of the biceps. *Journal of Shoulder and Elbow Surgery*, 26(8), 1484–1492. doi:10.1016/j.jse.2017.03.002.A

6. Anderton, M, Ede, MN. &and Holt, E. (2018). Normal range of motion of the shoulder: An imprecise benchmark. *Orthopaedic Proceedings*, 94(B), SUPP_XXXIX

7. Konin, J. (2006). *Special Tests for Orthopedic Examination*, 3rd edition. SLACK, Thorofare, NJ.

8. Chronopoulos, E, Kim, TK, Park, H Bin, Ashenbrenner, D and McFarland, EG. (2004). Diagnostic value of physical tests for isolated chronic acromioclavicular lesions. *American Journal of Sports Medicine*, 32(3), 655–661. doi:10.1177/0363546503261723

9. Sgroi, M, Loitsch, T, Reichel, H and Kappe, T. (2018). Diagnostic value of clinical tests for supraspinatus tendon tears. *Arthroscopy – Journal of Arthroscopic and Related Surgery*, 34(8), 2326–2333. doi:10.1016/j.arthro.2018.03.030

10. Walch, G, Boulahia, A, Calderone, S and Robinson, AH. (1998). The "dropping" and "hornblower's" signs in evaluation of rotator-cuff tears. *The Journal of Bone and Joint Surgery*, 80(4), 624–628.

11. Yoon, JP, Chung, SW, Kim, SH and Oh, JH. (2013). Diagnostic value of four clinical tests for the evaluation of subscapularis integrity. *Journal of Shoulder and Elbow Surgery*, 22(9), 1186–1192. doi:10.1016/j.jse.2012.12.002

12. van Kampen, DA, van den Berg, T, van der Woude, HJ, Castelein, RM, Terwee, CB and Willems, WJ. (2013). Diagnostic value of patient characteristics, history, and six clinical tests for traumatic anterior shoulder instability. *Journal of Shoulder and Elbow Surgery*, 22(10), 1310–1319. doi:10.1016/j.jse.2013.05.006

13. Kim, SH, Park, JC, Park, JS and Oh, I. (2004). Painful jerk test: A predictor of success in nonoperative treatment of posteroinferior instability of the shoulder. *American Journal of Sports Medicine*, 32(8), 1849–1855. doi:10.1177/0363546504265263

14. Tzannes, A and Murrell, GAC. (2002). Clinical examination of the unstable shoulder. *Sports Medicine*, 32(7), 447–457. doi:10.2165/00007256-200232070-00004

15 Instruments and Implants in Hand Surgery

Anil K Bhat, Ashwath M Acharya and Mithun Pai G

CONTENTS

INTRODUCTION

The human hand is an exquisite and delicate organ used to carry out complicated tasks generated by the brain. Pathological afflictions of the hand require a dedicated team of hand surgeons who use a unique set of instruments and implants to address the problems on the operating table. The current modern-day hand surgeon uses various instruments ranging from the most basic tools to incredibly complex gadgets. Awareness about some of the commonly used instruments is vital to enable useful and informative interaction among the surgical staff to achieve optimum results.

For the novice in hand surgery, information on various instruments, implants, and uses may be an uphill task. As surgical techniques develop and improve, new instruments and implants will only continue to add to the already bewildering armamentarium available to hand surgeons. Even though there are countless surgical instruments and implants in hand surgery, it becomes easier once we realize that they are classified by the type of utility during the procedure as specific tools are required for each surgical operation.

This chapter provides basic information on some of the essential instruments and implants used by hand surgeons during hand surgical procedures. The list provided in this chapter is by no means a comprehensive description. However, it provides an insight into the fascinating variety of tools and their applications. The reader is guided on identifying instruments and implants for hand surgery, starting with the basic hand surgery set that contains most of the commonly used instruments required for most procedures. The other instrument and implant sets are described subsequently.

BASIC HAND SURGERY SET

1. **Skin hook and cat's paw**: These are used for retracting the skin and subcutaneous tissue (Figure 15.1A,B).

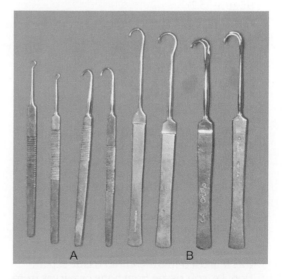

Figure 15.1 A) Skin hooks; B) Cat's paw.

2. **Langenbeck's retractor**: These are used to retract the soft tissues and wound edges

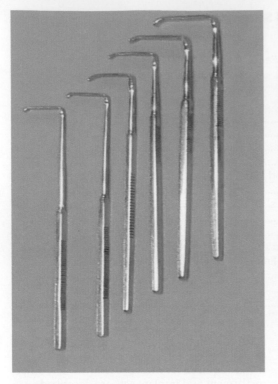

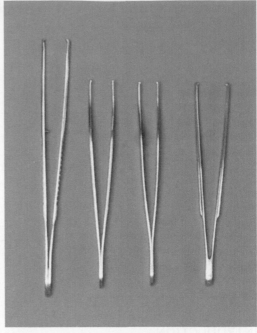

Figure 15.3 Adson's forceps.

Figure 15.2 Langenbeck's retractor.

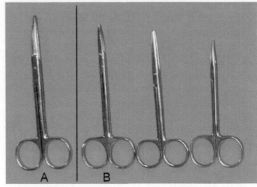

Figure 15.4 A) Mayo scissors; B) Metzenbaum scissors.

to visualize deeper structures. They were designed by the German surgeon Bernhard von Langenbeck for urological procedures (Figure 15.2).

3. **Adson's forceps**: These are used to hold and lift the soft tissues and muscles, facilitating meticulous dissection. They have narrow tips that are used for holding and manipulating delicate tissues. These forceps have a wide, flat thumb grasp area that is commonly serrated (Figure 15.3).

1. **Mayo scissors**: These are heavy scissors available in multiple designs. Straight scissors are used for cutting sutures ("suture scissors"), while curved scissors are used for cutting heavy tissue (e.g. Fascia) (Figure 15.4A).**Metzenbaum scissors**: These are lighter scissors used for cutting delicate tissues and for blunt dissection (Figure 15.4B).

5. **McDonald double-ended dissector/elevator:** It is used in differential tissue separation, i.e. soft tissue from bone or nerves from soft tissue, thereby increasing the field of vision and avoiding damage to vital structures (Figure 15.5).

6. **Trethowan bone levers**: These are used for deeper retraction in a perpendicular plane leading to better exposure (Figure 15.6).

7. **Hofmann bone lever of varying sizes**: These are used for deeper retraction in a perpendicular plane leading to better exposure (Figure 15.7).

8. **Bone curettes of varying sizes**: These are available in various sizes and are used to curette out the marrow or hematoma. They are also used as part of the debridement to clear out the dirt and slough from bone and soft tissues (Figure 15.8).

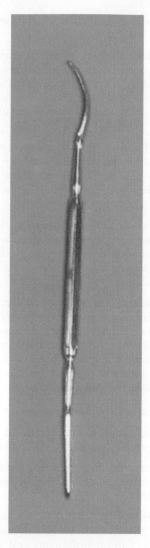

Figure 15.5 McDonald double-ended dissector/elevator.

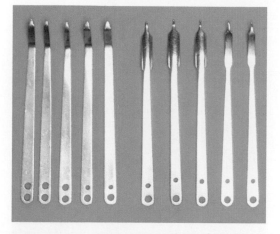

Figure 15.7 Hohmann bone lever of varying sizes.

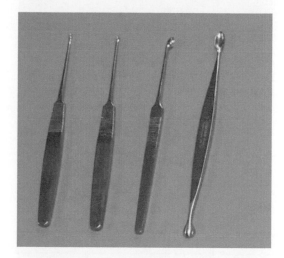

Figure 15.8 Bone curettes of varying sizes.

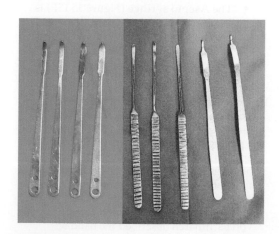

Figure 15.6 Trethowan bone levers.

9. **Mayo Hegar needle holder**: Available in various sizes to hold needles of different sizes to facilitate meticulous suturing of skin and deeper tissues (Figure 15.9).

10. **Suction tip and suction tube**: This is used to drain blood providing a better field of exposure facilitating dissection and avoiding injuries to vital structures (Figure 15.10).

11. **Mono polar cautery**: This electrosurgical unit (ESU) utilizes a high-frequency electric current for cutting, coagulating, desiccating and fulgurating tissues. To achieve these effects, a probe electrode applies the electrosurgical energy to the target tissue. The current then passes through the patient to a return pad and back to the ESU generator to complete the circuit. (Figure 15.11A)

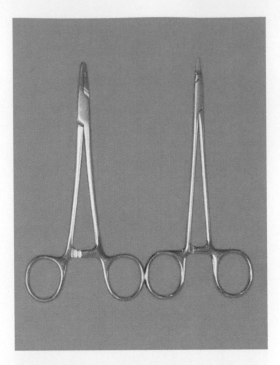

Figure 15.9 Mayo Hegar needle holder.

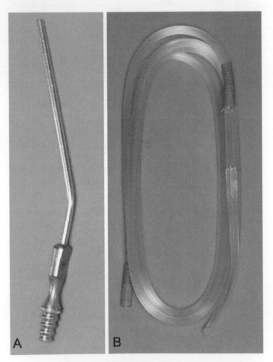

Figure 15.10 A) Suction tip; B) Suction tube.

Bipolar cautery: In contrast, the bipolar ESU uses a set of forceps where the current passes from one side of the forceps through the target tissue to the other side of

the forceps and then back to the generator (Figure 15.11B).

Cautery holder: It is safe to keep the cautery tips in the cautery holder to avoid any inadvertent complications to the patient. It also prevents the cautery from falling off the operating area and becoming unsterile (Figure 15.11C).

12. **Curved and straight artery forceps:** These are used as a hemostat, to facilitate accurate approximation of knots and also in soft tissue dissection around vital structures (Figure 15.12).

13. **Bard packer knife handle with blades:** These are used for making skin incisions and deeper dissections (Figure 15.13). The knife blades come in varying sizes like 10, 11, 15, 22.

14. **Stainless steel wires and twister:** Stainless steel wires are available in sizes 16–24 and used as encirclage wire in small bone fixation and whenever tension band principle is being used (Figure 15.14A). Wire twisters are used to twist the SS wires to achieve adequate tension (Figure 15.14B).

15. **Preparation and debridement set:**

- Towel clips are used to anchor the drapings before surgery (Figure 15.15A).

- Sponge holding forceps is used for painting the limb post scrubbing (Figure 15.15B).

- A kidney tray (Figure 15.15C) and surgical bowl (Figure 15.15D) are used to collect and maintain any grafts (tendon, bone) and also to keep the saline required for debridement.

- The Asepto syringe (Figure 15.15E) is used for wash outs in debridement. The pressure generated by the syringe is adequate to wash out the contaminants without causing damage to viable and vital tissues.

16. **Tourniquet cuff and Eschmarch bandage** The upper limb is exsanguinated using an Eschmarch bandage (Figure 15.16B), and a pneumatic tourniquet (Figure 15.16A) is applied around the upper arm to obtain a bloodless field during surgery. Lister was the first surgeon to use the tourniquet to provide a bloodless field for excision and arthrodesis of the tuberculous wrist joint. Later, Johann von Eschmarch described the bandage made of Indian rubber, which was fastened

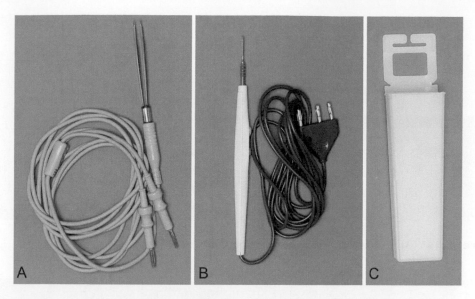

Figure 15.11 A) Monopolar cautery; B) Bipolar cautery; C) Cautery holder.

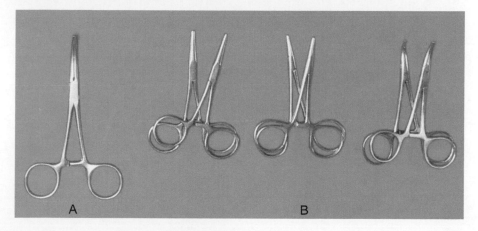

Figure 15.12 A) Curved and B) Straight artery forceps.

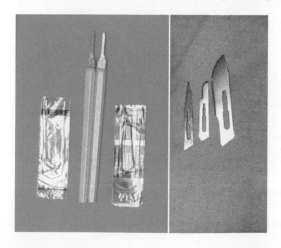

Figure 15.13 Bard packer knife handle with blades of size 11, 15, 22.

by a hook and brass chain. The Eschmarch bandage later came to be used as a tourniquet as well as for exsanguination. Harvey Cushing in 1906 invented the pneumatic tourniquet developing it from the standard Riva Rocci blood pressure apparatus. He initially described its use for craniotomies, but soon it was used for operations for limbs. The width of the cuff should be 20 per cent greater than the diameter of the upper arm, and the pressure should be 50 mm of mercury higher than the systolic pressure. One-and-a-half hours is considered the safe time of inflation, and it should not exceed two hours. In cases where re-inflation is warranted, a minimum gap of 20 minutes is given between the next inflation.

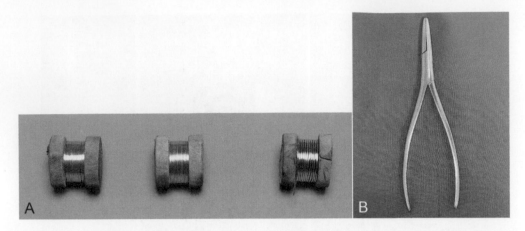

Figure 15.14 A) Stainless steel wires of varying size; B) Wire twister.

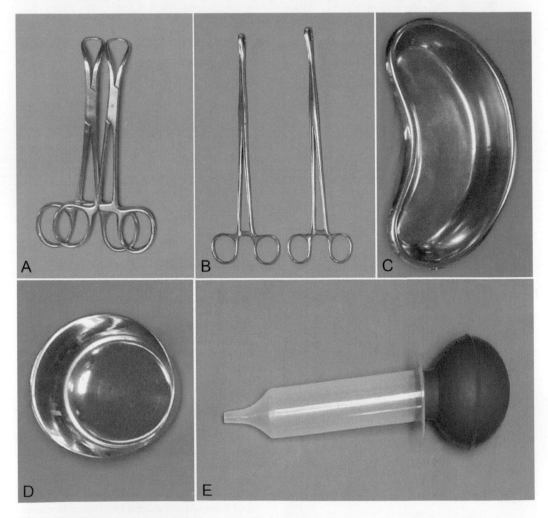

Figure 15.15 A) Towel clips, B) Sponge holding forceps; C) Kidney tray; D) Surgical Bowl; E) Asepto syringe.

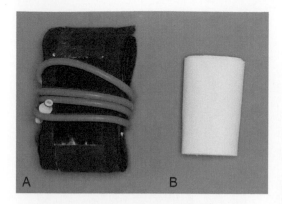

Figure 15.16 A) Tourniquet cuff; B) Eschmarch bandage.

BONE INSTRUMENTS SET

17. **Fine osteotomes of varying size:** These are used for performing osteotomies and smoothening the bone surface. A selection of sharp osteotomies of varying width is necessary to avoid injury to surrounding soft tissue when performing osteotomies of phalanges/metacarpals (Figure 15.17).

18. **Bone cutter and bone nibbler:** The delicate blades of the bone cutter are used to cut the bones precisely without damaging the surrounding tissue. The nibbler is used the nibble the cartilage from bone or fibrous tissue and to freshen the bone edges during fixation (Figure 15.18A,B).

19. **Bone impactor:** These are used to press-fit the cortical or cancellous grafts in the

treatment of fracture non-union like scaphoid or to punch in loose fragments of bone (Figure 15.19).

20. **Bone mallet:** A bone mallet is used along with an osteotome to mallet the bone, to freshen the bone ends before fusion, and for various wedge osteotomies (Figure 15.20).

21. **Periosteum elevator:** The periosteum elevator is used to elevate the periosteum or

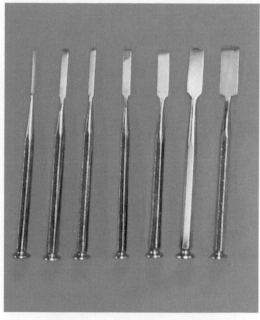

Figure 15.17 Fine osteotomes of varying size.

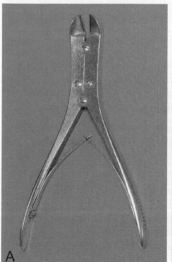
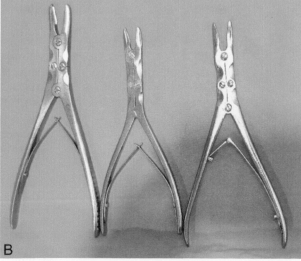

Figure 15.18 A) Bone cutter; B) Bone nibbler.

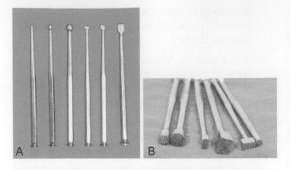

Figure 15.19 A) Bone impactor; B) End on view.

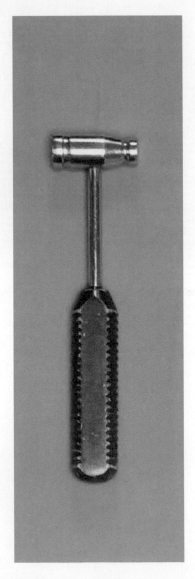

Figure 15.20 Bone mallet.

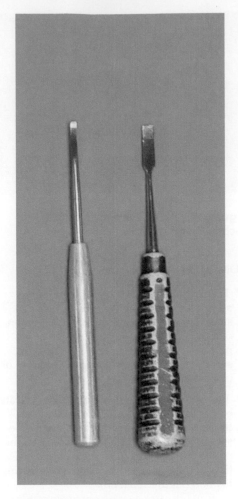

Figure 15.21 Periosteum elevator.

muscle attachments for exposing the bone surface before internal fixation and clearing the soft tissues attached to the bone (Figure 15.21).

22. **Bone awl**: The awl is used for creating an entry point for the intramedullary fixation, specifically in metacarpal fractures to pass the K wires (Figure 15.22).

23. **Bone gouge**: These are used to cut and core out portions of bone, especially cancellous bone used in bone graft harvest (Figure 15.23).

24. **Bone reduction forceps**: These are used in the temporary stabilization of bone fragments during fracture fixation. They are also used to compress fragments during the reduction of fractures (Figure 15.24).

25. **Bone rasp**: These are also known as rotatory files. These are small cutting tools

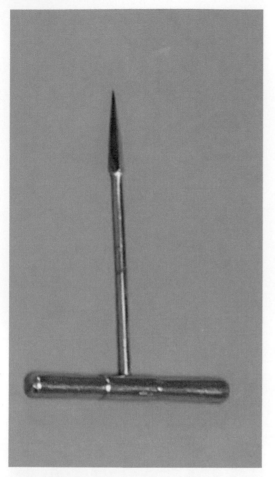

Figure 15.22 Bone awl.

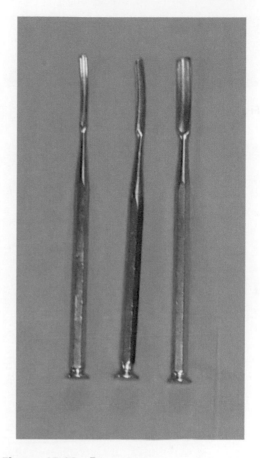

Figure 15.23 Bone gouge.

creating an even bony surface and smoothening sharp edges (Figure 15.25).

26. **Plate/bone holding forceps**: These forceps help in firmly holding the plate to the bone facilitating fracture reduction and screw fixation (Figure 15.26).

27. **Pneumatic oscillating bone saw and drill**: A power saw is used to cut the bone during osteotomies and amputation (Figure 15.27A). A power drill is used to drill the bone for making a pilot hole for applying screws to the plate for fracture stabilization. It is also used to drive K wires and guidewire as a part of internal fixation like cannulated screws and headless screw (Figure 15.27B,C).

28. **Kirschner wire set**: In 1909 Martin Kirschner introduced a smooth pin which is now as Kirschner or K wires. K wires are available in varying sizes ranging

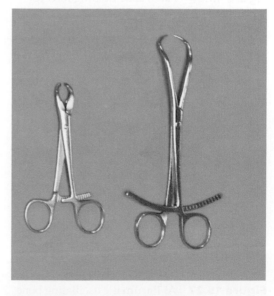

Figure 15.24 Bone reduction forceps.

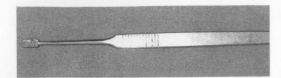

Figure 15.25   Bone rasp.

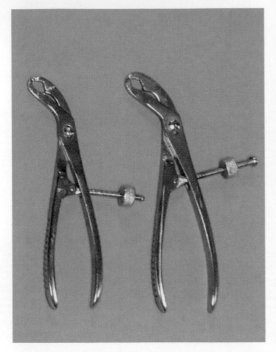

Figure 15.26   Plate/bone holding forceps.

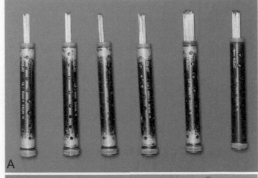

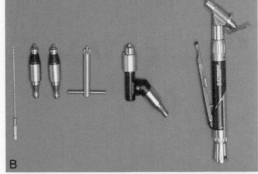

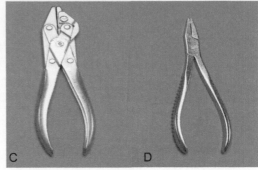

Figure 15.28   A) Kirschner wire sets of various diameters. B) K-wire pen drive and K-wire driver with various couplings. C) K-wire bender; D) K-wire cutter.

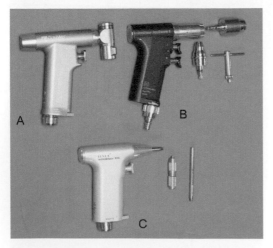

Figure 15.27   A) Pneumatic oscillating bone saw; B) Pneumatic drill; C) Kirschner (K) wire drive.

from 0.9 to 15 mm in diameter (0.035, 0.045, 0.062 inches) (Figure 15.28A), mainly used to fix the bone fragments together. Wires are also of varying lengths which may vary in the end construct. K wire could be a trocar tip, threaded tip or a diamond cut tip. The trocar tip is better suited for penetrating the cortical bone and later able to be braced against the endosteal surface of bone cortex or applicable to lodging in cancellous bone. Some may have one spatulated end without a point. Threaded wires are also available which are referred to as screw tips. These wires are driven

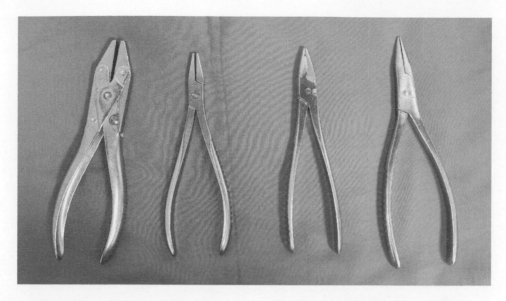

Figure 15.29   Nose pliers of varying size.

into the bone through the skin using a K wire driver. One of the advantages of K wires is the ease of atraumatic percutaneous insertion leading to less damage to soft tissue and tendons. Percutaneous fixation achieves stable fixation after adequate reduction and allows early mobilization thereby avoiding stiffness. Once driven, the wires are bent externally using a wire bender to avoid injury to surrounding structures. This also prevents proximal migration which is considered as one of the complications. Pin tract infection can be prevented by avoiding repeated drilling and optimal pin tract dressing. Burying the wire inside the skin can also be employed and at times requires a secondary procedure to remove them.

K wires are very versatile and are used for definitive fixation in metacarpal and phalangeal fractures which are removed usually after 3–4 weeks. They are also used as intramedullary fixation as a part of the bouquet technique in the case of the 5th metacarpal neck fracture. They are used in distal radius fracture fixation and temporary fixation in complex fractures of upper and lower limbs as well.

K wire driver: K wires are drilled with a dedicated K wire driver for optimal rotations per minute (RPM) and to prevent damage to the underlying structures (Figure 15.28B). The wires are to be bent and cut using a good quality wire bender and

wire cutter for an optimal finish (Figure 15.28C,D).

29. **Nose pliers of varying size**: The pliers are used to remove K wires. They are also used for bending the sharp edge of K wire and SS wire (Figure 15.29).

SKIN GRAFTING SET

In 1936 Humby described a "modified graft cutting razor," discarding the original large frame to steady the skin and returning to a solid blade that required sharpening. This knife had a rod with two screws on the upper surface to control the thickness of the graft and the roller smoothed out the skin in front of the cutting edge. The width of the graft was determined by the pressure on the knife [1] on either side to create a flat surface (Figure 15.30).

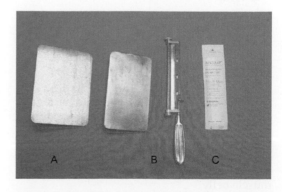

Figure 15.30   A) Spreader; B) Humby's graft handle; C) Blade.

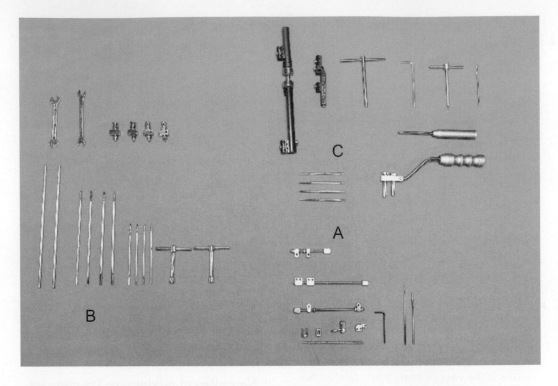

Figure 15.31   A) JESS fixator; B) AO fixator; C) Orthofix fixator.

THE EXTERNAL FIXATOR SYSTEM USED FOR FOREARM AND HAND

- The Joshi external stabilizing system (JESS) is commonly used for hands and includes multiple k wires, distractors, link joints, connecting rods, Z rods, L rods and a J-shaped Allen key (Figure 15.31A).

- When distraction across the wrist is required, an AO external fixator is used with 3/2.5 mm Schanz pins, AO clamps, and connecting rods to form the construct (Figure 15.31B).

- Bone lengthening and fracture fixation systems with a joint are also available with Orthofix fixators (Figure 15.31C).

TENDON SURGERY SET

The tendon stripper (Figure 15.32) and tunneler (Figure 15.33) are used in tendon transfer and grafting surgery. The tendon stripper is used to separate the tendon from its muscle belly. The free end of the tendon is threaded into the sleeve of the tendon stripper and the sleeve gently separates it from the main muscle belly.

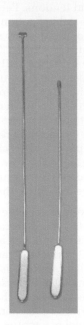

Figure 15.32   Tendon stripper.

The tendon tunneler (Figure 15.33) is used to create a pathway for the donor tendon and the forcep-like end will grasp the tendon and guide it to the recipient tendon in tendon transfers.

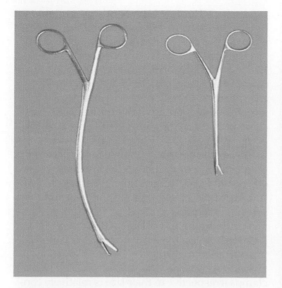

Figure 15.33 Anderson's tendon tunneler.

MICROSURGERY SET

Jassinowski described end-to-end anastomosis of vessels using suture materials, needles and instruments and in the year 1987 Murphy first attempted anastomosis of human vessels.

Microsurgery requires specific instruments to handle delicate vessels without inducing trauma. These instruments are essential right from the dissection of individual vessels from the pedicle to their preparation for anastomosis to an actual anastomosis (Figures 15.34–15.36) [2].

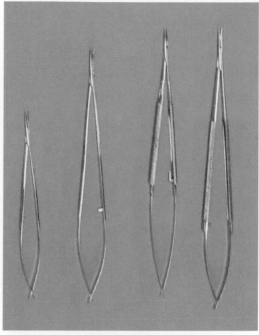

Figure 15.35 Micro scissors.

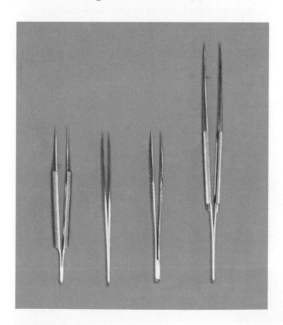

Figure 15.34 Jeweller's forceps.

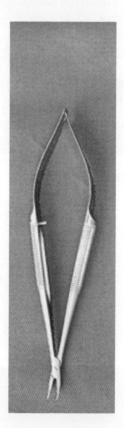

Figure 15.36 Needle holder.

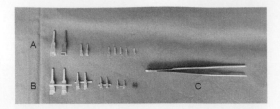

Figure 15.37 A,B) Acland's clamps and C) clamp applicator.

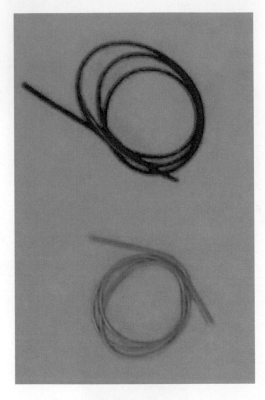

Figure 15.38 Vessel loop.

Jeweler's forceps: Number three straight and fine-tipped forceps are used for holding vessel wall and for tying sutures with the precision of 1/1000th of an inch which is the diameter of 10-0 nylon suture. The tip should be in uniform contact for a length of 3 mm to firmly hold the suture. Angled forceps are also available which facilitate going under the vessels especially branches, tying knots, and checking the patency of vessels (Figure 15.34).

Microscissors: Sharp tipped straight scissors are used for trimming of adventitia and vessel edges and for cutting sutures whereas curved rounded tip sutures are used for dissecting vessels (Figure 15.35).

Needle holder: Available with or without lock for holding the suture needles to avoid uncontrolled movements (Figure 15.36).

Vascular clamps: The pressure exerted by all clamps irrespective of their size is relatively constant which is 5 g/mm² on the largest vessel and 15 g/mm² on the smallest vessel (Figure 15.37A,B).

Single clamps are mainly applied over the proximal vessel when there is a leak after anastomosis that needs to be sealed by another suture (Figure 15.37A).

Double approximator clamps are commonly used to facilitate anastomosis of which Ackland's clamps are commonly used These can be of A and V patterns. V pattern is for all-purpose clamp, used for all veins and most arteries whereas A pattern is mainly for thick-walled vessels (Figure 15.37B).

A clamp applicator is used to open the clamps while adjusting vessel ends during anastomosis (Figure 15.37C).

Vessel loops are used to delineate the vital structures (artery and nerve) following skeletonisation to facilitate easy dissection (Figure 15.38).

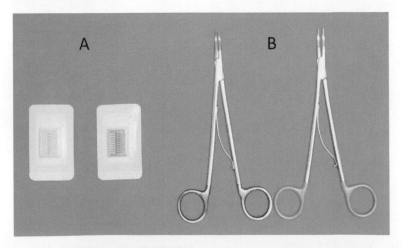

Figure 15.39 A) Liga clip; B) Applicator.

Liga clips and clip applicator are used to seal off the arterial branches and veins to achieve haemostasis (Figure 15.39 A). Liga clips are applied using liga clip applicator (Figure 15.39B).

Surgical loupes: These are divided into Galilean and Prismatic loupes. Galilean loupes use multiple lenses with intervening air spaces which allow an adjustment of magnification and working distance. It is not possible to achieve a high-quality image with Galilean loupes above 3.5 times magnification [3].

Prismatic loupes are optically advanced which are longer and heavier containing Pechan's or Schmidt's prisms with a series of mirror reflections within the loupes providing high resolution throughout the field of vision (Figure 15.40).

WRIST ARTHROSCOPY SET

Yung–Cheng Chen was the first to describe wrist arthroscopy. He used a 1.7 mm arthroscope and carried out procedures through dorsal portals in cadavers and amputated arms [4]. Standard equipment includes a 2.4 mm, 30° angled arthroscope (1.9 and 2.7 mm scopes are also used), a 3 mm hook probe and overhead traction. Instruments that are used in the treatment of intra-articular pathology include a radiofrequency ablation probe and a mechanical shaver. The shaver may be necessary to clear the wrist of synovitis or degenerative soft tissue changes to perform a comprehensive diagnostic evaluation of the wrist (Figures 15.41 and 15.42).

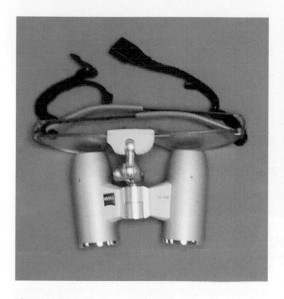

Figure 15.40 Surgical loupe.

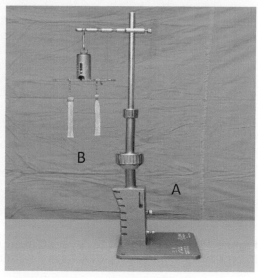

Figure 15.41 Traction tower (A) with Chinese finger traps (B).

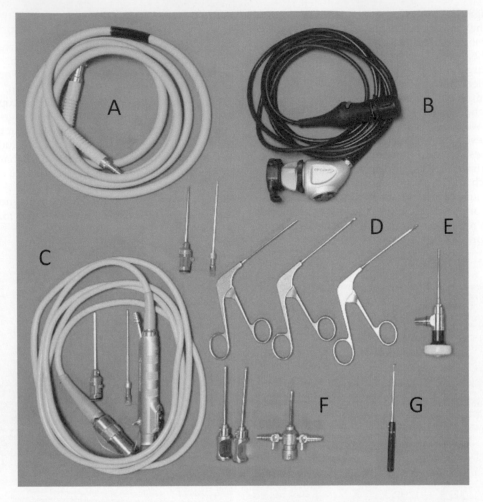

Figure 15.42 Wrist arthroscopy set: Camera (A) with the light source (B), shaver (C), basket forceps and grasping forceps (D), 2.4 mm wrist arthroscope (E), trocar (F) and probe (G).

ENDOSCOPY SET FOR CARPAL TUNNEL RELEASE

In 1987, Okutsu, a Japanese Orthopaedic surgeon, and his colleagues first reported the use of an endoscope to incise the transverse carpal ligament in patients with carpal tunnel syndrome. He developed a system called "The Universal Subcutaneous Endoscopic System" [5].

A 3.0 mm eyepiece endoscope is connected to a standard camera connector and light source [3]. A small hamate finder is used to create a path for the blade assembly. Dilators of various sizes are available for serial dilatation to facilitate the passage of a synovial dissector which has a blade to incise the transverse metacarpal ligament (Figure 15.43).

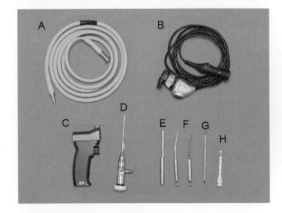

Figure 15.43 Carpal tunnel endoscopy set: A) Light source; B) Camera; C,D) Endoscope with handle; E) Hamate finder; F) Serial dilators; G) Synovial dissector; H) Endoscopy blade.

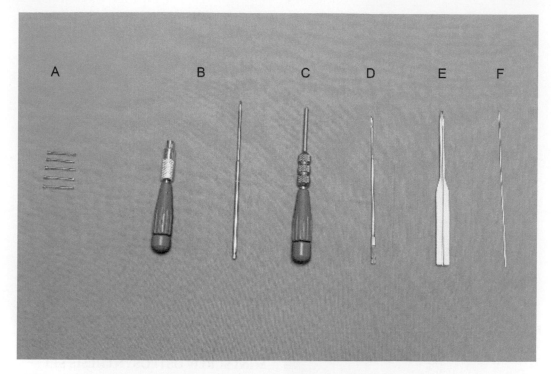

Figure 15.44 Headless compression screw set: A) 2.4 mm self-drilling self-tapping cannulated headless compression screw; B) Cannulated stardrive screwdriver shaft with handle; C) Compression sleeve with handle; D) 2 mm cannulated drill bit; E) Measuring device; F) 1.1 mm guidewire.

HEADLESS COMPRESSION SCREW SET

Headless compression screws are available in 2.4 mm and 3 mm sizes. They consist of a threadless central shaft with threads of differential pitch on either end promoting fracture compression. The proximal threads increase the bone purchase and screws are available in long threaded and short threaded configurations. They are canulated for precise insertion using a guidewire (Figure 15.44). The 2.4 mm screws are indicated for fixation of fracture of scaphoid, phalanges and metacarpals and also non-union of small bones like scaphoid. The 3 mm screws are indicated for fixation of intra-articular fractures.

LOCKING COMPRESSION PLATE SET FOR DISTAL RADIUS FRACTURE

The locking nature of the distal radius screw plate construct gives the extra edge in case of bone defects, comminution and osteoporotic bone and facilitates an early range of motion. The locking plates also provide indirect reduction of the distal fragment thereby achieving the necessary parmal tilt.

Distal radius locking compression plates (LCP) are available as volar and dorsal plates.

With the advent of a new fixed angle screw plate design, volar fixation has become the standard approach for intra-articular distal radius fractures. Also, dorsal plate complications such as stiffness and tendon attritions are relatively less.

Volar plates fall into four main categories [6]:

1) Buttress plates.

2) Fixed angle locking plates.

3) Poly axial locking plates.

4) Fragment specific plates.

Volar buttress plates are traditional plates used to treat shear fractures with no communition.

Fixed angle locking plates lock at a fixed trajectory. The locking screws provide good subchondral support and allow the direct purchase of bone fragments.

A 2.4 system of fixed angle LCP is commonly used.

A 1.8 mm drill bit is used for the threaded hole for locking screws and a 2.4 mm drill bit for the gliding hole in case of cortical screws. 2.4 mm locking screws are commonly used in the distal portion of dorsal or volar plates and

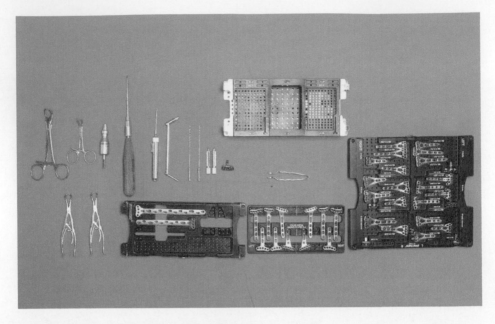

Figure 15.45 Distal radius fracture fixation set.

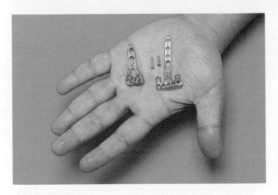

Figure 15.46 Distal radius plates: Variable angle LCP and 2.4 system two column volar distal radius plates.

2.4 mm locking or 2.4 mm cortical screws in the shaft of dorsal or volar plates (Figures 15.45 and 15.46).

Poly axial locking plates have the additional advantage of matching the distal fixation to variable geometry and surface contour of the distal radius. Here each intra articular fragment can be addressed independently. These plates usually have a thicker profile and tend to be prominent and it is here where the concept of placing the plate proximal to watershed line comes into play.

Fragment specific plates are designed to independently address each major fracture component. They have the added advantage of providing increased rigidity by placing the contract in the orthogonal plane.

MINI SCREW OSTEOSYNTHESIS SET

A mini screw osteosynthesis set (Figures 15.47 and 15.48) consists of plates of various shapes with a mini screw set.

They are available as LCP Compact Hand 1.0, 1.3, 1.5, 2.0 & 2.4.

They are used in the fixation of small fragments, avulsion fractures and fractures of distal and middle phalanges. They are used for arthrodesis of the phalanges and metacarpals. They are also used for fractures of the phalanges, metacarpals, wrist bones and arthrodesis of the interphalangeal joints (Figure 15.46).

The plates are available in various configurations such as

1) Low profile plates with fully countersunk screws.

2) Anatomically pre-contoured.

3) Rotation correction plate.

4) LCP combi-hole.

This table depicts an overview of the screws available and drill bit used:

Screw size(in mm)	Drill Bit Cancellous/Cortical
1.3	1/1.3
1.5	1.1/1.5
2	1.5/2
2.4	1.8/2

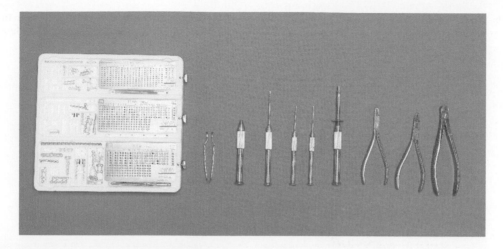

Figure 15.47 Mini screw osteosynthesis set.

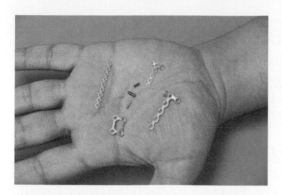

Figure 15.48 Mini plates for metacarpals and phalangeal fractures.

SUTURE ANCHORS

The bioabsorbable suture anchors are now made either of Poly-L-lactic acid, Poly-L/D-lactic acid (PLDLA), poly (lactide-co-glycolide) or a combination of these polymers (Figure 15.49).

Braided polyester sutures (e.g. Ethibond) were widely used in the past but improved, stronger suture materials, such as Fiberwire, made of ultrahigh molecular weight polyethylene (UHMWPE) are now available. The Orthocord suture is made of a UHMWPE sleeve and a polydioxanone (PDS) core with polyglactin 910 coating is also available [7].

In the wrist, suture anchors can be used for scapholunate and lunotriquetral ligament repair, as well as for triangular fibrocartilage repair. Suture anchors are also used in the repair of ulnar collateral ligament injuries of the thumb, as well as collateral ligament injuries of the finger metacarpophalangeal and interphalangeal joints. Ruptures of the flexor digitorum profundus tendon are commonly repaired using suture anchors.

REFERENCES

1. Ameer F, Singh AK and Kumar S. Evolution of instruments for the harvest of skin grafts. *Indian J Plast Surg.* 2013; 46:28–35.

2. Acland RD and Sabapathy SR. *Acland's Practice Manual for Microvascular Surgery*, 3rd edition. 2008.

3. Mohan R. Magnification tools: Surgical operating microscope and magnifying loupe in dental practice. *Int J Eng Res Tech.* 2013; 2:14–22.

4. Michelotti BF and Chung KC. Diagnostic wrist arthroscopy. *Hand Clin.* 2017 Nov; 33(4):571–583.

5. Bhat AK, Acharya AM, Mane PP, Babu S and Madi S. Our experience in first 100 cases of endoscopic carpal tunnel release: An Indian perspective. *J Arthrosc Joint Surg.* 2018; 5(1):51–55.

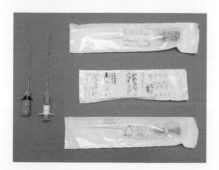

Figure 15.49 Suture anchors.

6. Loisel F, Kielwasser H, Faivre G, Rondot T, Rochet S, Adam A, Sergent P, Leclerc G, Obert L and Lepage D. Treatment of distal radius fractures with locking plates: an update. *Eur J Orthop Surg Traumatol*. 2018 Dec; 28(8):1537–1542.

7. Wiedrich TS. The use of suture anchors in the hand and wrist. *Oper Tech Plast Reconstr Surg*. 1997; 4(1):42–48.

16 Radiology of the Wrist and Hand

Anil K Bhat, Ashwath M Acharya and Mithun Pai G

CONTENTS

INTRODUCTION

When Wilhelm Conrad Rontgen created the radiograph of his wife Anna Bertha's hand in December 1895, the history of radiography and imaging of hand and wrist was born. Its first clinical application was also to detect pathology of the wrist, that is, Colles' fracture a year later. From a 20 minutes' exposure needed at that time for a radiograph to milliseconds exposure now, and from a plain radiograph to advanced imaging techniques available today, the understanding of hand and wrist imaging has leapt many folds [1].

16 projections of the wrist have been proposed by Graziani, in 1940, for its evaluation [2]. There has been addition of numerous other projections to increase the diagnostic accuracy which would further add to the complexity of topic The diagnostic modalities for hand and

wrist pathologies have attained rapid advancement over a decade. Despite these advancements, the humble radiograph remains the single most important imaging modality for hand and wrist. The wrist is a compact structure composed of eight carpal bones packed together in a relatively small space, which makes reading the wrist X-ray a daunting task but an interesting exercise worth mastering to minimise the use of costlier investigations. This conventional technique produces a two-dimensional representation of three-dimensional anatomical data on a photographic film. This is achieved by two views projected perpendicular to one another to obtain a three- dimensional perspective. Majority of the basic information could be obtained by the two standard projections of the wrist, i.e. the postero anterior (PA) and the lateral views, which would help

DOI: 10.1201/9781003125938-20

in diagnosing many clinical conditions. The special views are taken following a detailed history and clinical examination for specific clinical conditions Hence, an appropriate combination of these views will help the clinician better analyse the underlying pathology in the preliminary stages of investigations.

As mentioned earlier, standard projections for the wrist are posteroanterior and lateral views. Some authors also consider the oblique view as part of the standard views. The following section of this chapter describes the standard radiographic views first and proceeds to describe any ancillary views of the same and finally, dynamic studies using these projections.

POSTEROANTERIOR VIEW

The posteroanterior (PA) projection is obtained with the shoulder abducted 90° from the trunk. The elbow is flexed at 90° with the ulna perpendicular to the humerus and forearm in a pronated position (Figure 16.1). The wrist should be in a neutral position with no flexion, extension, or deviation. The hand should be palm down on the cassette with fingers extended.

In a true PA view of the wrist [3],

a) The ulnar styloid appears in its full profile on the medial most edge of the ulna head.

b) The extensor carpi ulnaris groove [4] (Figure 16.2) is radial to ulnar styloid and is well seen.

c) More than one half of lunate is in contact with the distal radius articular surface.

d) Second to fifth carpometacarpal joints are clearly visible.

e) The scaphoid ring occupies distal one-third of the scaphoid and is clear in its outline.

If the X-ray is taken in supination which is position of the forearm in an AP view

a) The ulnar styloid is seen in line with the pisiform at the middle of the ulnar head

The following characteristic features are also noted in the PA view.

1. The stability of the wrist is determined by the alignment and relationship between the carpal bones concerning each other. This can be assessed using the three principles as stated by *Gilula* which are *Arcs [5], spaces, and parallelism* (Figure 16.3)

The *arcs forming* the articular surfaces of the carpal bones should be parallel(*parallelism*), and the space between the joints should be about 2 mm wide (*spaces*). Any change in joint space or the shape of a carpal bone may indicate instability, subluxation, or dislocation.

Arcs of Gilula: These are drawn on the neutral PA view along the radiocarpal and midcarpal joints. Any discontinuity noted in the three arcs suggests carpal malalignment:

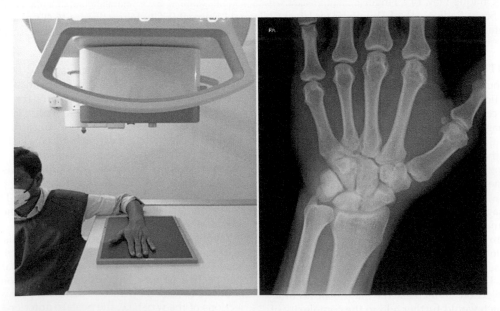

Figure 16.1 Posteroanterior view. The central beam is aligned vertically over a radial styloid 100 cm from the film.

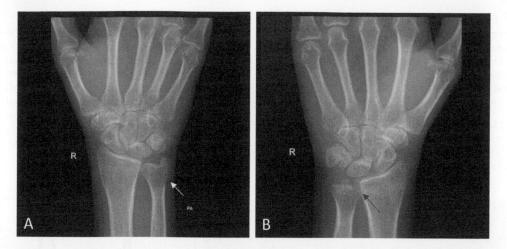

Figure 16.2 Comparison between the PA and AP views of the wrist. In the former, the ulnar styloid is seen arising from the most medial aspect of the ulna, and the ECU groove (yellow arrow) is radial to the ulnar styloid. In the latter (AP view), however, the ulnar styloid lies over the mid part of the ulnar head (red arrow).

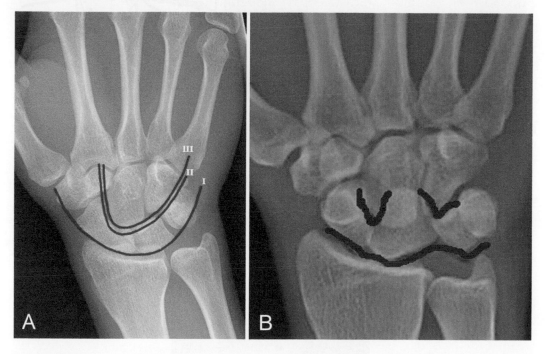

Figure 16.3 X-ray showing the Arc of Gilula (A) and its disruption (B) as seen in perilunate dislocation.

a) Arc along the proximal surfaces of the scaphoid, lunate, and triquetrum forming the proximal border of proximal carpal row.
b) Arc along the distal surface of the above mentioned carpal bones.
c) Arc along the the curvature of the capitate and hamate proximal surfaces forming the proximal border of distal carpal row.

The arcs do not apply to trapezium, trapezoid, and pisiform as they are overlapping structures on PA view [6]. Pathologies like perilunate dislocation or carpal instability can be diagnosed based on the continuity of these arcs.

2. **Scapholunate gap (S-L gap)**: The gap is measured at the centre of the scaphoid and lunate articulation (Figure 16.4). It can be diagnosed in either AP or PA views with the beam angled from the dorsal aspect of the wrist. Normally the S-L distance is about 2 mm[6].

3. **Ulnar variance**: Ulnar variance also known as Hulten line [2] is distance between line along the distal articular surface of the radius towards the ulna and the line along the distal articular surface of the ulna (Figure 16.5). It is a measures of the realtive postion of the radius and ulna distal articular surface. Neutral ulnar variance indicate that both articular surfaces are at the same level, positive indicate ulna being more distal and negative indicates that ulna is more proximal to the radius. Positive ulnar variance is associated with an ulnar abutment, and negative ulnar variance is thought to be associated with Kienbock's disease.

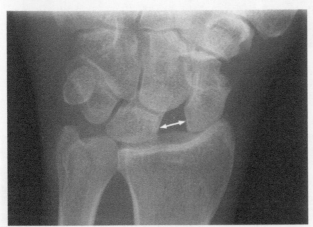 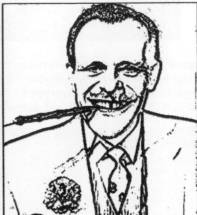

Figure 16.4 X-ray showing an increase in scapholunate space, the classical Terry Thomas sign named after a British comedian who had a gap between the front two teeth.

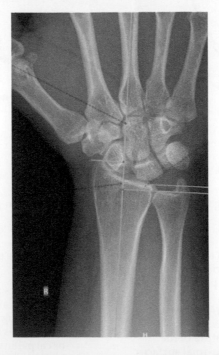

Figure 16.5 X-ray showing the assessment of ulnar variance with the methodology.

The ulnar variance depends on the elbow position during radiography which should be at shoulder height. If the elbow is kept lower than the shoulder height, the ECU groove overlaps the ulnar styloid. More adduction of the elbow towards the patient's side will make the ulna more positive. Hence, ulnar variance measurements should be done when the ECU groove [4] is in its proper place.

4. **Radial inclination**: It is an angle suspended by line along the distal radius articular surface with the line perpendicular to the shaft of the radius and varies between 20–23° (Figure 16.6). The radial inclination is one of the parameters which requires correction in distal radius fracture. Increased radial inclination leads to increased load over lunate and is associated with Kienbock's disease [6].

5. **Radial height**: It is measured as a distance between a line passing through the distal tip of the radial styloid perpendicular to long axis of the radius and a line drawn by intersecting the articular surface of the head of ulna (Figure 16.7). The normal range

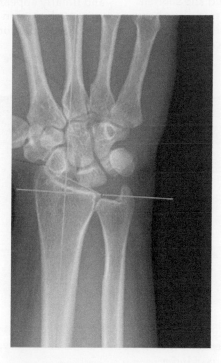

Figure 16.6 X-ray showing assessment of radial inclination with the methodology.

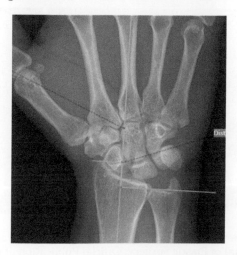

Figure 16.7 X-ray showing assessment of Radial height with the methodology

of radial height is 11-13mm. Radial height is one of the important parameters which needs to be restored in distal radius fracture fixation.

ANCILLARY PA VIEWS
Radiocarpal Joint View

This is a PA view obtained by angulating the beam by 25–30° towards the elbow, centred just distal to Lister's tubercle to better visualise radiocarpal articulation (Figure 16.8). This view will elongate the scaphoid and shorten the capitate and demonstrate minimum bony overlap with parallelism at the radiocarpal joint and provide more details of scaphoid abnormalities [1].

Dorsal Tilt View

This is a PA view with the central beam angled 25–30° towards the fingers, centred on the Capitate (Figure 16.9). This is useful when there is a suspicion of capitate waist fracture, as here, the capitate is elongated, and the scaphoid is foreshortened [1].

DYNAMIC PA VIEWS
PA in Ulnar Deviation

As the wrist is placed in ulnar deviation (Figure 16.10), the scaphoid rotates dorsally and ulnarly appearing elongated. This elongated position of the scaphoid allows for **easier detection of scaphoid fractures** [6]. The scaphoid can also be brought out to length much more by extending the wrist by

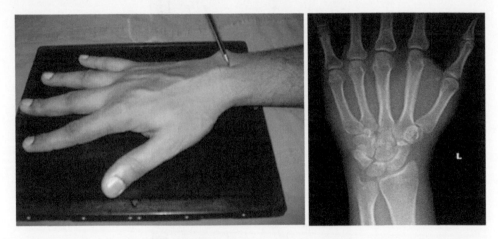

Figure 16.8 Radiocarpal joint view. The central beam is angled 25–30° towards the elbow, centred just distal to Lister's tubercle. © Indian Journal of Plastic Surgery: Official Publication of the Association of Plastic Surgeons of India

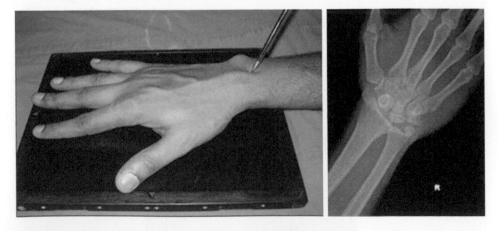

Figure 16.9 Dorsal tilt view. The central beam is angled 25–30° towards fingers, centred on the capitate. © Indian Journal of Plastic Surgery: Official Publication of the Association of Plastic Surgeons of India

20° or by angling the beam towards the wrist by 20°.

PA in Radial Deviation

Palmar flexion of the proximal carpal row occurs, and the distal pole of the scaphoid rotates into the palm as the wrist is radially deviated (Figure 16.11). This causes the normal scaphoid to appear foreshortened and exhibit a ring-like appearance (cortical ring) of its distal pole as the distal aspect of the scaphoid is seen end on. This view is used to visualise the ulnar-sided carpal interspaces. If the same view is taken with the wrist and hand resting on the ulnar surface by tilting 30° oblique and wrist

in maximum radial deviation, it becomes a PA radial flexion oblique view. This is an additional view for occult scaphoid fractures [1].

LATERAL VIEW

The lateral view (Figure 16.12) is critical in assessing the intercarpal alignment and instability. It is obtained with the elbow flexed to 90° and adducted against the trunk. The forearm should be mid prone, and the wrist should be in a neutral position. In the resulting radiograph, a straight line can be drawn through the axes of radius, lunate, capitate, and third metacarpal, or they should be coaxial within 10°. However, the range of capito-lunate angle is given to be 0–30°.

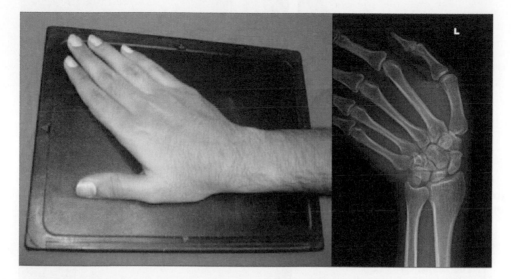

Figure 16.10 PA with ulnar deviation. The central beam is angled 20° longitudinal with the forearm, centred at the midcarpal region. © Indian Journal of Plastic Surgery: Official Publication of the Association of Plastic Surgeons of India

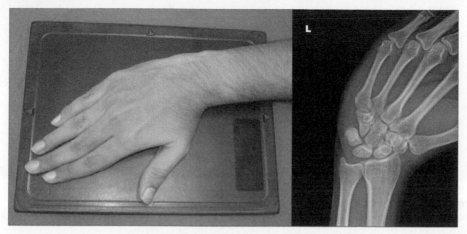

Figure 16.11 PA in radial deviation. The central beam is angled 20° longitudinal with the forearm, centred at the midcarpal region. © Indian Journal of Plastic Surgery: Official Publication of the Association of Plastic Surgeons of India

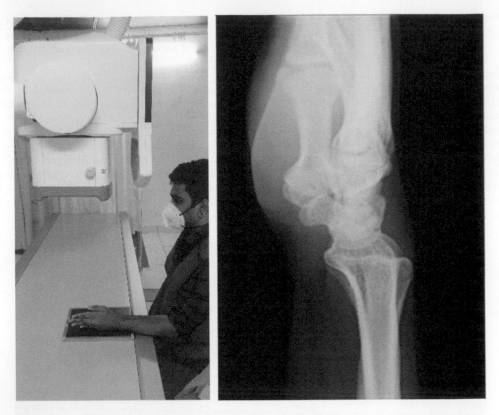

Figure 16.12 Lateral view: The central beam is aligned vertically over the radial styloid 100 cm from the film.

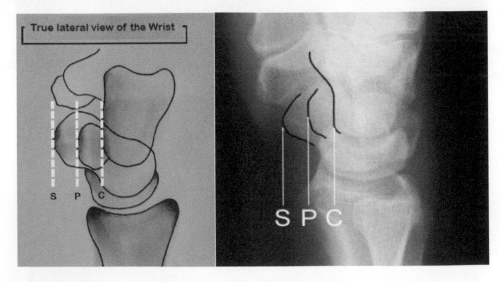

Figure 16.13 A true lateral view of the wrist as indicated by the position of the pisiform between the scaphoid and the capitate. The palmar cortex of the pisiform (P) lies midway between the palmar cortex of the capitate (C) and the scaphoid (S): SPC lateral.

The following features are to be noted in the lateral view.

a) The position of the scaphoid, pisiform and capitate tell us whether there was any wrist pronation or supination. In this view, the line of sight is when the palmar margin of the pisiform is projected midway between the palmar margins of the distal pole of the scaphoid and the capitate head. This is called **SPC lateral** [6] (Figure 16.13). More the supination of the wrist, more the pisiform projects palmar to the scaphoid. The lunate also falsely appears abnormally tilted dorsally. It is also to be borne in mind that evaluation of the position of the ulna with respect to the dorsal surface of radius is not an adequate standard to determine the true lateral view.

b) **The pronator fat pad** on the volar aspect of the distal radius. Subtle fractures of the distal radius can cause displacement or obliteration of the fat plane [2, 6] (Figure 16.14).

c) **Palmar tilt of distal radius**: It is an angle suspended by a line joining the volar & dorsal border of distal radius to the line drawn perpendicular to the long axis of the radius. The normal value is around 11–23° towards the palmar side in normal individuals (Figure 16.15). The dorsal angulation caused by the fracture in distal radius leads to loss of palmar tilt which needs to be restored [2].

d) **Teardrop angle**: Teardrop denotes the shape of the volar rim of the distal radius lunet facet. The teardrop angle is suspeded between a line through the central axis of the teardrop and a line through the central axis of the radius [3] (Figure 16.16).

The normal angle is around 45–70°. This angle is reduced to less than 45° in facture involving lunate fossa and also in di punch fracture of distal radius. Restoration of the teardrop angle needs accurate reduction and appropriate fixation of the ulnar die-punch fragment.

e) **Scapholunate angle**: The scapholunate angle denotes the angle suspended between the scaphoid and lunate in the lateral view. Normal angle ranges from 30–60°. The angle is suspended between the long axis of the lunate and the tangential line drawn connecting the volar tips of the proximal and distal poles of the scaphoid. This line is said to parallel the central axis of the scaphoid. The long axis of the lunate is perpendicular to the line connecting the palmar and dorsal distal articular tips of the lunate (Figure 16.17).

An angle of more than 60° indicates that the scaphoid is flexed indicating a DISI (dorsal intercalated segmental instability) deformity known to occur in scapholunate ligament injury. An angle of less than 30°

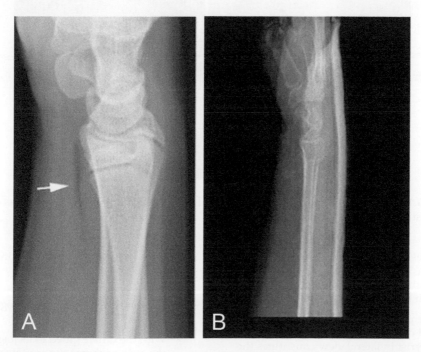

Figure 16.14 X-ray depicting the pronator fat pad (A), which can get obliterated in subtle distal radius fracture (B).

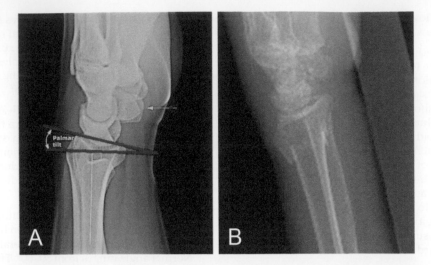

Figure 16.15 Normal volar or palmar tilt (A) of the distal radius articular surface with loss of palmar tilt seen in distal radius fracture (B).

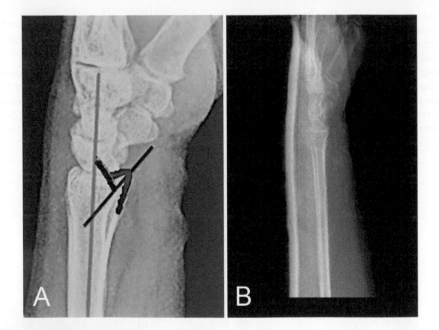

Figure 16.16 Normal teardrop angle of the distal radius articular surface (A) and loss of teardrop in distal radius fracture (B).

indicates that the scaphoid is extended indicating a VISI (volar intercalated segmental inostability) deformity which is known to occur in lunotriquetral ligament injuries [5].

f) **Lunate pathologies:** In the columnar concept of the wrist, the central column of the wrist in lateral view constitutes the third metacarpal, capitate, lunate and distal radius in single straight longitudinal axis (Figure 16.18 A).

The position of the lunate in this central column describes various pathological terminologies [5].

• With the lunate glued to its fossa in the radius wheras the capitate with other carpal bones move out of the axis

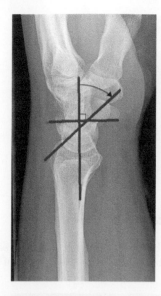

Figure 16.17 depicting the normal scapholunate angle.

describes the Peri-lunate dislocation (Figure 16.18 B,C).

- The lunate is dislocated out of this longitudinal axis which is classically described as spilled teapot sign is seen in lunate dislocation (Figure 16.18D).

ANCILLARY LATERAL VIEWS

a) **Carpal boss view or off-lateral view**: This lateral view is taken with the ulnar side of the wrist resting on the cassette, in minimal ulnar deviation and 30° supination. The central beam passes tangent to the dorsal prominence (Figure 16.19).

This view shows the dorsal carpal boss on a tangent. It enables distinction of (1) a separate os styloideum; (2) a bony prominence attached to the second or third metacarpal base or apposing surface of the trapezoid or capitate bones; (3) degenerative osteophytes; and (4) a fracture of the dorsal prominence of the second or third metacarpal [1].

b) **Lateral scaphoid view**: This is the same as the standard lateral view except that the wrist is kept in a 30° extension, and the beam is centred on the waist of the scaphoid (Figure 16.20). The distal pole and waist of the scaphoid are visualised.

DYNAMIC LATERAL VIEW

Lateral Flexion and Extension View

In these views, the central beam is directed perpendicular to the film and centred on the waist of the scaphoid. The wrist should be in the true lateral position on both radiographs. The extension and flexion of the wrist(maximum) are recognised by observation of the long axis of the third metacarpal extended dorsally (Figure 16.21) and flexed volar (Figure 16.22), respectively, relative to the long axis of the radius and ulna. These views demonstrate extension and flexion at the radiocarpal and midcarpal joints in normal wrists and can be further used to evaluate carpal instability patterns. In particular, these views can assist in distinguishing between a true instability pattern versus normal variance.

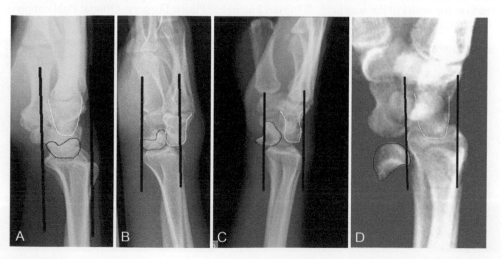

Figure 16.18 (A,B,C,D) Showing the profile of the carpal bones in the lateral view and the common disruption patterns.

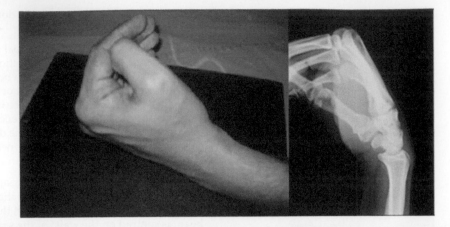

Figure 16.19 Carpal boss view. The central beam passes through or tangent to the dorsal prominence. © Indian Journal of Plastic Surgery: Official Publication of the Association of Plastic Surgeons of India

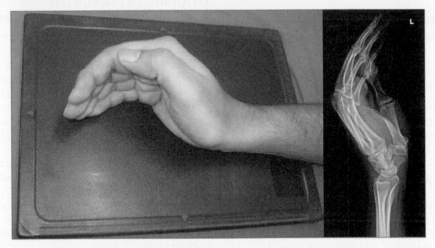

Figure 16.20 Lateral scaphoid view. The central beam is directed perpendicular to the film and centred on the waist of the scaphoid. © Indian Journal of Plastic Surgery: Official Publication of the Association of Plastic Surgeons of India

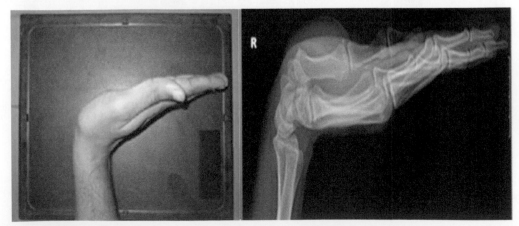

Figure 16.21 Lateral extension view. © Indian Journal of Plastic Surgery: Official Publication of the Association of Plastic Surgeons of India

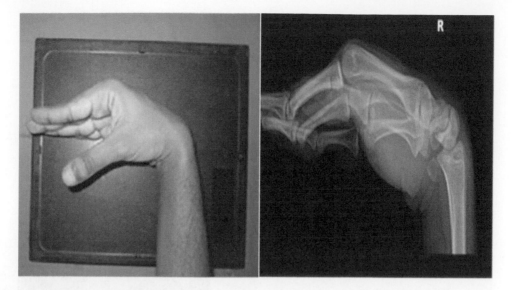

Figure 16.22 Lateral flexion view. © Indian Journal of Plastic Surgery: Official Publication of the Association of Plastic Surgeons of India

Oblique View

The oblique view uniquely reveals abnormalities and aids in better interpretation by increasing the confidence of the final radiographic diagnosis. This view is classically obtained by pronating the wrist by 45° from the lateral position (Figure 16.23) and can be made easy for the patient by using a step wedge to steady the wrist and hand. The oblique view is particularly useful in evaluating the wrist's radial corner, including the base of the thumb and the scapho-trapezio-trapezoidal joint. It also provides an additional view for scaphoid tuberosity and waist when the ulnar deviation is added to the same view. It also shows dorsal triquetral margin fractures.

ANCILLARY OBLIQUE VIEWS

a) **Semi supination oblique view (pisiform, pisotriquetral view) (Figure 16.24):** The pisiform, palmar aspect of triquetrum, palmar ulnar surface of the hamate, and pisotriquetral joint are better visualised by this view which is taken by seating the patient as in for lateral view. The wrist is supinated until it forms an angle of 45° from the true lateral position. The synonymous names for

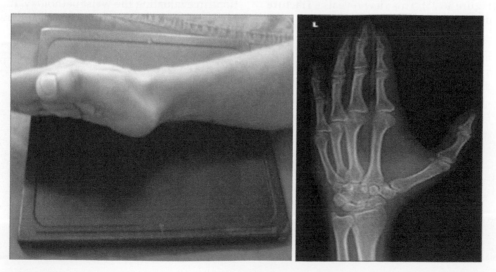

Figure 16.23 Oblique view of the wrist. © Indian Journal of Plastic Surgery: Official Publication of the Association of Plastic Surgeons of India

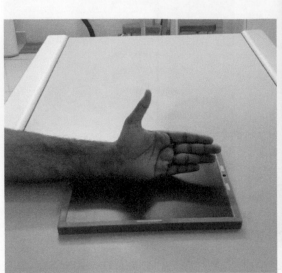

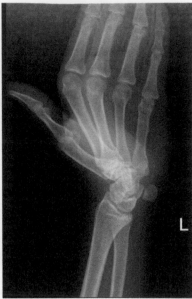

Figure 16.24 Semi supination oblique view.

this view include the Norgaard view, the ball catcher's view, or the "You are in good hands with Allstate" view [6].

The Norgaard view is optimal for evaluating early erosive changes in the hands and wrist of patients with inflammatory arthritis.

b) **Semi oblique lateral view (radial deviated, thumb abducted lateral view):** Here, the patient's wrist is in maximal radial deviation and thumb in maximum abduction. The forearm is kept at 45° supinations (Figure 16.25). This view reveals a **fracture of the hook of hamate**.

c) **Axial oblique view:** Also known as trapezium view where the thumb in kept in radial abduction laterally on cassette. The X-ray beam is kept perpendicular to the cassette aligned to the distal third of the carpus (Figure 16.26). The trapezium and trapezoid bones are clearly seen in its full profile useful in diagnosing the metacarpal base fracture and first CMC joint arthritis.

ANTEROPOSTERIOR VIEW

The anteroposterior or AP view or supinated view (Figure 16.27) has its specific applications in evaluating the wrist pathology. It profiles the scapholunate and lunotriquetral

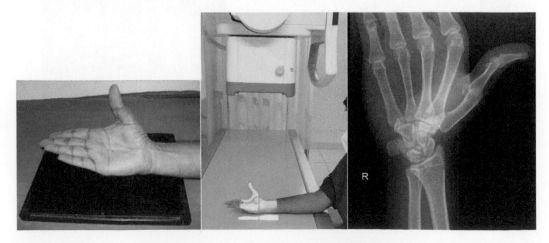

Figure 16.25 Semi oblique lateral view. The central beam is centred on the web space between the thumb and the index finger.

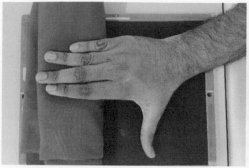
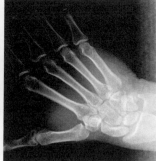

Figure 16.26   Axial oblique view.

carpal interspaces best and hence, is used in evaluating them. It is also used when the patient cannot pronate, and fingers cannot be fully extended. The dorsum of the wrist and hand are flat against the film, and the beam is centred over the capitate head. In the AP view, the ulnar styloid projects from the centre of the ulnar head, which has been described earlier.

DYNAMIC AP VIEW (CLENCHED FIST VIEW, CARPAL COMPRESSION OR POWER GRIP VIEW)

The AP view can be used dynamically (Figure 16.28) by asking the patient to clench the fist actively when the film is taken. This will demonstrate any scapholunate diastasis effectively. The clenched fist creates enough forces of the contracting muscles to drive the capitate towards the scapholunate joint and bring out the diastasis in a dynamic mode. It is best taken of both the wrists together in both

AP and PA (Figure 16.29) projection to compare and contrast if the other wrist is considered normal [5, 6].

The clinical correlation of pain and tenderness at the scapholunate joint should guide the radiographic evidence as wrists with lax ligaments can show the widening on routine radiographs. It is prudent to obtain both wrists radiograph as it is a comparative measurement of SL space.

- Compare the width of the adjacent capitolunate joint to provide a reference.

- The third CMC joint should also be looked at to see its profiling. If the CMC joints are not profiled, the wrist was in extension or flexion, and the scapholunate width measurement is inaccurate. This is because the scapholunate joint is wider at the dorsal and palmar portions than the central portion.

- Lastly, both AP and PA clenched fist views are to be taken when suspecting

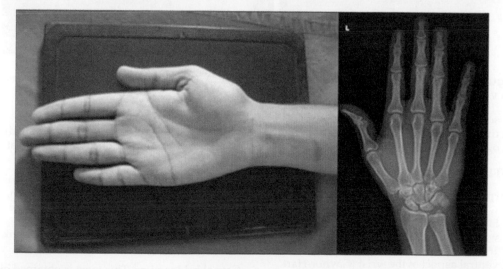

Figure 16.27   Anteroposterior view. © Indian Journal of Plastic Surgery: Official Publication of the Association of Plastic Surgeons of India

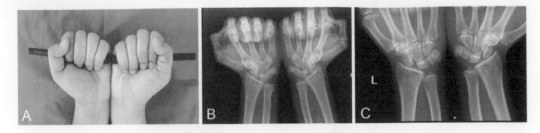

Figure 16.28 Anteroposterior clenched fist view. The central beam is directed perpendicularly at the level of the midcarpal region (A and B), scapholunte gap noted in a AP view (C).

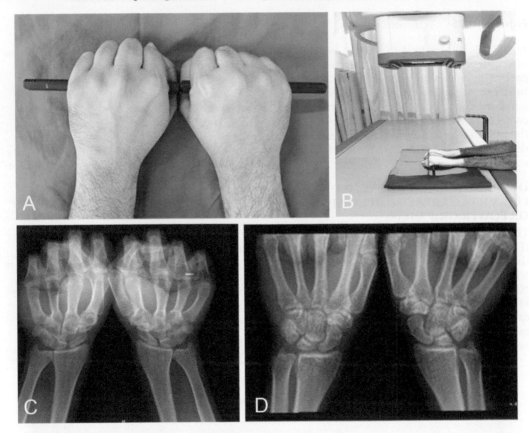

Figure 16.29 Dynamic PA view (clenched fist view). (A, B and C) with scapholunate gap seen in PA view (D).

scapholunate instability strongly, as sometimes the PA view might show the pathology rather than the AP view.

OTHER SPECIAL VIEWS

Carpal tunnel view: This view is obtained with the wrist in dorsiflexion, and the hand is hyperextended by grasping the fingers with the other hand by the patient (Figure 16.30A,B). Another method is placing the ventral aspect of the wrist (Gaynor-Hart method) or the palm on the film cassette (Figure 16.30C). The beam is angled to

profile the carpal tunnel by directing it along the volar aspect to a point 2.5 cm distal to the base of the fourth metacarpal at an angle of 25^0-$30°$ to the long axis [1].

This view shows the palmar soft tissues and the palmar aspects of the trapezium, scaphoid tuberosity, capitate, hook of the Hamate, triquetrum and the entire pisiform. Mainly useful identifying in a hook of hamate fracture.

Carpal bridge view: This view is obtained by placing the dorsum of the wrist on the film and palmar flexing the wrist by 90° approximately (Figure 16.31). The beam is angulated by 45° in a supero inferior direction towards the wrist. There is a tangential view of the dorsal aspect of the scaphoid, lunate, and triquetrum on a properly taken view. The superimposed capitate should be visible. This view helps in evaluating dorsal surface fractures of the scaphoid and dorsal fractures of other carpal bones, lunate dislocation and also demonstrates calcifications and foreign bodies in the dorsal soft tissues.

Brewerton view:

With the MCP joints flexed to 65°, the dorsum of the fingers is placed in contact with the cassette. The central beam is directed at an angle of 15° ulnar to radial at the apex of the web space. The angulated beam helps in clearly visualising the head of the second metacarpal [6] (Figure 16.32). This view is useful in diagnosing metacarpal heads pathologies, especially in patients with rheumatoid arthritis (Figure 16.32).

RADIOLOGY FOR SUSPECTED SCAPHOID FRACTURE [6]

Scaphoid, being an obliquely placed bone in the wrist, is not visualised easily in the standard PA and lateral views, and hence, additional views may be required.

Whenever there is a clinical suspicion of scaphoid fracture, one should ask for four standard views: posteroanterior (PA) with ulnar deviation of the wrist (A), lateral (B), semi pronated or 45° pronation oblique views (C) and semi supinated oblique views (D) (Figure 16.33).

The PA and lateral view help study the proximal pole, waist, and full length of the scaphoid. The 45° semi pronated oblique view helps to study the distal pole along with the STT joint. The 45° semi supinated oblique view helps to study the scaphoid's proximal pole and assess the flexion deformity seen in scaphoid non-union.

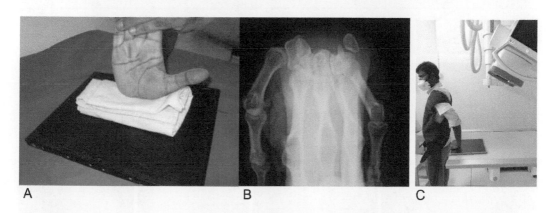

Figure 16.30   The classical Carpal tunnel view (A,B) and the Gaynor-Hart method (C).

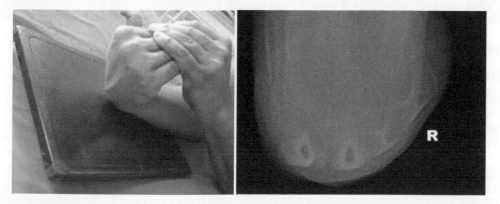

Figure 16.31   Carpal bridge view. The central beam is directed to a point 45° supero inferior to the wrist joint. © Indian Journal of Plastic Surgery: Official Publication of the Association of Plastic Surgeons of India

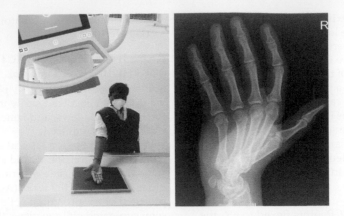

Figure 16.32 Position of the hand and direction of the x-ray beam for obtaining a Brewerton view.

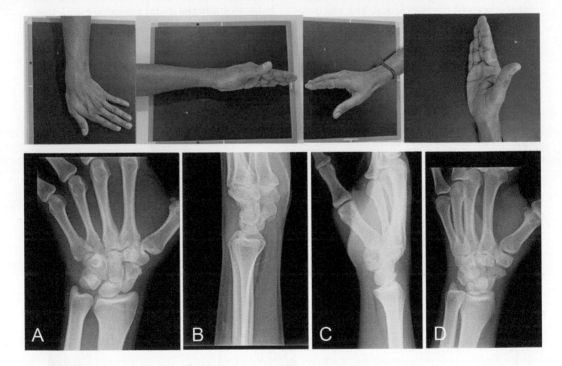

Figure 16.33 (A,B,C,D) The four sequential views form the scaphoid series.

OTHER SPECIAL VIEWS FOR SCAPHOID

a) **Stetcher's projection view [3, 6]** is to visualise the full length of the scaphoid. The pronated forearm and hand are placed on the cassette with the clenched fist in ulnar deviation (Figure 16.34).

b) **Bridgeman's view:** The pronated forearm and hand are placed on the cassette with the wrist in 17° dorsiflexion using a folded sheet. This aligns the central beam perpendicular to the waist of the scaphoid and parallel to the fracture plane. Mainly used to visualise the proximal pole and scaphocapitate joint (Figure 16.35).

c) **Shreck's projection view** is an oblique pronated quill holding position view with the wrist held in a 45° extension to visualise scaphoid tuberosity better (Figure 16.36).

d) **Hyper pronation view:** The forearm and hand are held in pronation and ulnar deviation with the wrist in 30° extension. This view is used to visualise the full length of the scaphoid (Figure 16.37).

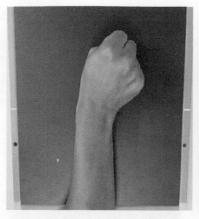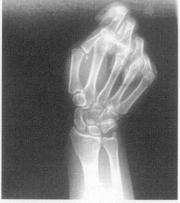

Figure 16.34 Stetcher's projection.

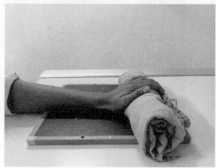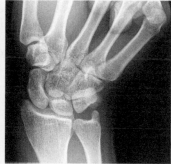

Figure 16.35 Bridgeman's projection.

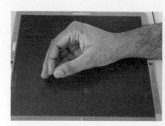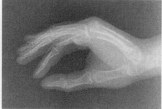

Figure 16.36 Shreck's projection view.

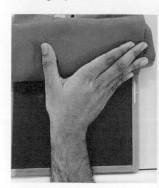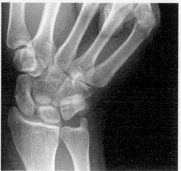

Figure 16.37 Hyper pronation view.

RADIOGRAPHY OF THE HAND

Standard projections for the hand are posteroanterior, oblique, and lateral views. The following section of this chapter describes the standard radiographic views in the hand and their clinical implications.

Posteroanterior View

The posteroanterior view is taken in the sitting position, with the entire palm touching the cassette and fingers and thumb slightly opened. The beam is centred over the third metacarpal. In a PA view of the hand, the metacarpal and proximal phalanges are best exposed, the distal phalanges are overexposed, and the carpal bones are underexposed (Figure 16.38).

Oblique View

The palm is placed semi prone on the cassette, and the beam is centered over the metacarpals. The oblique view is to visualise the metacarpals when they tend to overlap in a true lateral view [2] (Figure 16.39).

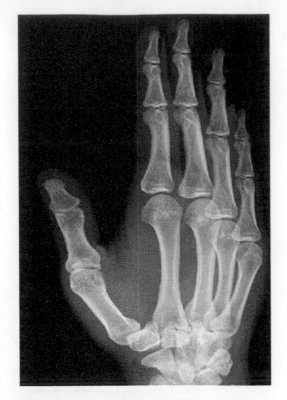

Figure 16.39 Oblique view of the hand.

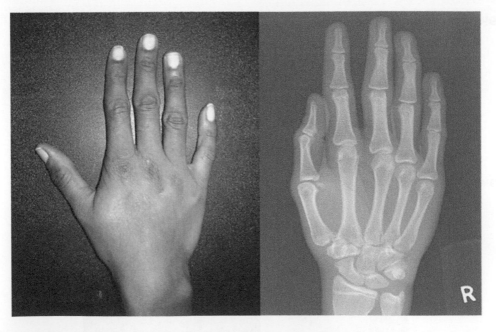

Figure 16.38 The posteroanterior view of the hand.

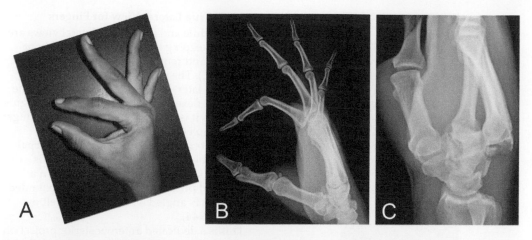

Figure 16.40 Splaying lateral view (A,B). True lateral view showing CMC dislocation (C).

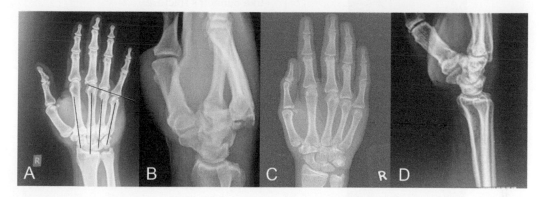

Figure 16.41 A) Anteroposterior view show obliteration of carpometacarpal joint space and loss of metacarpal cascade (line along the axis of metacarpal should meet at a point) and loss of oblique metacarpal line (line along the 3rd, 4th and 5th metacarpal head) suggestive of metacarpal shortening. B) The true lateral view of hand confirming 2nd to 5th CMC joint dislocation. C) Post reduction anteroposterior X-ray showing restoration of metacarpal cascade line, M lines, oblique metacarpal line, (D) confirmation of reduction on a true lateral X-ray.

True Lateral View

This is also known as the splayed finger view (Figure 16.40A,B). The palm is placed 90° mid prone over the cassette with splaying of all the digits. This is used to visualise the phalanges of all the digits and mainly the carpometacarpal joints (CMC). The true lateral view is used to visualise CMC joint dislocations and carpal bossing (Figure 16.40C).

Evaluating Carpometacarpal joint dislocation [7]

Subtle CMC joint dislocation may be missed if proper Xray views are not taken. True lateral view helps in indentifying the direction of dislocation. Obliteration of CMC joint space,

loss of metcarpal cascade and loss of oblique metacarpal line are some of the signs suggesting CMC dislocation (Figure 16.41).

RADIOGRAPHY OF THE FINGERS

Standard projections for the fingers are posteroanterior, oblique, and lateral views. The beam is centred over the point of interest which may be the proximal interphalangeal or distal interphalangeal joint.

Posteroanterior View

The posteroanterior view is taken in a sitting position, with the volar side of the finger touching the cassette and all digits abducted from the center (Figure 16.42).

True Lateral View for Fingers

Index, middle and little finger lateral views are taken by keeping their respective MCP joint extended and remaining fingers flexed (Figure 16.43A,B,C). The exception is the ring finger, where the lateral view is taken by keeping the MCP joint flexed, as shown in the figure (Figure 16.44D), as it is difficult to extend the ring finger alone completely.

True lateral of the first carpometacarpal joint (Robert's view) of the thumb: This view is taken with the thumb placed in a horizontal position and hand hyperextended. The beam is angled 45° towards the elbow (Figure 16.44).

This is a dedicated anteroposterior projection with beam angulation for changes in the first CMC joint in arthritis or traumatic conditions like Bennett's fracture.

True lateral of the finger is also useful in diagnosing fracture-dislocation of PIP joint. In subtle fracture subluxation, the 'V' sign on a true lateral X-ray is diagnostic (Figure 16.45).

The true lateral view is also useful in determining the plane of dislocation, i.e. volar (Figure 16.46A) and dorsal (Figure 16.46B), dislocation based on the displacement of the distal fragment compared to the proximal.

The PIP fracture-dislocations can be completely evaluated to understand the fracture

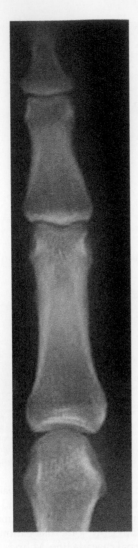

Figure 16.42 True PA view for finger.

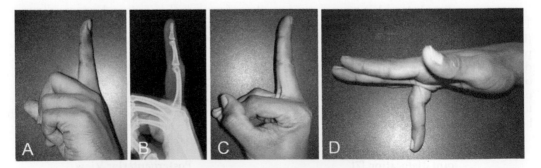

Figure 16.43 Finger lateral view for index (A,B), middle finger (C) and ring finger (D).

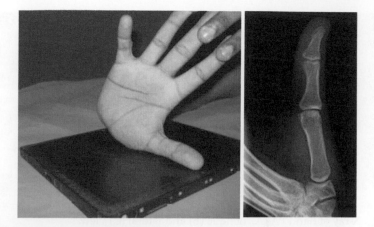

Figure 16.44   First carpometacarpal joint view.

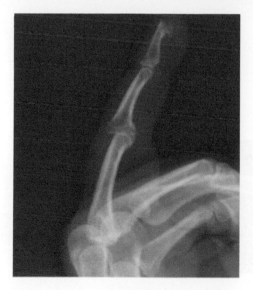

Figure 16.45   True lateral X-ray of index finger showing subtle fracture subluxation.

pattern if all three views are taken. The tendency to order an oblique instead of a true lateral view might be inadequate, and the actual degree of commination may be masked (Figure 16.47).

Oblique View of a Finger

Helpful in the assessment of joint injuries. The classical **double condyle** sign is seen in PIPJ fracture [3, 6] (Figure 16.48).

Stress Radiograph of Thumb [6] for Ulnar Collateral Ligament (UCL) Injury (Figure 16.49)

Used for identifying the Skier's thumb (acute ulnar collateral injury at MCP joint) or game-keeper's thumb (chronic ulnar collateral injury. It may or may not be associated with an avulsion fracture of the condyle. If ulnar collateral ligament (UCL) is injured, then PA view of thumb with stress on the radial side of MCP joint is to be taken. If the joint opening is more

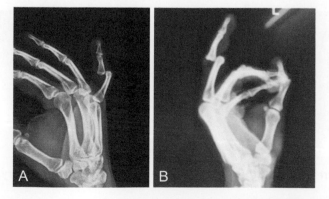

Figure 16.46   A) True lateral X-ray of the little finger showing volar proximal interphalangeal joint dislocation. B) True lateral X-ray of index finger showing dorsal proximal interphalangeal joint dislocation.

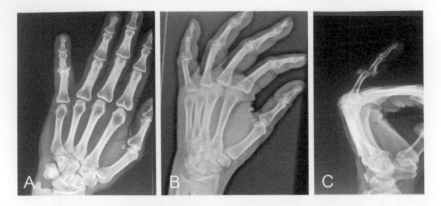

Figure 16.47 X-ray of hand PA (A), oblique (B) and lateral (C) view.

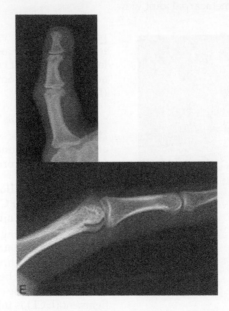

Figure 16.48 Oblique view demonstrating double condyle sign.

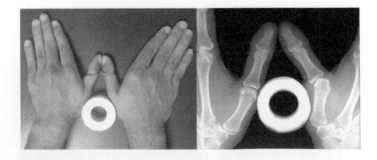

Figure 16.49 Stress view for the diagnosis of ulnar collateral ligament injury.

than 30^0 (or more than 15^0 compared to the normal side) it is considered near or complete ligament avulsion.

REFERENCES

1. Bhat AK, Kumar B and Acharya A. Radiographic imaging of the wrist. *Indian J Plast Surg.* 2011; 44:186–196.

2. Schmitt R and Lenz U. *Diagnostic imaging of the hand.* New York: Thyme, 2008.

3. Laredo RA, Surge DG and Garcia G. Radiographic evaluation of the wrist: A vanishing art. *Sem Roentgenol.* 2005; 40:248–289.

4. Lewis CM, Yang Z and Gilula LA. Validation of the extensor carpi ulnaris groove as a predictor for the recognition of standard posteroanterior radiographs of the wrist. *J Hand Surg.* 2002; 27A:252.

5. Wilson AJ, Mann FA and Gilula LA. Imaging of the hand and wrist. *J Hand Surg (Br)* 1990; 15(B):153–167.

6. Lindequist S and Marelli C. Modern imaging of the hand, wrist, and forearm. *J Hand Ther.* 2007; 20:119–137.

7. Bhardwaj P, Sivakumar BS, Vallurupalli A, Pai M and Sabapathy SR. Fracture dislocations of the carpometacarpal joints of the fingers. *J Clin Orthop Trauma* 2020; 11(4):562–569.

17 Congenital Hand

Takehiko Takagi

CONTENTS

DOI: 10.1201/9781003125938-21

When diagnosing congenital differences in the upper limbs, giving a diagnosis name has the same meaning as classifying the disease. In order to make a correct diagnosis, knowledge of diagnostic criteria is required. In addition, it is important that the classification method used is appropriate. Congenital differences occur at some point in the embryo due to genetic or extrinsic damage to the embryo or fetus. That is, the impairment caused by the pathological condition of the embryonic period are congenital differences. Therefore, it should be also classified based on the disorder of the embryonic period.

In 1976, Swanson published a taxonomy that incorporates knowledge of embryology. This classification method has been widely used as an improved classification method of the International Federation of Societies for Surgery of the Hand (IFSSH) [1]. In 2010, Oberg et al. presented a new classification for congenital upper-limb differences [2]. In 2013, the older Swanson classification for congenital hand differences was replaced by a new system, proposed by Oberg, Manske and Tonkin (OMT) at the recommendation of the IFSSH Committee for Congenital Conditions [3], with the rapid progression of knowledge in limb development and clinical genetics, although its limitations were immediately highlighted in the 2013 review by the IFSSH

committee with recommendations of three yearly reviews to allow updates of knowledge, changes in groupings and additions of new categories [3]. Recently, the 2020 OMT classification was provided an update [4]. Compared with the Swanson classification, the OMT classification allows upper-extremity anomalies to be specifically placed under their respective diagnoses [4]. Lam et al., wrote that the classification has several advantages of its simplicity, flexibility, comprehensiveness, logic and educational benefits [5]. The OMT App, the OMT classification mobile app, under the educational recourses on the IFSSH website was developed as a free tool that allows easy reference to the system, and gave additional information on etiologies, photographs, easy keyword search function and the Online Mendelian Inheritance of Men (OMIM) links. The clinical examinations about the representative congenital differences are outlined along with the OMT classification (Table 17.1).

MALFORMATIONS

Poland Syndrome (OMT Classification, I. A. 1. ii. a.)

It is characterized by brachydactyly/syndactyly and hypoplastic breast with hypoplasia of the costosternal portion of the pectoralis major muscle and pectoralis minor muscle or ribs 2–5

Table 17.1: OMT Classification of Congenital Hand [4]

I.Malformations

  A. Entire upper limb: Abnormal axis formation (early limb patterning)

    1. Proximodistal axis

      i. Brachymelia

      ii. Symbrachydactyly spectrum (with ectodermal elements)

        a) Poland syndrome

        b) Whole limb excluding Poland syndrome

          (various levels: Humeral to phalangeal)

      iii. Transverse deficiency (without ectodermal elements)

        a) Amelia

        b) Segmental (various levels: Humeral to phalangeal)

      iv. Intersegmental deficiency (phocomelia)

        a) Proximal (humeral: Rhizomelic)

        b) Distal (forearm: Mesomelic)

        c) Proximal plus distal (hand to thorax)

      v. Whole limb duplication/triplication

    2. Radioulnar (anteroposterior) axis

      i.   Radial longitudinal deficiency

      ii. Ulnar longitudinal deficiency

      iii. Ulnar dimelia

      iv. Radiohumeral synostosis

      v.   Radioulnar synostosis

      vi. Congenital dislocation of radial head

      vii. Forearm hemiphyseal dysplasia, radial (Madelung deformity), or ulnar

    3. Dorsoventral axis

      i. Ventral dimelia

      ii. Dorsal dimelia

    4. Unspecified axis

      i. Shoulder

        a) Undescended (Sprengel)

        b) Abnormal shoulder muscles

      ii. Upper to lower limb transformation

  B. Hand plate: Abnormal axis differentiation (late limb patterning/differentiation)

    1. Proximodistal axis

      i.   Brachydactyly

      ii. Symbrachydactyly (with ectodermal elements)

      iii. Transverse deficiency (without ectodermal elements)

      iv. Cleft hand (split hand/foot malformation)

    2. Radioulnar (anteroposterior) axis

      i.   Radial longitudinal deficiency, hypoplastic thumb

      ii. Ulnar longitudinal deficiency, hypoplastic ulnar ray

      iii. Radial polydactyly

      iv. Triphalangeal thumb

        a) Five-finger hand

      v. Ulnar dimelia (mirror hand)

      vi. Ulnar polydactyly

    3. Dorsoventral axis

      i. Dorsal dimelia (palmar nail)

      ii. Ventral dimelia (hypoplastic/aplastic nail)

(Continued)

Table 17.1 (Continued): OMT Classification of Congenital Hand [4]

    4. Unspecified axis

      i. Soft tissue

        a) Cutaneous (simple) syndactyly

      ii. Skeletal

        a) Osseous (complex) syndactyly

        b) Clinodactyly

        c) Kirner deformity

        d) Synostosis/symphalangism

      iii. Complex

        a) Syndromic syndactyly (e.g., Apert hand)

        b) Synpolydactyly

        c) Not otherwise specified

II. Deformations

  A. Constriction ring sequence

  B. Not otherwise specified

III. Dysplasias

  A. Variant growth

    1. Diffuse (whole limb)

      i. Hemihypertrophy

      ii. Aberrant flexor/extensor/intrinsic muscle

    2. Isolated

      i. Macrodactyly

      ii. Aberrant intrinsic muscles of hand

  B. Tumorous conditions

    1. Vascular

      i. Hemangioma

      ii. Malformation

      iii. Others

    2. Neurological

      i. Neurofibromatosis

      ii. Others

    3. Connective tissue

      i. Juvenile aponeurotic fibroma

      ii. Infantile digital fibroma

      iii. Others

    4. Skeletal

      i.   Osteochondromatosis

      ii. Enchondromatosis

      iii. Fibrous dysplasia

      iv. Epiphyseal abnormalities

      v.   Pseudoarthrosis

      vi. Other

  C. Congenital contracture

    i. Arthrogryposis multiplex congenita

      a) Amyoplasia

      b) Distal arthrogryposis

      c) Other

    ii. Isolated

(Continued)

Table 17.1 (Continued): OMT Classification of Congenital Hand [4]

    a) Camptodactyly

    b) Thumb in palm deformity

    c) Other

IV. Syndromes*

  A. Specified

    1. Acrofacial dysostosis 1 (Nager type) (MIM 154400)

    2. Apert (MIM 101200)

    3. Al-Awadi/Raas-Rothschild/Schinzel phocomelia (MIM 276820)

    4. Baller-Gerold (MIM 218600)

    5. Bardet-Biedl (21 types)

    6. Beals (MIM 121050)

    7. CLOVES (MIM 612918)

    8. Carpenter (MIM 201000)

    9. Catel-Manzke (MIM 616145)

    10. Cornelia de Lange (5 types)

    11. Crouzon (MIM 123500)

    12. Down (MIM 190685)

    13. Ectrodactyly-ectodermal dysplasia-clefting (MIM 129900)

    14. Fanconi pancytopenia (MIM 227650)

    15. Freeman Sheldon (MIM 193700)

    16. Fuhrmann (MIM 228930)

    17. Goltz (focal dermal hypoplasia) (MIM 305600)

    18. Gorlin (basal cell nevus syndrome) (MIM 109400)

    19. Greig cephalopolysyndactyly (MIM 175700)

    20. Hajdu-Cheney (MIM 102500)

    21. Hemifacial microsomia (Goldenhar syndrome) (MIM 164210)

    22. Holt-Oram (MIM 142900)

    23. Lacrimoauriculodentodigital (Levy-Hollister) (MIM 149730)

    24. Larsen (MIM 150250)

    25. Laurin-Sandrow (MIM 135750)

    26. Leri-Weill dyschondrosteosis (MIM 127300)

    27. Liebenberg syndrome (MIM 186550)

    28. Moebius sequence (MIM 157900)

    29. Multiple synostoses (4 types)

    30. Nail-patella (MIM 161200)

    31. Noonan (2 types)

    32. Oculodentodigital dysplasia AD (MIM 164200);
       AR (MIM 257850)

    33. Orofaciodigital (18 types)

    34. Otopalatodigital spectrum (filamin A)

    35. Pallister-Hall (MIM 146510)

    36. Pfeiffer (MIM 101600)

    37. Pierre Robin (4 subtypes)

    38. Poland (MIM 173800)

    39. Proteus (MIM 176920)

    40. Roberts (MIM 268300)

    41. SC phocomelia (MIM 26900)

    42. Rothmund-Thomson (MIM 268400)

(Continued)

Table 17.1 (Continued): OMT Classification of Congenital Hand [4]

43. Rubinstein-Taybi (2 types)

44. Saethre-Chotzen (MIM 101400)

45. Split hand-foot malformation (7 types)

46. Thrombocytopenia absent radius (MIM 274000)

47. Townes-Brock (2 types)

48. Trichorhinophalangeal (3 types)

49. Ulnar-mammary (MIM 181450)

50. VACTERL association (3 types)

B. Others

*Specified syndromes are those considered most relevant; however, many other syndromes have a limb component categorized under "B. Others."

[6, 7]. It is thought that there may be an interruption of early embryonic blood supply in the subclavian or vertebral arteries, resulting in unilateral upper limb differences and unilateral chest wall deformities [6].

Phocomelia (OMT Classification, I. A. 1. iv.)

Phocomelia is considered a transverse, intercalated segmental dysplasia [8]. The diagnosis of phocomelia came into common usage in the early 1960s with the markedly increased incidence of congenital malformations related to the use of thalidomide in early pregnancy [9, 10]. Sulamaa et al., had proposed that the clavicle was turned in the direction of the arm and fixed to the bony rudiments of the arm [11]. The recent development of the prostheses is hopefully applied for the differences.

Whole Limb Duplication/Triplication (OMT Classification, I. A. 1. v.)

The duplication of the entire upper limb, the upper limb dimelia, is a very rare congenital difference [12]. Several etiological theories have been proposed for this clinical presentation. An amniotic constriction band disruptive event is theoretically possible given the presence of the epidermoid, such as occurs in syndactyly associated with constriction band syndrome [13]. It was treated with a simple amputation of the inferior limb resulting in cosmetic improvement and maintenance of range of motion in the preserved limb [12].

Radial Longitudinal Deficiency (OMT Classification, I. A. 2. i., I. B. 2. i.)

Radial longitudinal deficiency is a spectrum of malformations affecting the structures of the radial side of the forearm, including hypoplasia of the bones and joints, muscles and tendons ligaments, nerves and blood vessels [14]. Radial ray deficiency is an uncommon condition, although it is the most common type of longitudinal failure of formation [15]. Although the molecular basis of isolated radial ray deficiency is still unknown, individuals with radial ray deficiency have a high incidence of medical and musculoskeletal anomalies that increase with increasing severity of the deficiency. Children with bilateral and severe radial ray deficiency have considerable functional impairment as a result of thumb dysfunction, wrist instability and short upper extremities. Independent performance of activities of daily living, such as fastening buttons and zippers or accomplishing personal hygiene, is difficult. Objective reproducible hand function testing awaits the development and identification of function tests suitable for children with these malformations [16].

Ulnar Longitudinal Deficiency (OMT Classification, I. A. 2. ii., I. B. 2. ii.)

Ulnar longitudinal deficiency usually affects the entire upper limb, including the elbow, forearm and wrist. Angulation of the wrist occurs but is typically not as severe as seen in radial longitudinal deficiency. The wrist remains resting in 5–40° of ulnar deviation [17]. Unlike radial longitudinal deficiency, patients with ulnar longitudinal deficiency rarely have heart or hematopoietic anomalies, although the patients may have associated musculoskeletal disorders such as proximal femoral focal deficiency, scoliosis, clubfeet and spina bifida [18].

Ulnar Dimelia (OMT Classification, I. A. 2. iii., I. B. 2. v.)

Ulnar dimelia (mirror hand with double ulna) is a rare congenital difference in which both forearm bones develop as a normal ulna and polydactyly is present in the hand, the thumb and radius bone being absent [19]. Elbow reconstruction improves activities of daily living with better forearm range of motion [20].

Radioulnar Synostosis (OMT Classification, I. A. 2. v.)

Congenital radioulnar synostosis is mostly fixed in pronation on the forearm [21]. This may cause severely disabling functional impairment such as inability to scoop up water in the hands or to drink water from a glass [22]. Successful mobilization of congenital proximal radioulnar synostosis with a free vascularized adipofascial flap has been reported [23, 24]. On the other hand, simple rotational osteotomy as a reliable, satisfactory and safe procedure has also had good clinical results with daily activities [21, 22].

Madelung Deformity (OMT Classification, I. A. 2. vii.)

Madelung deformity is caused by growth disturbance in the palmar and ulnar portions of the physis. The Vickers ligament covers the palmar side of the wrist from the distal end of the pronator quadratus muscle [25]. A variety of osteotomies to correct the complex deformity based on plain radiographs have been reported [26, 27]. Computed tomography imaging and recent computer software techniques are used to accurately evaluate the 3D deformity in the bones and to perform 3D corrective osteotomy using customized surgical guides [28, 29].

Symbrachydactyly (with Ectodermal Elements) (OMT Classification, I. B. 1. ii.)

Symbrachydactyly presents with a variety of findings including digital hypoplasia, aplasia or deficiency of the hand or forearm. The absent fingers are represented by "nubbins" with/without nail remnants [30]. The defect is believed to be mesodermal, which explains the remaining distal finger ectodermal structures [31].

Transverse Deficiency (without Ectodermal Elements) (OMT Classification, I. B. 1. iii.)

The most common level of transverse deficiency is at the proximal part of the forearm, followed by transcarpal, distal forearm and transhumeral failure [32]. The recent development of a prostheses is hopefully applied for the deficiency.

Cleft Hand (Split Hand and Foot Malformations) (OMT Classification, I. B. 1. iv.)

The manifestation of cleft hand may vary from only a very minor cutaneous cleft without absence of the finger to a severe form in which only the little finger remains. The condition may involve the feet [31]. Cleft hand is commonly inherited as an autosomal dominant trait and is associated with syndromes such as split-hand/split-foot or ectodactyly, ectodermal dysplasia and cleft lip/palate (EEC) syndrome [33, 34].

Radial Polydactyly (OMT Classification, I. B. 2. iii.)

Radial polydactyly is documented in high proportions in Native American and Asian populations [35]. Most cases are unilateral, sporadic and without systemic problems [36]. The Wassel classification is most widely used, although the true nature of the thumbs is usually not apparent because the skeletons are immature in the children. Wassel type IV is the most common type and recently subtyped into type IVA (hypoplastic type), IVB (ulnar deviated type), IVC (divergent type) and IVD (convergent type) [37]. A radially deviated type should be also considered [38]. In triplicate digit, a rare type of polydactyly, the most developed proximal components and most developed distal components are often in different rays, therefore the ray transfer is needed for the surgery [39].

Cutaneous (Simple) Syndactyly (OMT Classification, I. B. 4. i. a)

Osseous (Complex) Syndactyly (OMT Classification, I. B. 4. ii. a)

Syndactyly is defined as the fusion of the cutaneous (simple) or osseous (complex) elements of adjacent digits. Cutaneous (simple) syndactyly has only skin or soft tissue connections. The joints, tendons and digital neovascularity are usually normal and independent. Osseous (complex) syndactyly has skeletal fusions. The incidence of tendon and neurovascular anatomy are usually complexed in the syndactyly [31].

Clinodactyly (OMT Classification, I. B. 4. ii. b)

Clinodactyly typically presents as radial deviation of the little finger and is often bilateral. The thumb and ring finger are the next most frequently affected digits [6]. The delta phalanx is the result of early complete ossification of a C-shaped bracket and results in the most severe deformities [40].

DEFORMATIONS
Constriction Ring Sequence (OMT Classification, II. A.)

Constriction ring sequence is characterized by partial or complete circumferential constrictions around limbs, digits or other body parts [41]. The constrictions may be amputation or near amputation with distal oedema and may also produce fusion of the digits to those adjacent of nonadjacent digits, producing a complicated syndactyly/arcosyndactyly with a distal fusion of the digits [31].

DYSPLASIAS
Macrodactyly (OMT Classification, III. A. 2. i.)

Macrodactyly consists of a significant increase in the length and girth of most or all digits. Both the soft tissue and skeletal elements are diffusely enlarged in the affected digits. It is often associated with lipofibromatosis. The growth of the enlarged digit may be disproportionate (progressive type), or the digits may maintain a consistent proportion to the remainder of the hand (static type) [31].

Neurofibromatosis (OMT Classification, III. B. 2. i.)

Neurofibromatosis is characterized by multiple café-au-lait spots under the skin. Pseudarthrosis of the bone and the scoliosis may also be present. Congenital pseudarthrosis is most common in the tibia. It may occasionally involve the ulna or the radius, usually in the distal or middle third, is replaced by fibrous tissue with a progressive forearm deformity [42, 43]. The vascularized fibula graft is applied, but the creation of a one-bone forearm is an option available to restore forearm stability [44, 45].

Osteochondromatosis (OMT Classification, III. B. 4. i.)

Osteochondromas grow from the physes of long bones, the pelvis, ribs, scapula or vertebrae. Forearm osteochondromas frequently cause a discrepancy in length of the radius and ulna [46]. Early removal of osteochondroma may retard or prevent progressive growth disturbance [47, 48]. Ulnar lengthening may be performed in a single stage or by gradual distraction osteogenesis [32].

Arthrogryposis Multiplex Congenita (OMT Classification, III. C. i.)

Arthrogryposis is the general term given to conditions characterized by multiple joint contractures resulting in substantial disability most frequently found in childhood [49].

The most common pattern of deformity is internal rotation of the shoulder with weak or absent shoulder girdle muscles; extension contracture of the elbow with weak or absent biceps and brachialis muscles; pronated, flexed and ulnarly deviated wrists, with weak or absent wrist extension and rigid digits with thumb and palm deformity [6]. The osteotomy, tendon transfer or capsular release is considered, if after nonoperative treatment functional independence is still not possible. The elbow is most critical in terms of achieving passive mobility to gain hand-to-mouth function [49, 50].

Camptodactyly (OMT Classification, III. C. ii. a)

Bilateral deformities occur in approximately two-thirds of cases and the little finger is usually involved. Multiple digits can be affected, with less frequent involvement of the radial digits [6]. Abnormalities of almost every structure around the PIP joint including the flexor digitorum superficialis or the intrinsic musculature have been described [51].

SYNDROMES

The syndromes category has been expanded with Mendelian Inheritance in Man (MIM) numbers and the name of the syndrome as found on the OMIM. Syndromes and the main clinical features of the hand/upper extremity [6] are as follows:

Acrofacial Dysostosis 1 (Nager Type) (MIM 154400)

Radial deficiency (hypoplastic/aplastic thumb), clinodactyly, syndactyly, elbow contracture.

Apert (MIM 101200)

Acrosyndactyly ("mitten hand"), radial deviation of the thumb, clinodactyly.

Al-Awadi/Raas-Rothschild/Schinzel Phocomelia (MIM 276820)

Oligodactyly/monodactyly with nail dysplasia, hypoplasia/aplasia of the elbow joint, reduction of the radius/ulna to a single bone [52].

Baller-Gerold (MIM 218600)

Radial deficiency (hypoplastic/aplastic thumb).

Bardet-Biedl

Postaxial polydactyly.

Beals (MIM 121050)

Arachnodactyly with joint contractures [53].

CLOVES (MIM 612918)

Macrodactyly with lipomatous overgrowth/ vascular malformations [54].

Carpenter (MIM 201000)

Brachydactyly with clinodactyly and syndactyly, broad bifid thumbs.

Catel-Manzke (MIM 616145)

Clinodactyly, polydactyly, index finger hyperphalangy [55].

Cornelia de Lange

Oligodactyly, ulnar deficiency [56].

Crouzon (MIM 123500)

Carpal fusions.

Down (MIM 190685)

Clinodactyly of the little finger.

Ectrodactyly-Ectodermal Dysplasia-Clefting (MIM 129900)

Cleft hand with polydactyly, syndactyly and camptodactyly [57].

Fanconi pancytopenia (MIM 227650)

Hypoplastic/aplastic thumb [58].

Freeman Sheldon (MIM 193700)

Ulnar deviation of the fingers, camptodactyly, first web space contracture and hypoplasia of the thumb [59].

Fuhrmann (MIM 228930)

Symmetrical fingernail deficiency [60].

Goltz (Focal Dermal Hypoplasia) (MIM 305600)

Split hand deformity [61].

Gorlin (Basal Cell Nevus Syndrome) (MIM 109400)

Hypoplastic thumb [62].

Greig Cephalopolysyndactyly (MIM 175700)

Preaxial/postaxial polydactyly, syndactyly.

Hajdu-Cheney (MIM 102500)

Shortening of the fingers (transverse osteolysis involving distal phalanx [acro-osteolysis]) [63, 64].

Hemifacial Microsomia (Goldenhar Syndrome) (MIM 164210)

Radial deficiency [65].

Holt-Oram (MIM 142900)

Brachydactyly, syndactyly, occasional involvement of shoulder girdle.

Lacrimoauriculodentodigital (Levy-Hollister) (MIM 149730)

Split hand deformity, polydactyly, syndactyly, little finger clinodactyly.

Larsen (MIM 150250)

Multiple joint contractures, wide distal phalanx at the thumb [66, 67].

Laurin-Sandrow (MIM 135750)

Polysyndactyly, mirror hand [68].

Leri-Weill Dyschondrosteosis (MIM 127300)

Madelung deformity [69].

Liebenberg Syndrome (MIM186550)

Brachydactyly, dysplasia of the elbow, forearm, wrist and hands with Joint deformities/contractures [70, 71].

Moebius Sequence (MIM 157900)

Brachydactyly, oligodactyly.

Multiple Synostoses

Brachydactyly, cubital valgus with elbow joint dysplasia.

Nail-Patella (MIM 161200)

Poorly developed fingernails, contracture of the elbows with arthrodysplasia.

Noonan

Cutaneous syndactyly, cubitus valgus, hand oedema.

Oculodentodigital Dysplasia AD (MIM 164200); AR (MIM 257850)

Ulnar syndactyly, clinodactyly [72].

Orofaciodigital

Preaxial/postaxial polysyndactyly [73, 74].

Otopalatodigital Spectrum (Filamin A)

Camptodactyly, hypoplastic thumb [75].

Pallister-Hall (MIM 146510)

Mesoaxial/postaxial polydactyly, syndactyly.

Pfeiffer (MIM 101600)

Brachydactyly, syndactyly, radially deviated thumb.

Pierre Robin
Syndactyly, brachydactyly [76].

Poland (MIM 173800)
Unilateral brachydactyly, syndactyly, oligodactyly [77].

Proteus (MIM 176920)
Macrodactyly with hamartomas composed primarily of lipomatous tissue [78].

Roberts (MIM 268300)
Clinodactyly, syndactyly, joint contractures [79].

SC Phocomelia (MIM 26900)
Phocomelia [80].

Rothmund-Thomson (MIM 268400)
Radial deficiency, brachydactyly, clinodactyly.

Rubinstein-Taybi
Brachydactyly, broad thumb with radial deviation, clinodactyly.

Saethre-Chotzen (MIM 101400)
Brachydactyly, clinodactyly, 2–3 syndactyly.

Split Hand-Foot Malformation
Cleft hand, brachydactyly [81].

Thrombocytopenia Absent Radius (MIM 274000)
Hypoplastic/aplastic thumb.

Townes-Brock
Distal deviation of thumb, hypoplastic thumb, preaxial polydactyly.

Trichorhinophalangeal
Brachydactyly, clinodactyly, short metacarpals phalanges [82].

Ulnar-Mammary (MIM 181450)
Postaxial polydactyly [83].

VACTERL (vertebral defects, anal atresia, cardiac defects, tracheo-esophageal fistula, renal anomalies and limb abnormalities) Association
Radial deficiency with hypoplastic/aplastic thumb [84].

REFERENCES

1. Swanson AB. A classification for congenital limb malformations. *J Hand Surg Am* 1976;1:8–22.

2. Oberg KC, Feenstra JM, Manske PR and Tonkin MA. Developmental biology and classification of congenital anomalies of the hand and upper extremity. *J Hand Surg Am* 2010;35:2066–2076.

3. Ezaki M, Baek GH, Horii E and Hovius S. IFSSH Scientific Committee on Congenital Conditions. *J Hand Surg Eur* 2014;39:676–678.

4. Goldfarb CA, Ezaki M, Wall LB, Lam WL and Oberg KC. The Oberg-Manske-Tonkin (OMT) classification of congenital upper extremities: Update for 2020. *J Hand Surg Am* 2020;45:542–547.

5. Lam WL, Oberg KC and Goldfarb CA. The 2020 Oberg-Manske-Tonkin classification of congenital upper limb differences: updates and challenges. *J Hand Surg Eur* 2020;45:1117–1119.

6. Burke LW and Laub Jr DR. Incidence and syndromes associated with congenital anomalies of the upper limb. In: Laub Jr DR (ed.), *Congenital Anomalies of the Upper Extremity*. New York, NY: Springer; 2015, pp. 27–38.

7. Bainbridge LC, Wright AR and Kanthan R. Computed tomography in the preoperative assessment of Poland's syndrome. *Br J Plast Surg* 1991;44:604–607.

8. Goldfarb CA, Manske PR, Busa R, Mills J, Carter P and Ezaki M. Upper-extremity phocomelia reexamined: A longitudinal dysplasia. *J Bone Joint Surg Am* 2005;87:2639–2648.

9. Somers GS. Thalidomide and congenital abnormalities. *Lancet* 1962;1:912–913.

10. Speirs AL. Thalidomide and congenital abnormalities. *Lancet* 1962;1:303–305.

11. Sulamaa M and Ryoeppy S. Early treatment of congenital bone defects of the extremities: Aftermath of thalidomide disaster. *Lancet* 1964;1:130–132.

12. Takagi T, Nojiri A, Seki A, Takayama S and Watanabe M. Upper limb dimelia. *J Hand Surg Am* 2017;42:575 e1–e5.

13. Shah C, Manske PR and Goldfarb CA. A child with longitudinal cleavage of the upper extremity: Treatment and etiology considerations. *J Hand Surg Am* 2010;35:1762–1767.

14. James MA, McCarroll HR, Jr and Manske PR. The spectrum of radial longitudinal deficiency: A modified classification. *J Hand Surg Am* 1999;24:1145–1155.

15. Takagi T, Seki A, Takayama S, Watanabe M. Current Concepts in Radial Club Hand. Open Orthop J, 11:369-377, 2017.

16. Goldfarb CA, Wall L and Manske PR. Radial longitudinal deficiency: The incidence of associated medical and musculoskeletal conditions. *J Hand Surg Am* 2006;31:1176–1182.

17. Elhassan BT, Biafora S and Light T. Clinical manifestations of type IV ulna longitudinal dysplasia. *J Hand Surg Am* 2007;32:1024–1030.

18. Bauer AS, Bednar MS and James MA. Disruption of the radial/ulnar axis: Congenital longitudinal deficiencies. *J Hand Surg Am* 2013;38:2293–2302; quiz 302.

19. Harrison RG, Pearson MA and Roaf R. Ulnar dimelia. *J Bone Joint Surg Br* 1960;42-B:549–555.

20. Takagi T, Seki A and Takayama S. Elbow and forearm reconstruction in patients with ulnar dimelia can improve activities of daily living. *J Shoulder Elbow Surg* 2014;23:e68–e72.

21. Ogino T and Hikino K. Congenital radio-ulnar synostosis: Compensatory rotation around the wrist and rotation osteotomy. *J Hand Surg Br* 1987;12:173–178.

22. Satake H, Kanauchi Y, Kashiwa H, Ishigaki D, Takahara M and Takagi M. Long-term results after simple rotational osteotomy of the radius shaft for congenital radioulnar synostosis. *J Shoulder Elbow Surg* 2018;27:1373–1379.

23. Kanaya F and Ibaraki K. Mobilization of a congenital proximal radioulnar synostosis with use of a free vascularized fascio-fat graft. *J Bone Joint Surg Am* 1998;80:1186–1192.

24. Tsumura T, Matsumoto T, Matsushita M, Kishimoto K, Murase T and Shiode H. A three-step method for the treatment of radioulnar synostosis with posterior radial head dislocation. *J Hand Surg Asian Pac* 2021;26:118–125.

25. Vickers D and Nielsen G. Madelung deformity: Surgical prophylaxis (physiolysis) during the late growth period by resection of the dyschondrosteosis lesion. *J Hand Surg Br* 1992;17:401–407.

26. dos Reis FB, Katchburian MV, Faloppa F, Albertoni WM and Laredo Filho J, Jr. Osteotomy of the radius and ulna for the Madelung deformity. *J Bone Joint Surg Br* 1998;80:817–824.

27. Potenza V, Farsetti P, Caterini R, Tudisco C, Nicoletti S and Ippolito E. Isolated Madelung's deformity: Long-term follow-up study of five patients treated surgically. *J Pediatr Orthop B* 2007;16:331–335.

28. Imai Y, Miyake J, Okada K, Murase T, Yoshikawa H and Moritomo H. Cylindrical corrective osteotomy for Madelung deformity using a computer simulation: Case report. *J Hand Surg Am* 2013;38:1925–1932.

29. Yanagisawa S, Takagi T, Murase T, Kobayashi Y and Watanabe M. Open wedge osteotomy with ulnar shortening for madelung deformity using a computer-generated template. *J Hand Surg Asian Pac* 2017;22:538–543.

30. Miura T, Nakamura R and Horii E. The position of symbrachydactyly in the classification of congenital hand anomalies. *J Hand Surg Br* 1994;19:350–354.

31. Kay SP, McCombe DB and Kozin SH. Deformities of the hand and fingers. In: Wolfe SW (ed.), *Green's Operative Hand Surgery*, 7th ed. Philadelphia, PA: Elsevier; 2017, pp. 1217–1288.

32. James MA and Bauer AS. Malformations and deformities of the wrist and forearm. In: Wolfe SW (ed.), *Green's Operative Hand Surgery*, 7th ed. Philadelphia, PA: Elsevier; 2017, pp. 1328–1364.

33. Ianakiev P, Kilpatrick MW, Toudjarska I, Basel D, Beighton P and Tsipouras P. Split-hand/split-foot malformation is caused by mutations in the p63 gene on 3q27. *Am J Hum Genet* 2000;67:59–66.

34. Qumsiyeh MB. EEC syndrome (ectrodactyly, ectodermal dysplasia and cleft lip/palate) is on 7p11.2-q21.3. *Clin Genet* 1992;42:101.

35. Kozin SH. Deformities of the thumb. In: Wolfe SW (ed.), *Green's Operative Hand Surgery*, 7th ed. Philadelphia, PA: Elsevier; 2017, pp. 1289–1364.

36. Ezaki M. Radial polydactyly. *Hand Clin* 1990;6:577–588.

37. Hung L, Cheng JC, Bundoc R and Leung P. Thumb duplication at the metacarpophalangeal joint. Management and a new classification. *Clin Orthop Relat Res* 1996;31–41.

38. Ogino T, Ishii S and Minami M. Radially deviated type of thumb polydactyly. *J Hand Surg Br* 1988;13:315–319.

39. Takagi T, Takayama S and Mochida J. Ray transfer for triplicate digit. *J Hand Surg Eur* 2016;41:772-773.

40. Jones GB. Delta Phalanx. *J Bone Joint Surg Br* 1964;46:226–228.

41. Guzman-Huerta ME, Muro-Barragan SA, Acevedo-Gallegos S, et al. Amniotic band sequence: Prenatal diagnosis, phenotype descriptions, and a proposal of a new classification based on morphologic findings. *Rev Invest Clin* 2013;65:300–306.

42. Ramelli GP, Slongo T, Tschappeler H and Weis J. Congenital pseudarthrosis of the ulna and radius in two cases of neurofibromatosis type 1. *Pediatr Surg Int* 2001;17:239–241.

43. Sellers DS, Sowa DT, Moore JR and Weiland AJ. Congenital pseudarthrosis of the forearm. *J Hand Surg Am* 1988;13:89–93.

44. Vitale MG, Guha A and Skaggs DL. Orthopaedic manifestations of neurofibromatosis in children: An update. *Clin Orthop Relat Res* 2002:107–118.

45. Peterson CA, 2nd, Maki S and Wood MB. Clinical results of the one-bone forearm. *J Hand Surg Am* 1995;20:609–618.

46. Shapiro F, Simon S and Glimcher MJ. Hereditary multiple exostoses. Anthropometric, roentgenographic, and clinical aspects. *J Bone Joint Surg Am* 1979;61:815–824.

47. Arms DM, Strecker WB, Manske PR and Schoenecker PL. Management of forearm deformity in multiple hereditary osteochondromatosis. *J Pediatr Orthop* 1997;17:450–454.

48. Masada K, Tsuyuguchi Y, Kawai H, Kawabata H, Noguchi K and Ono K. Operations for forearm deformity caused by multiple osteochondromas. *J Bone Joint Surg Br* 1989;71:24–29.

49. Takagi T, Seki A, Kobayashi Y, Mochida J and Takayama S. Isolated Muscle Transfer to Restore elbow flexion in children with arthrogryposis. *J Hand Surg Asian Pac* 2016;21:44–48.

50. Van Heest A, James MA, Lewica A and Anderson KA. Posterior elbow capsulotomy with triceps lengthening for treatment of elbow extension contracture in children with arthrogryposis. *J Bone Joint Surg Am* 2008;90:1517–1523.

51. McFarlane RM, Classen DA, Porte AM and Botz JS. The anatomy and treatment of camptodactyly of the small finger. *J Hand Surg Am* 1992;17:35–44.

52. AlQattan MM, AlAbdulkareem I, Ballow M and Al Balwi M. A report of two cases of Al-Awadi Raas-Rothschild syndrome (AARRS) supporting that "apparent" Phocomelia differentiates AARRS from Schinzel Phocomelia syndrome (SPS). *Gene* 2013;527:371–375.

53. Viljoen D. Congenital contractual arachnodactyly (Beals syndrome). *J Med Genet* 1994;31:640–643.

54. Bloom J and Upton J 3rd. CLOVES syndrome. *J Hand Surg Am* 2013;38:2508–2512.

55. Wilson GN, King TE and Brookshire GS. Index finger hyperphalangy and multiple anomalies: Catel-Manzke syndrome? *Am J Med Genet* 1993;46:176–179.

56. Mehta D, Vergano SA, Deardorff M et al. Characterization of limb differences in children with Cornelia de Lange Syndrome. *Am J Med Genet C Semin Med Genet* 2016;172:155–162.

57. Seno H, Yanai A, Sugino H, Inoue M, Takei T and Miyake I. Ectrodactyly, ectodermal dysplasia, and cleft lip syndrome. Case report. *Scand J Plast Reconstr Surg Hand Surg* 1996;30:227–230.

58. Webb ML, Rosen H, Taghinia A et al. Incidence of Fanconi anemia in children with congenital thumb anomalies referred for diepoxybutane testing. *J Hand Surg Am* 2011;36:1052–1057.

59. Kalliainen LK, Drake DB, Edgerton MT, Grzeskiewicz JL and Morgan RF. Surgical management of the hand in Freeman-Sheldon syndrome. *Ann Plast Surg* 2003;50:456–462; discussion 63–70.

60. Lipson AH, Kozlowski K, Barylak A and Marsden W. Fuhrmann syndrome of right-angle bowed femora, absence of fibulae and digital anomalies: Two further cases. *Am J Med Genet* 1991;41:176–179.

61. Al Kaissi A, Safi H, Ghachem MB and Grill F. Split hand/split foot deformity with focal

dermal hypoplasia (Goltz syndrome). *J Coll Physicians Surg Pak* 2010;20:770–772.

62. Kansal A, Brueton L, Lahiri A and Lester R. Hypoplastic thumb in Gorlin's syndrome. *J Plast Reconstr Aesthet Surg* 2007;60:440–442.

63. Jimenez I, Medina-Gontier J, Caballero J and Medina J. Hand deformities in Hajdu-Cheney syndrome: A case series of 3 patients across 3 consecutive generations. *J Hand Surg Am* 2021;46:73 e1–e5.

64. Palav S, Vernekar J, Pereira S and Desai A. Hajdu-Cheney syndrome: A case report with review of literature. *J Radiol Case Rep* 2014;8:1–8.

65. Avon SW and Shively JL. Orthopaedic manifestations of Goldenhar syndrome. *J Pediatr Orthop* 1988;8:683–686.

66. Laville JM, Lakermance P and Limouzy F. Larsen's syndrome: Review of the literature and analysis of thirty-eight cases. *J Pediatr Orthop* 1994;14:63–73.

67. Steel HH and Kohl EJ. Multiple congenital dislocations associated with other skeletal anomalies (Larsen's syndrome) in three siblings. *J Bone Joint Surg Am* 1972;54:75–82.

68. Lohan S, Spielmann M, Doelken SC et al. Microduplications encompassing the Sonic hedgehog limb enhancer ZRS are associated with Haas-type polysyndactyly and Laurin-Sandrow syndrome. *Clin Genet* 2014;86:318–325.

69. Kozin SH and Zlotolow DA. Madelung deformity. *J Hand Surg Am* 2015;40:2090–2098.

70. Mennen U, Mundlos S and Spielmann M. The Liebenberg syndrome: In depth analysis of the original family. *J Hand Surg Eur* 2014;39:919–925.

71. Abdel-Ghani H, Mansour A, Mahmoud M and Ez-Elarab M. Liebenberg syndrome: Case report and insight into molecular basis. *J Hand Surg Am* 2013;38:459–465.

72. Jones C, Baldrighi C, Mills J, Bush P, Ezaki M and Oishi S. Oculodentodigital dysplasia: Ulnar-sided syndactyly and its associated disorders. *J Hand Surg Am* 2011;36:1816–1821.

73. Malekianzadeh B, Vosoughi F and Zargarbashi R. Orofaciodigital syndrome type II (Mohr syndrome): A case report. *BMC Musculoskelet Disord* 2020;21:793.

74. Sakai N, Nakakita N, Yamazaki Y, Ui K and Uchinuma E. Oral-facial-digital syndrome type II (Mohr syndrome): Clinical and genetic manifestations. J Craniofac Surg 2002;13:321–326.

75. Robertson SP. Otopalatodigital syndrome spectrum disorders: Otopalatodigital syndrome types 1 and 2, frontometaphyseal dysplasia and Melnick-Needles syndrome. *Eur J Hum Genet* 2007;15:3–9.

76. Wood VE and Sandlin C. The hand in the Pierre Robin syndrome. *J Hand Surg Am* 1983;8:273–276.

77. Al-Qattan MM. Classification of hand anomalies in Poland's syndrome. *Br J Plast Surg* 2001;54:132–136.

78. Barmakian JT, Posner MA, Silver L, Lehman W and Vine DT. Proteus syndrome. *J Hand Surg Am* 1992;17:32–34.

79. Freeman MV, Williams DW, Schimke RN, Temtamy SA, Vachier E and German J. The Roberts syndrome. *Birth Defects Orig Artic Ser* 1974;10:87–95.

80. Maheshwari A, Kumar P, Dutta S and Narang A. Roberts-SC phocomelia syndrome. *Indian J Pediatr* 2001;68:557–559.

81. Gane BD and Natarajan P. Split-hand/feet malformation: A rare syndrome. *J Family Med Prim Care* 2016;5:168–169.

82. Forys-Dworniczak E, Zajdel-Cwynar O, Kalina-Faska B, Malecka-Tendera E and Matusik P. Trichorhinophalangeal syndrome as a diagnostic and therapeutic challenge for paediatric endocrinologists. *Pediatr Endocrinol Diabetes Metab* 2019;25:41–47.

83. Joss S, Kini U, Fisher R et al. The face of Ulnar Mammary syndrome? *Eur J Med Genet* 2011;54:301–305.

84. Carli D, Garagnani L, Lando M et al. VACTERL (vertebral defects, anal atresia, tracheoesophageal fistula with esophageal atresia, cardiac defects, renal and limb anomalies) association: Disease spectrum in 25 patients ascertained for their upper limb involvement. *J Pediatr* 2014;164:458-62 e1–2.

Index

Note: Page numbers with *t* and *f* in *Italic* refer to tables and figures.

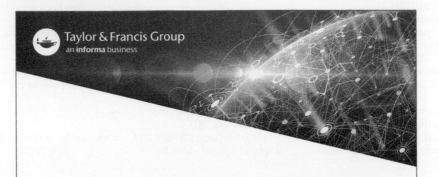

Printed and bound by CPI Group (UK) Ltd, Croydon, CR0 4YY

24/10/2024

01778298-0006